GW00656854

A VETERINARY BOOK FOR DAIRY FARMERS

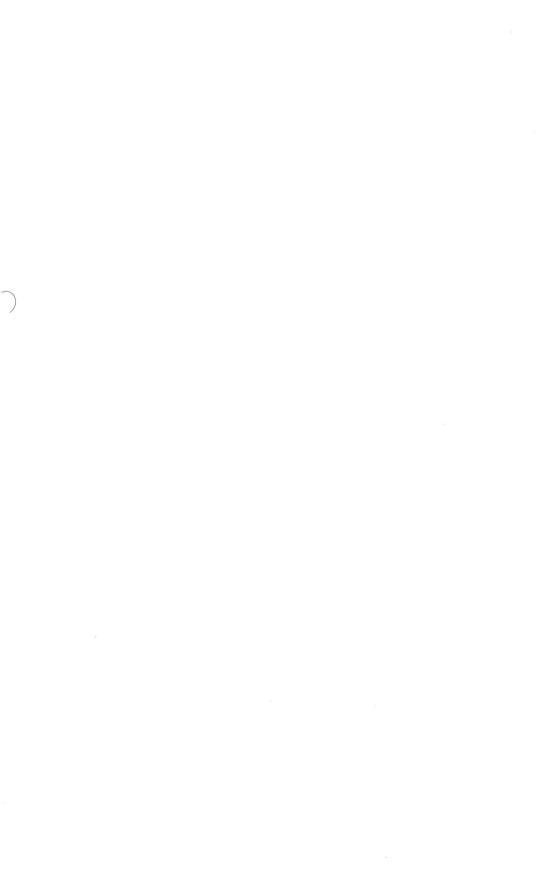

A VETERINARY BOOK FOR DAIRY FARMERS

R. W. BLOWEY, B.Sc., B.V.Sc., MRCVS

FARMING PRESS LIMITED
Wharfedale Road, Ipswich, Suffolk IP1 4LG

First published 1985

British Library Cataloguing in Publication Data

Blowey, R. W.
A veterinary book for dairy farmers.
1. Dairy cattle—Diseases
I. Title
636.2′142   SF961

ISBN 0-85236-151-3

Phototypeset by Galleon Photosetting, Ipswich
Printed in Great Britain by Page Bros. (Norwich) Ltd.

Contents

Colour Plates

Plates

Plates (*contd*)

Figures

Acknowledgements

Thanks must go to the farmers around Gloucester who have given me my experience and training over the past fifteen years and more recently to those who have had to pause while I photographed various cases. I would like to acknowledge my many colleagues who have been pestered for photographs, tables, drawings and information generally and I am grateful to Mrs Catherine Girdler for typing and proof-reading. Thanks are also due to Kate Bazeley, James Booth, James Greenwood, Diane Powell and George Chancellor, all of whom commented on the initial script. Finally I must acknowledge and apologise to my wife Norma and to my family for the many hours that I have had to spend locked away from them during the preparation of this book.

Photograph credits

Beecham Animal Health, colour plates 6, 7, 10, 11, 12.
Dairy Farmer magazine, Ipswich, plates 4.1, 4.3, 6.1, 7.5, 7.14, 9.29, 10.3, 12.11, 3.17, 13.18, 13.19, 13.20(b), 13.21.
Dr Donaldson, Animal Virus Research Institute, Pirbright, colour plates 14, 15, 16.
Dr P. Francis, CVL, Weybridge, colour plates 9, 10.
Mike Girdler, plates 2.3, 2.5, 2.6, 3.6, 9.11, 9.19, 9.22, 9.28, 9.30, 13.14, 13.15, 13.16; colour plate 13.
I.R.A.D., Compton, plates 5.7, 5.8, 5.9, 5.10, 5.13; colour plates 4, 5 (Dr K. Hibbitt).
M.M.B., plates 7.2, 7.4, 13.30.

Diagrams

Louise Dunn, figures 2.3, 4.1, 5.7, 8.5, 8.15, 9.1, 9.4, 9.12, 12.9.
Keith Pilling, prepared figures throughout the text.

Preface

OVER THE past ten years progressively tighter financial constraints, and particularly the imposition of dairy quotas, have led to two important changes in livestock farming. Firstly, because the number of dairy holdings is gradually decreasing but the total number of cows has remained approximately static, animals are being kept in much larger groups. Secondly, farmers are looking very carefully at their costs, and veterinary services are certainly no exception. The consequence of these changes is that a single herdsman will be in charge of many more animals and therefore more likely to meet a wide range of disease conditions. Intense stocking can even precipitate disease. Some ailments will be seen quite regularly and the herdsman will soon learn to recognise them. At the same time financial pressures will be such that, rather than call for veterinary assistance, he will also be expected to deal with these ailments himself.

The overall effect therefore is that the stockman and the farmer now have both the opportunity and the need to carry out a wide range of clinical tasks, many of which were once considered to be the province of the veterinarian. However, some of their increased involvement in animal health and veterinary techniques has not always been matched by an improvement in their knowledge and understanding of the basic principles of the subject. It is this gap between practical knowledge and theoretical background which I have attempted to bridge in this book. Take the chapter on mastitis as an example. First the mechanisms of milk synthesis and milk let-down in a normal cow are described. Then the changes which take place as the result of an infection of the udder are shown, including the defences of the cow against such an infection. With these principles firmly understood, the reader should then be able to appreciate the various control measures described for mastitis and the reason why they are applied.

The emphasis of this book is on the causes and prevention of cattle diseases, particularly where husbandry measures can be applied as a means of control. Treatment of the various conditions is much more of a veterinary matter and although treatments are mentioned, these tend to be given in outline only. Lists of differential diagnoses are provided at the end of the text, but the reader should use these with considerable caution. A full diagnosis is only made after careful consideration of the age of the animal, its environment, its likely exposure to infection and many other factors, not simply on the most prominent clinical signs seen.

Although the title is *A Veterinary Book for Dairy Farmers* I am sure that there are sections of interest to those involved in other aspects of cattle husbandry, particularly calf rearing and beef production. I have provided a detailed and comprehensive index for ease of reference and I hope that the book will be of value to farmer, agriculturalist and adviser. With a better understanding of the mechanisms and effects of disease, the farmer and his stockman should be able to work in parallel with their veterinary surgeon, appreciating the benefits that an efficient veterinary service can provide. The co-operative efforts of all three parties could result in an improvement in animal health, welfare and productivity, and if this book goes a small way towards achieving this goal, I shall be well pleased.

MINSTERWORTH, GLOUCESTER   ROGER W. BLOWEY
May 1985

Chapter 1

A CONCEPT OF DISEASE

FOR SOME diseases there is a simple relationship between the infection, the animal and the treatment needed. Examples include foul of the foot, caused by a bacterial infection and treated with antibiotics, or ringworm, a mycotic infection which can be treated with antifungal drugs. However, many of the more common conditions seen on farms today are due to an interaction between the animal, its environment and a wide range of infectious organisms. Probably the best example is calf pneumonia and this will be referred to again later in the chapter. Another example of the complexity of disease is milk fever. In early lactation the cow's calcium requirements for milk production may exceed her capabilities to provide the mineral, although she has ample reserves in her skeleton. The clinical symptoms are due to a deficiency of calcium in the blood and this is known as a metabolic disorder or a production disease.

Both the farmer and his veterinary surgeon must thoroughly understand the mechanisms of disease if we are to reduce some of the enormous losses that are incurred, and I would urge the reader to spend a short while studying this first chapter before embarking on the main text. The chapter describes the nature of the infectious agents associated with disease, some of the ways in which the animal protects itself, and finally it shows how infection, immunity and environment interact in a clinical situation. The concept of metabolic disease is slightly different and this is elaborated in Chapter Six.

THE INFECTIOUS AGENTS

There are a range of living organisms which, when growing on or inside the animal, can cause adverse effects on that animal. These effects are known as the clinical signs of disease, and the most common organisms involved are the bacteria, viruses and parasites.

Bacteria

A typical bacterium is shown in figure 1.1. It is a single cell, and consists of a thick outer structure, the cell wall, inside which there is a protein membrane

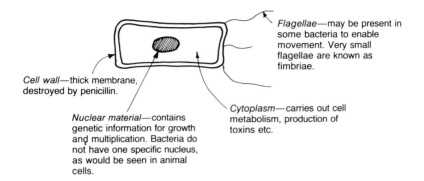

Cell wall—thick membrane, destroyed by penicillin.

Flagellae—may be present in some bacteria to enable movement. Very small flagellae are known as fimbriae.

Nuclear material—contains genetic information for growth and multiplication. Bacteria do not have one specific nucleus, as would be seen in animal cells.

Cytoplasm—carries out cell metabolism, production of toxins etc.

Figure 1.1   A typical bacterial cell. Even the largest bacteria (e.g. anthrax) are only 0.005 mm long. They multiply by dividing into two; and under favourable conditions this may occur every 30 minutes, so that one bacterium could produce 17 million offspring in twelve hours!

enclosing the cytoplasm and the nuclear material. The nuclear material contains the genetic components, the DNA, and by a complex arrangement of molecules, DNA functions as the regulator for all cell processes, determining the size and shape of the cell and the activities that take place within its cytoplasm. These 'activities' are the processes of reproduction and growth. Nutrients are absorbed through the cell wall, metabolised in the cytoplasm and waste products are excreted back out from the cell. It is often these waste products which cause the adverse effects on the animal that are the signs of disease. Bacteria are therefore individual discrete units of life. Given ideal conditions of warmth, nutrients and moisture most of them can also multiply outside the animal's body. Under adverse conditions some bacteria can turn themselves into a very resistant spore form, which can survive for many years. The classic example is that of anthrax, whose spores can persist in the soil for up to forty years. Other examples of bacterial infections include the majority of the causes of mastitis, the clostridial diseases of blackleg and tetanus, and conditions producing pus, such as navel ill and calf diphtheria.

Viruses

Viruses are much smaller than bacteria and in fact they may even infect and cause disease in bacteria. They cannot be seen with a normal light microscope; electron microscopy is required. They consist simply of central nuclear material, which may be DNA or RNA, and this is surrounded by a capsule of fat and protein (figure 1.2). Because viruses have no cytoplasm or proper nucleus, they cannot carry out their own metabolic functions of growth and reproduction and they are therefore unable to multiply outside the animal's living cells. For their survival away from the animal and hence their transfer from one animal to another viruses must be protected, for example in sputum

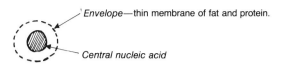

Figure 1.2   A virus particle. A virus is very much smaller than a bacterium. It uses the processes of metabolism within the animal cell for its own multiplication and growth, and as such it cannot live a separate existence away from the animal. This is very different from bacteria.

(pneumonia viruses), milk (foot and mouth virus) or blood (EBL virus). Once inside the animal, viruses penetrate the animal's cells and use the metabolic processes within the cytoplasm of those cells for their own purposes of multiplication and growth. When a cell is packed full of viruses, it bursts and virus particles are released to penetrate and infect adjacent animal cells. It is the bursting of these cells which generally causes the detrimental effects on the animal and hence the signs of disease, although some viruses (e.g. those causing teat warts, see page 195, or EBL, page 283) induce a proliferation or excessive multiplication of animal cells to produce a tumour.

Both bacteria and viruses may be very specific in the site they choose to infect. For example, certain groups will grow only in the respiratory tract— and these cause the clinical signs of a cold, influenza or pneumonia. Others can live only in the intestine and they will cause scouring. It is by this mechanism that we associate particular strains of bacteria or viruses with specific diseases. Different strains of bacteria and viruses vary considerably in shape and size, in the same way that the different species of animal or bird are so variable. Thus it is often possible to identify the type of bacteria or virus in a sample simply by examining them with a microscope. Electron microscopy is used for viruses.

Parasites

Parasites vary enormously in size from the very small single-celled protozoa-like coccidia in the intestine, or babesia which lives inside red blood cells and causes redwater in cattle, to much larger and multicellular parasites such as the mange mites and intestinal worms. The larger species all have their own metabolism systems, and may be capable of living for a considerable length of time outside the animal's body, although generally they must return to the animal to feed. The word parasite means an organism which takes nutrients from its host for its own purposes of growth and multiplication, but contributes nothing to the host animal in return.

The bacteria, viruses and parasites are the main classes of infectious agents. There are others, such as mycoplasmas, which are close relatives of bacteria, and the mycotic agents or fungi, which include ringworm and aspergillus, a possible cause of abortion. If the animal had no defences against these agents, contact of animal with infection would always produce disease and often rapid death. We know that this is rarely the case, however, and this is because the animal has many defence mechanisms to counteract the infections. These defences are described in the following section.

IMMUNITY AND OTHER DEFENCES

The animal has two major defence mechanisms. Firstly there are physical barriers which simply prevent infections from gaining access to susceptible animal cells, and secondly there are the processes of immunity, which actively seek out and destroy the infections. There are of course additional genetic factors interacting between the infection and the animal, and this explains why foot and mouth virus never infects dogs, and also why distemper/hardpad virus is not a problem in cattle.

Physical Defences

The skin must be the best example of a physical barrier. It consists of a thick layer of epithelial cells, with a dead and keratinised (or reinforced) surface, and it is certainly not a good medium for viral or bacterial multiplication. Should the skin get very dirty, however, or if it is broken by physical damage, then bacteria may gain entry, the infection may become established and pus or abscesses may form. Bacteria retard healing and this is why wounds and cuts should always be cleaned and washed with antiseptic, thus preventing the bacteria from becoming established. Pus is an accumulation of dead white blood cells, dead cells from animal tissue and bacteria. Skin is also covered by a film of fatty acids which help to prevent bacterial multiplication. Excessive washing, and especially with detergents, removes these acids and thus renders the skin more susceptible to infection. This is of particular relevance to teats, and is one reason why 'chapping' is so common unless emollients are added to the teat dip.

The air passages (trachea, bronchi, etc.) and the intestine could be termed external surfaces because they come into contact with materials (air and food) from outside the animal's body. In the nose there are hairs which prevent large particles from being inhaled into the lungs. Their function is supported by a microscopic layer of cilia, small, finger-like projections lining the surface of the trachea, which move in a wave motion to propel bacteria and other smaller particles back up towards the mouth, where they can be swallowed or coughed away. In addition mucus glands produce a sticky secretion to line the airways, thus trapping any bacteria or viruses which happen to land and this prevents them from reaching the susceptible tissues of the lungs.

The mouth and oesophagus have a thick horny lining, like skin, and this helps to prevent bacterial penetration. The stomach, on the other hand, produces mucus and acid, partly to assist digestion, but also helping to prevent bacterial growth, whereas the upper small intestine is very alkaline, again inhibiting bacterial growth. These extremes of acid and alkaline conditions should perhaps be considered as chemical rather than physical defence mechanisms. Vaginal secretions are also acid.

The eye has some interesting and rather unique defences. The eyelids close rapidly when an object is approaching, and this protects the eyeball from physical damage. If a foreign body does land on the eye however, tears are produced to wash it away and rapid blinking helps to move the object to the corner of the eye where it can cause less damage. If the surface of the eye does become damaged blood vessels grow across the cornea to supply antibodies and rebuilding materials. This is known as *pannus* formation, and is described in more detail on page 84.

The final type of physical defence is provided by the bacteria which *normally* live in and on the animal as 'commensals', that is they live there without causing disease. However, they compete with disease-causing (pathogenic) infections for both nutrients and space. If these normal microbe populations are disturbed, for example by a prolonged course of antibiotics by mouth, it is possible that the more serious pathogenic infections may proliferate and cause disease.

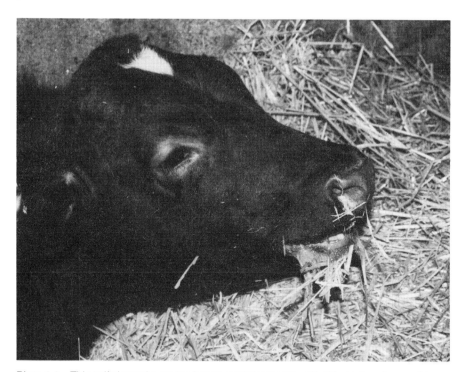

Plate 1.1   This calf showed a severe hypersensitivity reaction 15–20 minutes after receiving a penicillin injection. Note the swollen eyelids, and the drooling and frothing from the mouth denoting laboured breathing. Treatment with cortisone and antihistamines produced a dramatic recovery.

Cellular Defences

If infection manages to penetrate the physical defences of the animal, an alarm signal goes out and large numbers of cells are sent, via the blood, to the point where the infection is trying to establish its own colony. Some of these cells (neutrophils and macrophages) actually engulf the invading organisms, while others produce chemicals (e.g. histamine) to destroy them. On occasions, the chemicals are produced in excess, the body over-reacts and an allergic or hypersensitivity reaction occurs. A typical example is shown in the calf in plate 1.1. It was given an injection of long-acting penicillin because it had a mouth infection. Twenty minutes later it was found collapsed, panting, frothing at the mouth and with its eyelids and anus swollen. Cortisone, antihistamines and adrenalin were given to counteract the reaction, and the calf was almost back to normal three hours later.

These are a few examples of the animal's defences to infection and they are summarised in table 1.1 Acting in conjunction with these physical and cellular barriers there is a whole system of *immunity*, specific defences from within the animal.

Table 1.1   Some of the ways in which an animal can counteract disease

Physical	Skin	—toughened epithelium + film of fatty acids
	Digestive system	—epithelium and extremes of pH
	Respiratory system	—hairs in nose —cilia in trachea —mucus glands
	Eye	—lid closure, tears, pannus formation
	Normal bacteria	—on skin, mouth, vagina, intestine etc.
Cellular	Cells from the blood attempt to eliminate the invading organisms	
Immunity	Active antibodies Passive antibodies Cell-mediated immunity	—produced in response to antigens —obtained preformed in colostrum

The Immune System

Immunity can be roughly subdivided into two parts, cellular immunity and antibodies, although within the animal the two systems will work very much in conjunction with one another to counteract disease. Although I shall be dealing with the immune response to disease-causing organisms, the reader should appreciate that an identical immune reaction is evoked against any material which the animal recognises as being 'foreign' to its system. This is very important in the human fields of allergy and organ transplant rejection. Any material which the animal recognises as foreign is called an *antigen*, and antigens evoke both a cellular and an antibody response.

Antibodies

Antibodies are large protein molecules produced by the animal to combine with, and hence neutralise, the invading agents. The most interesting feature of antibodies is that they are very specific. Whereas all the other defence mechanisms we have discussed so far will be effective against any bacteria, viruses or even dust, there has to be a separate and specific antibody for every type of infectious agent. Thus antibodies effective against one type of E. coli bacteria may not have any action against a slightly different strain of E. coli. A type of white blood cell, the lymphocyte, is the cell which recognises substances as being antigenic to the cow. When they are enlarged and carrying antibodies they are known as plasma cells. Other lymphocytes are able to specifically attack microbes in a complex procedure known as cell-mediated immunity.

Antibodies are acquired by the animal in two separate ways known as 'active' and 'passive'. Active immunisation is the process whereby the animal produces its own antibodies following exposure to an antigen. The cow can produce antibodies however and supply them preformed to the calf during the first few hours of its life via the colostrum. Because the calf has not produced the antibodies itself, they are called 'passive' antibodies and they provide immediate protection against infections present in the environment.

Before an animal can produce its own active antibody defences against a particular infection, it must have been exposed to that infection at some time in the past, recognised it as foreign (viz as an antigen) and stored the information in a type of memory, ready to produce antibodies to overcome subsequent challenges. This initial exposure may be by vaccination, but it is much more likely to be the result of natural infection. A low dose of disease organisms which is not sufficient to cause visible symptoms will be quite adequate to stimulate antibody production and provide active immunity. This process is occurring throughout the animal's life, and re-exposure to infections helps to boost immunity levels. Vaccines will be used only when there is a risk of a heavy challenge from a specific infection, and especially if the animal has not had previous exposure to that infection. A vaccine consists of the infectious agent which has been altered in some way. When administered to the animal it stimulates the processes of recognition and antibody production, but it cannnot cause disease. Vaccines may either be living, when only one dose may be required, or killed, when two doses will be needed at an interval of approximately four weeks. The presence of passive immunity, that is antibodies acquired from the mother, may prevent the calf from responding to the vaccine and this is why the instructions will state that animals under a certain age should not be vaccinated, or perhaps that if young animals are vaccinated, then an additional dose may be necessary at a later date. Passive immunity generally persists until the animal is two to three months old, depending on the amount of antibody received in the colostrum, and on the type of infection. Vaccination should therefore be carried out at an age such that the period between passive and active protection is minimal, but not too early so that there is a risk of a poor vaccine 'take' due to persistence of passive colostral immunity.

It is because of antibodies and other defence mechanisms that an animal can have bacteria living in it without succumbing to disease. The situation can rapidly change however if we mix groups of animals, for example calves from different sources. Calves from one farm may be carrying infection 'A' and have antibodies to 'A'. Calves from a second farm have infection 'B' and the corresponding 'B' antibodies. When the two groups are mixed, calves from 'A' farm are exposed to infection 'B', but they only have antibodies to 'A'. If the dose of 'B' infection is large enough (for example if the groups were mixed and crowded into a poorly ventilated building) then 'B' disease may occur in 'A' calves before they are able to build up sufficient antibodies against 'B' for protection. This is shown diagrammatically in figure 1.3.

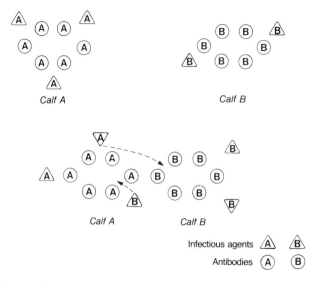

Figure 1.3   Each calf can exist in the presence of infection A or B provided it has antibodies against A or B. Problems occur when they are mixed because infection B may produce disease in calf A before it can develop antibodies against B.

THE BALANCE OF DISEASE

Having described the types of infectious agents and the physical and immune defence mechanisms of the animal, their interaction can now be examined and related to the production of disease. Take a case of humon typhoid. The disease itself does not matter and the figures used are not accurate, but it serves to illustrate the point very well. Putting one typhoid bacterium on the tongue of a healthy person would probably have no effect on him at all. Give him a hundred bacteria and he may feel rather off-colour and would probably get diarrhoea. Using a dose of a thousand bacteria, our 'guinea-pig' would develop a severe illness, with sickness, diarrhoea and generalised symptoms.

Now if, before we started our dosing regime, this same man had been drinking heavily, had lost his way home and had spent twenty-four hours in the cold without food and was suffering from exposure, in this case we would expect different results. Possibly one bacterium would cause mild diarrhoea, a hundred would cause a severe illness and a dose of a thousand would be fatal.

The example serves to illustrate two extremely important points, namely that the severity of a disease is dependent upon:

1. the dose of infection received;
2. the state of health of the animal being infected.

This situation is extremely common in animal disease, where there is often a multiplicity of factors affecting the severity and spread of a condition. It is more easily understood by saying that health and disease are on each side of a *balance*, with the animal acting as the pivot of that balance. This is illustrated in figure 1.4. Along each arm of the balance can be 'hung' various items which will either boost health or exacerbate disease. Provided the animal can be maintained with the balance in the level position, it can cope quite happily with infection, living with it but suffering relatively few adverse effects. This is the basis of preventive medicine. There is a risk of certain diseases occurring on every farm, and so it is necessary to take various husbandry and other preventive measures to minimise those risks. One of the best diseases to illustrate this point is enzootic pneumonia (sometimes called virus pneumonia) of calves, although E. coli and the other causes of environmental mastitis would serve as an equally good example, as would lameness in dairy cows. The diseases are dealt with in detail in later chapters and so I will mention here just a few of the factors involved in the 'balance' of pneumonia. Calf pneumonia is caused by a wide range of infections, and these are shown in

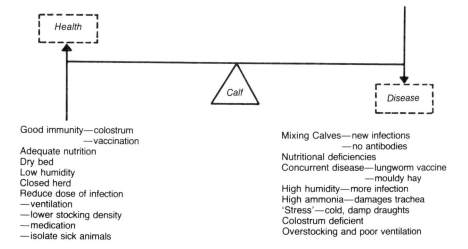

Good immunity—colostrum
　　　　　　—vaccination
Adequate nutrition
Dry bed
Low humidity
Closed herd
Reduce dose of infection
—ventilation
—lower stocking density
—medication
—isolate sick animals

Mixing Calves—new infections
　　　　　　—no antibodies
Nutritional deficiencies
Concurrent disease—lungworm vaccine
　　　　　　—mouldy hay
High humidity—more infection
High ammonia—damages trachea
'Stress'—cold, damp draughts
Colostrum deficient
Overstocking and poor ventilation

Figure 1.4　The balance of disease—using calf pneumonia as an example.

Table 1.2 Some of the infectious agents known to be associated with calf pneumonia

Viruses	Bacteria	Others
Respiratory Syncytial Virus RSV		Moulds
Parainfluenza type 3 P.I.3.	Pasteurella	Mycoplasma
Bovine Viral Diarrhoea BVD	Haemophilus	Acholeplasma
Infectious Bovine Rhinotracheitis IBR	C. Pyogenes	Ureaplasma

table 1.2. Viruses, mycoplasmas and bacteria may be involved, and the condition can be exacerbated by fungal spores from mouldy hay or even lungworm larvae (e.g. following husk vaccination). Important features on the positive side of the disease balance (in figure 1.4), that is acting to reduce the incidence and severity of calf pneumonia, are:

1. Avoid mixing calves from different sources. This ensures that all calves will have antibodies against the infections to which they will be exposed.
2. Make sure the young calf suckles its colostrum and therefore starts life with a good level of passive immunity.
3. Vaccination. Several commercial vaccines are available. They contain some, but by no means all, of the infectious agents known to be involved in pneumonia, and they may be used in older calves or where calves are mixed.
    Ensuring adequate colostrum intake and vaccination are two ways of boosting antibody levels.
4. Maintain adequate ventilation. If there is a good flow of air through the building, infection coughed up by the calves is carried away and the overall challenge dose of infection is thus reduced.
5. Isolate the individually sick animal. Not only is this good nursing, but it also eliminates a major source of infection from the remainder of the calves.
6. Keep different age-groups of calves in separate air-spaces. Again this is to ensure that a calf is exposed to the minimum level of infection at any one time. Large 'umbrella'-type buildings are poor because they allow the air to circulate freely from one group to another, thus transferring infection.
7. Provide a dry bed. Dampness leads to chilling, a stress which would render the calf more susceptible to any disease. In addition dampness can increase the ammonia fumes in the atmosphere and this will directly reduce the effectiveness of the cilia in the nose and trachea. A damp atmosphere also supports a much higher level of air-borne infectious agents than dry air. This is one reason why calf pneumonia is more common on foggy humid days than during the winter.
8. Strong, well-fed animals, which have not been weakened by attacks of scouring or other diseases, are much more capable of producing their own antibodies and overcoming pneumonia infection.
9. Medication. When an outbreak of pneumonia occurs, sick calves are coughing up infection and this raises the overall challenge of disease in

the environment. If the whole group is medicated, for example with antibiotics, infection levels may be reduced to the point which allows the calves to develop an active immunity without succumbing to clinical disease.
10. Avoid any other condition leading to lung damage—e.g. fungal spores from mouldy hay or lungworm vaccine—which may be sufficient to tip the animal into a disease state.

Figure 1.4 shows the wide range of factors which can influence the course of calf pneumonia. *All* calves will be carrying some of the infectious agents involved, but disease will occur only when the weight of adverse factors overcomes the 'health' factors. Often the simple correction of one adverse condition is sufficient to swing the balance towards health and allow the calf to overcome the other factors, using its own defence mechanisms. Minimising the challenge dose of infection and maximising the adequacy of the animal's defences are two of the most important facets of preventive medicine, and I would urge the reader to construct his own 'balance' diagrams for whatever disease condition he is considering.

Principles of Treatment

Details of treatment for each condition are described later in the book. As a general rule, however, treatment is of two types, namely nursing and therapy.

Nursing

A sick animal is less able to compete with the remainder of the group for food, water and even shelter, and there are many instances when it is best moved into a loose-box or a small pen of its own for a few days to convalesce. This allows more attention to be given and it is also much easier to monitor the animal's progress. Is it eating and drinking? Are its faeces normal? Special succulent food may be offered to tempt it to eat, and for the animal with a high temperature, a warm, well-bedded dry environment is essential. Any necessary medicines can be given much more easily and if medication is easily administered it is more likely to be given at the correct dose and with the correct frequency.

The other advantage of separating a diseased animal is that it reduces the risk of that animal spreading its infection to the remainder of the group; that is, its removal effectively reduces the challenge dose of infection to the others.

Therapy

This covers the general field of medication and can be divided into specific therapy and supportive measures.

Specific Therapy

There are some drugs which will specifically destroy the infectious agents and thus reduce the severity of disease. Obvious examples are antibiotics, anthelmintics and insecticides.

Antibiotics
Antibiotics are chemicals which destroy bacteria but have little or no adverse effect on the animal. Some act by actively killing the bacteria (e.g. penicillin, which damages their outer membrane) and these are called *bacteriocidal* antibiotics. Others simply prevent bacterial growth and multiplication (e.g. chloramphenicol interferes with their protein synthesis) and the bacteria then either die at a normal rate or are killed by the animal's defence mechanisms. These are known as *bacteriostatic* antibiotics. It is important to appreciate this difference. Bacteriocidal and bacteriostatic antibiotics should not be used simultaneously in an animal, since one counteracts the effects of the other. This is because the bacteriocidals work best against rapidly growing and dividing bacteria, whereas bacteriostatics actually inhibit bacterial growth and multiplication.

In addition, different antibiotics are effective against varying types of bacteria. Some, for example the tetracyclines and chloramphenicol, are known as 'broad-spectrum' antibiotics and are effective against most organisms. Others, such as penicillin, are only effective against staphylococci, streptococci and a few other groups. Even then, certain strains of staphylococci produce *penicillinase* which destroys penicillin and thus prevents its action. These strains of staphylococci are called penicillin resistant. Even when the correct antibiotic has been chosen to counteract the cause of the disease, consideration must still be given to the tissues within the body which are harbouring the infection. Following administration to the animal, some antibiotics (e.g. tylosin and lincomycin) are found in particularly high concentrations in the lungs and would therefore be effective as a pneumonia treatment. Others (e.g. ampicillin) achieve high levels in the urine and could be used to treat kidney and bladder infections. In both cases this assumes that the bacteria concerned are sensitive to lincomycin or ampicillin.

If antibiotics are used indiscriminately, and especially for prolonged periods at low levels, there is a danger of bacteria mutating into forms which are resistant to the particular antibiotic. Sometimes this resistance is 'infectious' and can spread extremely rapidly in the form of genetic material to other strains of bacteria which have not been exposed to the antibiotic. The particular genetic material is unusual in that it is not part of the nucleus of the cell. Chloramphenicol is currently one of the drugs of choice in the treatment of human typhoid and certain other enteric infections and, to maintain its effectiveness, it has been requested that its use in the veterinary field is restricted to only essential cases, thus decreasing the risk of bacterial resistance developing.

There are many other factors which must be taken into account when using antibiotics and these few examples were given merely as an illustration of the complexity of the subject. It was for reasons like these that antibiotics became 'prescription-only medicines' (POM), that is they may be used only under veterinary guidance and supervision. There are usually milk- and meat-withholding periods following the administration of antibiotics and these need to be carefully observed.

Anthelmintics

These are drugs which destroy helminths, that is intestinal worms, lungworms or liver fluke. As with antibiotics, each drug has its own spectrum of activity, some being effective against adult worms only, others treating 'arrested development' larval forms, while others are specifically against liver fluke. Table 1.3 gives an outline of the activities of the commonly used anthelmintics, although you should consult your veterinary surgeon for more specific details, including milk- and meat-withholding periods after treatment. There are several other drugs not listed which can be used. Only the chemical names have been given and you will need to read the small print to see which chemical is present in the particular commercial preparation you are using.

Table 1.3   The activities of some common anthelmintics

	INTESTINAL WORMS			LUNGWORMS		FLUKE	
	adults	larvae	arrested	adults	larvae	adults	immatures
Thiabendazole	+[5]	+/−	−	−	−	−	−
Cambendazole	+	+/−	−	+	+/−	−	−
Other benzimidazoles[1]	+	+	+	+	+	(+/−)[2]	−
Levamisole[3]	+	+	−	+	+	−	−
Ivermectins[4]	+	+	+	+	+	−	−
Oxyclozanide	−	−	−	−	−	+[5]	(+/−)[6]
Rafoxanide	−	−	−	−	−	+	+
Nitroxynil	−	−	−	−	−	+	+

Notes
1. Thiabendazole and cambendazole are part of this group. 'Others' includes fenbendazole, oxfendazole, albendazole.
2. Albendazole is effective against worms but only has any significant effect against fluke at double the normal dosage rate. Triclabendazole is a benzimidazole with good anti-fluke activity.
3. Available as a 'pour-on', drench or injection.
4. Ivermectins are also effective against lice, mange and warble. In addition they have a persistancy effect which prevents reinfestation with lungworms and stomach worms for up to three weeks after treatment. This property is not shared by any of the other anthelmintics.
5. The only product licensed for use in dairy cows.
6. Very limited activity.

Insecticides

This is the name given to the drugs which kill insects. The most commonly used are:

- Gamma benzene hexachloride (γ BHC)—also called 'Lindane'. It is the common constituent of louse powder, and is one of the 'chlorinated hydrocarbon' group of compounds or 'systemics'.

- Organo-phosphorus compounds—these are often available as 'pour-on' preparations, having been combined with a chemical which carries the drug through the skin of the animal and throughout its body via the blood. They are a common treatment for lice, mange and warbles, and are particularly effective because they give whole-body cover.
- Ivermectins—in addition to their anthelmintic properties, ivermectins are also effective against lice, mange and warbles.

Virus treatment
So far no mention has been made of the treatment of virus infections. There are *no* drugs currently available in animal medicine for the treatment of viral diseases and even in the human field the chemical *interferon* is used only rarely because of its expense. Treatment of viral infections is therefore largely a combination of nursing, the use of antibiotics to prevent secondary bacterial infection of tissues damaged by the virus, and supportive therapy. The animal must use its own immune defence mechanisms to neutralise the virus particles.

Supportive Therapy

This is aimed at treating the *effects* of the disease rather than its basic cause. The best example is undoubtedly the administration of fluids to the scouring calf. Fluids hasten the recovery and reduce the mortality from scouring and are often of greater benefit to the calf than the use of antibiotics to eliminate the infectious agents. Other examples of supportive therapy include B vitamins to assist in detoxification processes; cortisone to reduce the adverse effects of the inflammatory reaction, and antipyretics (e.g. aspirin) which reduce the temperature in a fevered animal. All of these treatments are designed to assist the animal to overcome the damage caused by the disease, to improve its feeling of 'well-being', to restore its appetite and hence return it to health.

Chapter 2

THE YOUNG CALF

THIS CHAPTER deals with the health of the calf from birth to weaning, that is until approximately six weeks old.

Current figures give a national calf mortality of approximately 5 per cent of live births. Taking the 1985 value of a calf at £100, this means a loss of £500 per annum to the average 100-cow dairy herd, and if there are 200,000 calves born each year, it represents a national annual loss of £20 million. There are many reasons why the young calf is particularly susceptible to disease. Its defence mechanisms will not be fully developed, it will be going through the transition from active to passive immunity, it may have several changes of diet, and on top of all this it has an additional route by which infection may enter the body, that is through the navel. As many of the diseases of young calves are the result of failures of proper housing, feeding and colostrum intake, these factors will be discussed in some detail before specific health problems are dealt with.

HOUSING

Undoubtedly the healthiest calves are those born outdoors, but this is impractical in the winter and presents its own problems of management (e.g. when assistance is required) in summer. Individual calving boxes are ideal, as it is then easier to ensure that the calf is not 'mis-mothered', that is, that it suckles its own mother first and therefore receives adequate colostrum. The majority of calves from dairy herds are moved into rearing quarters after a few days and the most important criteria for their housing are:

- a warm dry bed
- shelter from direct draughts and extremes of weather
- cleanliness
- preferably separation from other calves.

Although sub-zero conditions are best avoided, provided that the calf has a dry bed with ample straw, it is doubtful if house temperature is too important. However, ventilation as a pneumonia-preventive is vital. Individual penning is a great advantage in that feed intakes for each calf can be monitored and the slower drinker will not be penalised. Any sick calves are much more readily apparent and there is a reduced risk of the spread of disease, especially scouring. Pen size and construction will vary with the manufacturer but it is important to ensure that the calf has sufficient room to turn round easily. Although the majority of commercial pens have railed divisions, I prefer to see solid sides. This gives a greater freedom from draughts and a reduced risk of the spread of disease, but at the same time the calves can have some contact with each other during feeding times. The pens shown in plate 2.1 were constructed of 2.4 m by 1.2 m (8 ft × 4 ft) sheets of 95 mm marine ply and the fronts were home made. The whole assembly can be dismantled for cleaning out.

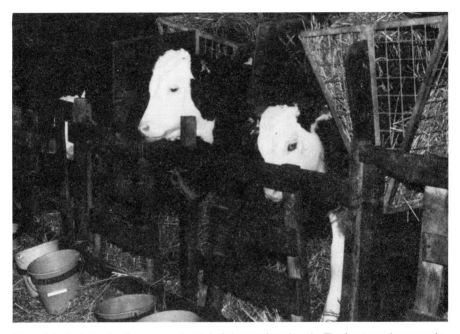

Plate 2.1   Individual calf pens constructed of sheets of marine ply. The fronts are home made.

Where fixing is required it is important to use bolts, screws or wire. String is best avoided. It will be sucked by the calves and even the most secure knots can come undone. They then chew and eat the string and may develop indigestion, or even a fatal obstruction from string in the gut.

Whatever the construction, it should be possible to dismantle the pens, take them outside for cleaning, then thoroughly clean out, wash, disinfect and rest the calf house. If calves are purchased, then they should be reared in groups preferably of the same age and size. When the first group is weaned, empty the whole house and clean it, then rest it for at least a week before introducing the next batch. This is known as the 'all in, all out' system and it is a most important factor in preventing the spread of disease between groups of calves. On dairy farms where calves may be born throughout the year, at least two different buildings should be used for calf rearing. As soon as the calves have been moved, dismantle the pens, remove all dung and bedding and give the pens and fittings a good soaking with water. Then thoroughly clean them using a detergent to remove the layer of fat which would otherwise remain as a thin film and obstruct the penetration of the disinfectant. Disinfect the pens and leave the building empty for at least a week, and preferably longer. Cleaning and disinfection must be carried out *before* the rest period to maximise its benefits and this routine should be followed even when healthy calves have been reared although it is of course more important if disease has been present. It is good preventive medicine. It is aimed primarily at reducing scouring and pneumonia but it will also improve growth rates generally.

THE IMPORTANCE OF COLOSTRUM

Colostrum, the first 'milk' produced by the cow at calving, has two very important properties. Firstly it is highly nutritious and secondly it contains antibodies. The difference in composition between milk and colostrum at the time of calving is shown in table 2.1. The total quantity of solids in colostrum is double that found in milk, and in addition to high levels of fat and protein, colostrum is also rich in the fat-soluble vitamins A, D and E. At birth the calf has very little of these vitamins and its liver stores come almost entirely from colostrum. Fat acts as a laxative, assisting the passing of *meconium*, the foetal dung, and it also provides a good source of energy for the calf, to boost its body temperature and assist in survival.

The production of antibodies was explained in Chapter One. In late pregnancy the cow concentrates antibodies in her colostrum, so that the calf can receive immediate preformed immunity to the diseases to which it

Table 2.1   Some of the differences between milk and colostrum, expressed on a fresh weight basis

	Colostrum	Milk
Total solids %	25	12.6
Fat %[1]	5.1	3.8
SNF %[1]	19.6	8.8
Protein %[1]	16.4	3.2
Lactose %[1]	2.2	4.7
Immunoglobulins (antibodies) g/kg[2]	60	0.9
Vitamin A μg/g fat[2]	45	8
Vitamin D μg/g fat[2]	23–45	15
Vitamin E μg/g fat[2]	100–150	20

[1] from Godsell, personal communication; [2] from J. H. B. Roy, *The Calf*.

will be exposed. The final concentration of antibodies in colostrum is much higher than that originally present in blood, and is the reason why the protein content of colostrum is so high. The immunity given to the calf is of course only related to the infections which the cow herself has contacted (see also page 96). If a cow is purchased and moved into a new herd only a few days before calving, then clearly there is a risk that the calf will be challenged by infections for which it has no colostral protection.

Antibodies are proteins and as such they would normally be digested (viz broken down) in the calf's intestine. However, during the first few hours of life the intestine has a special ability to absorb whole proteins. These pass into the calf's bloodstream and the amount of antibody absorbed can be measured in blood samples by means of the zinc sulphate turbidity test, ZST. Sometimes all purchased calves are blood sampled on arrival, to ensure that the farm of origin has been taking enough care in giving their calves colostrum. The absorption of colostral antibodies is of vital importance to the calf, not only for the first few days of life, but continuing for weeks and even months. Calves which have not received adequate colostrum have been shown to:

- have a higher overall death rate, especially from septicaemia and joint-ill
- be more likely to develop scouring (one trial reduced scouring from 12 per cent to 2 per cent by improving the supervision of colostrum intake)
- be more likely to develop pneumonia, even at two or three months old.

Colostrum therefore has a profound effect on subsequent calf performance and viability and it is important to have some idea of the factors involved in its absorption, especially when surveys have shown that up to 50 per cent of the calves in the UK do not receive adequate intakes. Whole antibodies are most efficiently absorbed during the first few hours of the calf's life, although the facility may persist at a reduced level for up to twenty-four or even thirty-six hours, *provided* that no other food is eaten. The antibody levels of the colostrum are highest in the very first milk and there is little point in transferring a calf to another cow which calved one to two days previously, especially if she has already been milked.

As a 'rule of thumb' I would suggest that a calf receives colostrum:

- at the rate of 6 per cent of its body weight
- within six hours of birth.

Half a litre of colostrum will protect a calf against septicaemia, but 5–7 litres are needed for protection against scour. It is not sufficient simply to leave the calf with its dam. Several studies have shown that inadequate colostral intakes may result. This could be because of a weakly calf, a nervous mother, or possibly an older cow with a pendulous udder and splayed teats. Wherever possible the calf should be lifted to suckle as soon as it is reasonably able to stand and suckling will need to continue for fifteen to twenty minutes. Because the first feed of colostrum stimulates the production of digestive enzymes, thus reducing the absorption of further antibodies, this first feed needs to be as large as possible. Colostrum does *not* need to clot in the abomasum, so there is little risk of overfeeding and producing digestive upsets, even if it is given by drench or stomach tube (see plate 2.16).

Mothering also has an effect on the uptake of colostral antibodies and on subsequent circulating blood levels. Ideally the calf should suckle colostrum from its own dam. However, if artificial feeding is necessary (e.g. if the cow is recumbent due to milk fever, injury or mastitis, or perhaps because she has been premilked), then antibody absorption is considered to be more effective in the presence of the cow, even when the colostrum is being given via a teat. When it is known that artificial feeding will be required, then every effort should be made to achieve this within the first six hours of life.

Finally it has been shown that there can be a considerable variation in the antibody content of the colostrum itself and cows which are in poor condition, affected by chronic mastitis, suffering from a debilitating disease (e.g. liver fluke) or which have been induced to calve prematurely using corticosteroids are simply unable to provide adequate protective antibodies for their offspring.

Colostrum retains its nutritive and antibody potency when frozen, and the deep-freeze can be a useful emergency store *provided* that the colostrum is reheated carefully. Boiling destroys the antibodies. Colostrum 'banks' can be set up by freezing it in the quantities which would be needed for an individual calf, viz a minimum of two litres (3½ pints). There is then always a supply available for those unexpected occasions of mastitis in all four quarters, death of the cow at calving, recumbency and other such unfortunate incidents, which would otherwise render the calf colostrum deficient.

DIGESTION

Figure 2.1 shows the essential anatomy of the digestive system of the calf. Food is taken into the mouth and swallowed, a process whereby the respiratory route is closed and the food is transferred into the oesophagus.

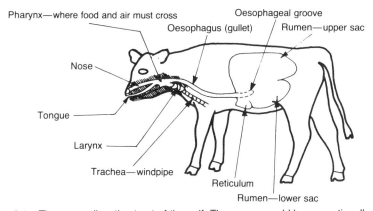

Figure 2.1   The upper digestive tract of the calf. The rumen would be proportionally much smaller than this in a young milk-fed calf.

Once in the oesophagus, the food is propelled downwards by *peristalsis*, which is the name given to a wave-like muscular activity which has a similar effect to the hand of a milker on a cow's teat. First the top of the teat is squeezed between the thumb and forefinger. Then, maintaining this pressure, the next finger is squeezed against the hand, then the next and so on. In this way milk is squeezed through the teat sphincter under pressure, with the first fingers preventing reverse flow back into the udder. Propulsion of food by peristalsis occurs throughout the digestive tract.

The calf is a ruminant and in common with other ruminants (e.g. sheep, goats and camels) it has four stomachs, namely the reticulum, rumen, omasum and abomasum. Plate 2.2 shows the stomachs of an adult as viewed from above, with the animal's head pointing forwards.

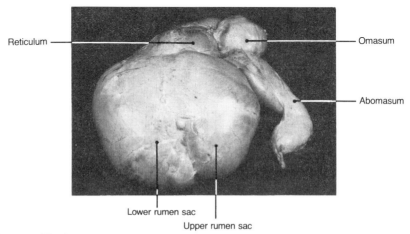

Plate 2.2   The four stomachs of an adult ruminant as if viewed from above and with the animal facing forward. The rumen would be proportionally very much smaller than this in a calf on an all-milk diet.

The very young calf uses only its fourth stomach, the abomasum, and functions essentially as a *monogastric* animal, that is an animal with a single stomach. Its rumen, reticulum and omasum would be proportionally much smaller than those in plate 2.2. Milk has to flow directly from the oesophagus into the abomasum, by-passing the rumen and reticulum, and this is done by a self-closing channel in the roof of the rumen, known as the *oesophageal groove*. Figure 2.2 shows the groove in transverse section, that is, as if you had cut through the wall of the rumen. When the groove is in the open position milk passing from the oesophagus would fall into the rumen, become sour and cause a digestive upset. When the groove closes, a 'pipe' is formed which transports milk directly through the omasum and into the abomasum.

Once in the abomasum, milk must 'clot'; that is the protein solidifies and then contracts, squeezing out the liquid whey which passes down into the duodenum and small intestine for digestion. The clotting is carried out under the influence of the enzyme renin, and the digestion of the remaining protein by the enzyme pepsin.

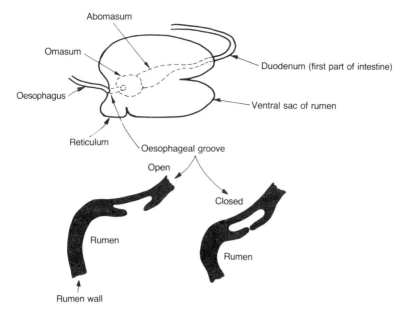

Figure 2.2 Function and position of the oesophageal groove. The rumen would be proportionally smaller than this in a calf on an all-milk diet.

The Oesophageal Groove Closure Reflex

When the calf suckles there is a reflex action, activated via the bicarbonate in its saliva, which results in muscular closure of the oesophageal groove. As it gets older, simply the thought of feeding and the sight, sounds and other stimuli associated with the arrival of its milk will be sufficient to provoke closure. It is most important that closure occurs prior to feeding and hence it can be seen that the establishment of a *feeding routine* is vital. Feeding times should be consistent each day and milk should be provided at the correct temperature and not in excessively varying amounts. Stressed calves, for example those which have just arrived from market or which have been frightened for some other reason, may not achieve groove closure and digestive problems could result. Calves should not be fed immediately after moving, handling or, for example, following dehorning. Similarly a sick calf being drenched may not achieve groove closure and it would therefore be better to use electrolyte and glucose solutions rather than milk for such cases. There will be little adverse effect if glucose enters the rumen.

Slow drinkers present a problem. While their milk is warm, the oeso-phageal groove remains closed. If the bucket is left in front of the calf however, the milk cools and if it is drunk later, oesophageal groove closure may be incomplete and some of the cold milk could spill into the rumen, producing a digestive upset.

The Abomasal Milk Clot

For whole milk and the majority of milk substitutes, formation of a milk clot in the abomasum is an essential first step in digestion. If the clot fails to form, whole milk passes into the small intestine. This provides an excellent medium for bacterial fermentation, and scouring results. Some of the adverse factors associated with poor clot formation are:

- irregular feeding times
- nervous or stressed calves
- milk fed at the wrong temperature
- milk substitute fed at the incorrect strength
- inflammation of the abomasum.

Some of the newer milk substitute powders, especially those associated with ad libitum acidified cold milk feeding, do not need to form an abomasal clot. Overfeeding, leading to improperly digested food passing into the intestine, is still important however, even though the acidified milk helps to prevent excessive bacterial growth.

Diseases of the Calf

Problems with young calves generally fall into two main categories. They are conditions affecting the navel and conditions affecting the digestive system, of which scouring is of course by far the most common. Pneumonia can also occur in preweaned calves, but as it is more common in the older animal, a full discussion of the condition has been left until the next chapter.

Conditions Affecting the Navel

During pregnancy the navel is the calf's 'life line', supplying it with nutrients from the placenta and removing its waste products. The structure of the placenta and the umbilical cord is explained in more detail on page 96 and figure 5.3. At birth the cord is the only part of the animal not covered with a protective layer of skin and it is therefore very susceptible to entry of infection. The blood vessels from the placenta originally passed directly into the liver, so once infection gains entry at the navel, there is a serious risk of liver abscesses or even generalised infection throughout the body.

Navel Ill

Navel ill is generally seen in calves in their first week of life and, despite very simple control measures, it is still an extremely common condition. In the early stages the calf may show no generalised signs of illness, but the navel cord feels enlarged and painful and the tip is generally moist and has a purulent smell. The calf's temperature will be raised. More advanced cases will be dull and reluctant to move, and pain makes them stand with an arched back, as shown in plate 2.3.

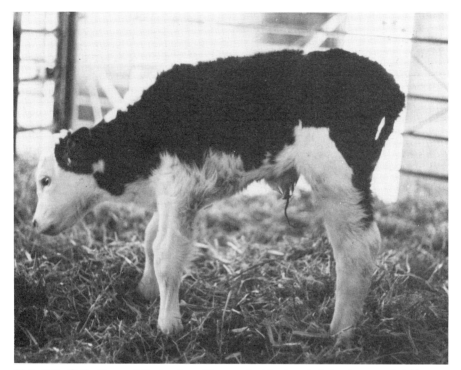

Plate 2.3   Calf with navel ill, standing with an arched back and obviously uncomfortable.

Treatment
Daily antibiotic injections should be given for several days (depending on the severity of the condition) and it is also useful to keep the moist end of the cord bathed in warm dilute disinfectant to encourage pus to drain out.

Prevention
Ensure that cows calve down in a clean environment and immediately after birth thoroughly spray the fleshy navel cord with an antibiotic/gentian violet aerosol, or dip it into iodine. This has two functions. Firstly it dries the cord, making it less attractive to bacteria and secondly it destroys any bacteria which may have already become established.

Joint Ill

We have already said that infection entering the navel at birth can pass along the cord to the liver and then spread around the body via the blood stream, and this is especially so in colostrum-deficient animals. The bacteria often localise in the joints, and this produces *joint ill*. Joint ill is seen at a later stage than navel ill, probably at two to four weeks old, and although the infection originally entered at the navel, calves with joint ill do not necessarily have an

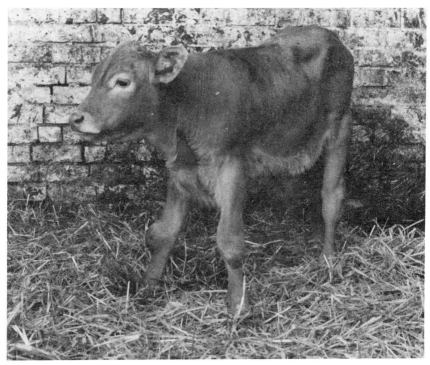

Plate 2.4 Calf with joint ill. Note the swollen front knees. Pus was drained from the knees using a needle and the calf eventually recovered.

associated navel ill. In the early stages calves are lethargic, they are reluctant to move and they have a raised temperature. Later, heat and a fluid swelling appears in one or more joints, and it is the hocks and knees which are particularly commonly affected. Because there is no blood flow into the joints, the condition is difficult to treat. If a case is caught in the early stages, then a prolonged course of antibiotic, for example up to three weeks, may produce a cure, and the Charolais calf in plate 2.4 was one such lucky case. Even so, pus had to be drained from its knees on two separate occasions. Once the calf has become totally recumbent from joint ill it is not worth treating. Probably half of the calves which develop serious joint ill die. Early treatment is essential. Prevention simply consists of dressing the navel at birth, as described for navel ill.

Umbilical Hernia (Navel Rupture)

The blood vessels from the placenta pass through a small hole in the skin and muscle of the calf's abdomen, and this should close at birth. Sometimes the hole in the muscle is larger than necessary however, and, after birth, this allows a segment of small intestine to prolapse through and lie between the skin and the muscle, producing a swelling in the navel region (plate 2.5). The

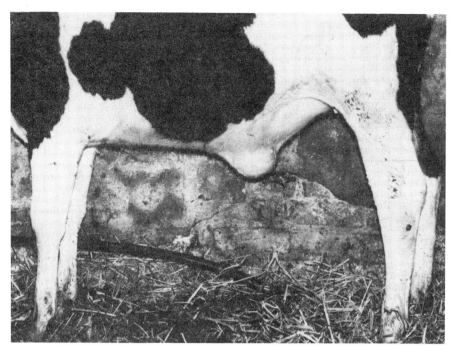

Plate 2.5   A large umbilical hernia.

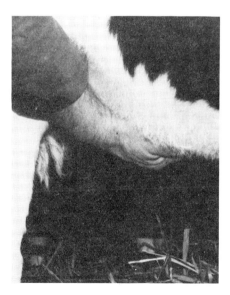

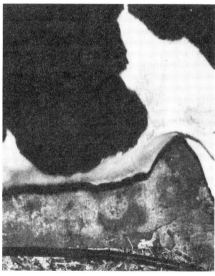

Plate 2.6   A hernia can easily be pushed back into the abdomen with your hand. A navel enlarged from infection cannot.

Plate 2.7   This is the same calf as plate 2.5, two weeks after its operation.

condition is correctly termed a hernia, because the intestine is prolapsing through a natural opening in the body wall. Although the term rupture is frequently used, this word should really be reserved for those cases where the body wall splits due to injury or excessive strain on the muscles, and intestine is then prolapsing through an artificial opening. Often the condition is not noticed until the calf is two months old or more. It differs from navel ill in that a navel hernia is soft, fluctuating and not painful; there is no temperature, the calf is not ill in any way and the swelling can easily be pushed back into the abdomen (plate 2.6). If the calf is sat upright on its tail the intestine returns to the abdomen and the swelling disappears. If the hernia is small, it will eventually resolve, since the hole in the body wall remains the same size, but the intestine enlarges with age until it is eventually unable to pass through the hernia. Other cases require surgery. The calf in plate 2.5 was four months old and there was no sign of the hernia regressing. A general anaesthetic was given, the body wall was closed with strong nylon tape and the excess skin removed and sutured. Plate 2.7 shows the same calf a week later. Some veterinary surgeons simply apply a metal clamp (plate 2.8) to the loose fold of skin, tightening the screws daily until the excess skin falls off due to lack of blood. This procedure was very successful for the calf shown in plate 2.9. The remaining skin is then much tighter along the body wall and keeps the intestine pushed back into the abdomen, although the hole remains.

On occasions I have seen large quantities of intestine prolapse through the fleshy navel cord immediately after birth, to lie exposed on the ground. This is a serious condition, but if the calf is operated on promptly it can be saved. You should keep it still, warm and quiet, and call for veterinary assistance.

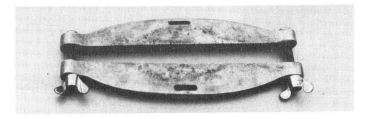

Plate 2.8   Metal clamp used to remove excess skin from a hernia.

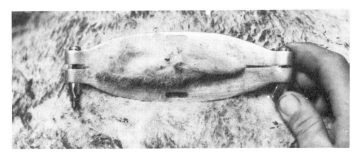

Plate 2.9   Hernia clamp applied to a calf. The two thumb screws have to be regularly tightened.

Conditions Affecting the Digestive Tract

Calf Diphtheria

This occurs mainly in the mouth, and may be seen in calves before and after weaning. Although the name is identical to the condition in man, the disease has a different cause and is far less serious. The bacterium concerned, *Fusiformis necrophorus*, gains entry to the soft tissues after the thick epithelial lining of the mouth has been damaged. Once established, the infection forms an ulcer covered by a layer of thick pus and this can be seen inside the calf's mouth. The common sites affected are the inside of the cheek and at the back of the tongue. The cheek form is probably caused by the calf accidentally biting the inside of its mouth and it is seen as a swelling of the skin between the upper and lower teeth (plate 2.10). This often causes little adverse effect on the calf, whereas the tongue form leads to difficulty in swallowing and affected calves are drooling and often frothing at the mouth (plate 2.11). When examined, they may have a mass of partially chewed hay at the front of the tongue and this needs to be removed in order to see the pus and blood associated with the diphtheria ulcer. These calves will also have a high temperature and often a foul-smelling breath. If left untreated, infection can pass down into the lungs and cause a fatal pneumonia. Occasionally the larynx ('voice box', figure 2.1) is the primary site of infection. Affected calves breathe extremely noisily, a 'roaring' or 'snoring' breathing, but they are not

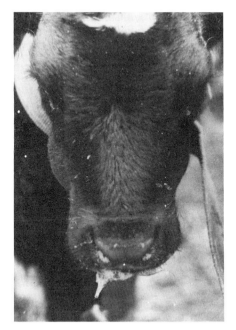

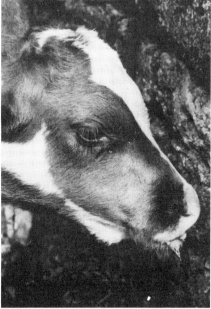

Plate 2.10 Calf with diphtheria—note the swelling of the cheeks on the left.

Plate 2.11 Calf with diphtheria on tongue, drooling badly and prolapsing its tongue.

particularly ill and their respiration rate is normal. This syndrome should not be confused with calf pneumonia, where breathing will be quieter but faster, and the calf will be very sick. Occasionally diphtheria infection also passes down into the rumen and produces a digestive upset.

Treatment
Antibiotic therapy by injection is needed and your vet will prescribe a suitable drug. If the calf is badly affected, it needs to be fed liquids, preferably three or four times daily and removed from the rest of the group, since it could act as a source of infection to the others.

Prevention
Avoid dirty feeding troughs and hay containing thistles or other sharp material which might damage the lining of the mouth.

Ruminal Bloat

In the preweaned calf this is caused by a defect in feeding, such that the oesophageal groove fails to close and milk passes into the rumen. As there are no digestive enzymes in the rumen, the milk 'sours' and ferments, producing gas which cannot be released because the immature rumen does not contract. This leads to bloat, the gas-filled rumen pushing out the skin on the left side of the calf. Affected calves are unthrifty, dull and poor feeders because of the pain associated with the ruminal distension. They may also develop a pasty scour, caused by sour milk passing from the rumen into the lower digestive tract. If left unattended, extreme pressure can develop inside the rumen leading to death from heart failure. On other occasions the bloat leads to acute colic and the calf may fall to the ground, kicking at its abdomen, some thirty to sixty minutes after feeding.

Treatment
In severe cases the first priority must be to relieve the gas, either by passing a stomach tube, or by inserting a large-bore needle through the skin and into the rumen. As with bloat in the adult animal (when a trocar and cannula would be used), the instrument must be pushed through the skin on the *left* side, at a point mid-way between the last rib and the edges of the vertebrae of the spine. The correct position is shown in figure 2.3. The needle or trocar (plate 12.7) is then pushed towards the direction of the right front leg, that is through the skin and into the rumen. The stomach of the calf can be lifted upwards with your knee to expel the remaining gas. This is an emergency procedure however. It will certainly save the life of a seriously blown calf, but I suggest that you then call for veterinary assistance to prevent peritonitis and other complications.

There is less risk associated with passing a stomach tube, and a length of flexible 15 mm garden hosepipe will suffice provided that it does not have sharp ends. If you reverse the calf into a corner, stand beside it and hold its mouth upwards as shown in plate 2.12 the stomach tube can be used quite

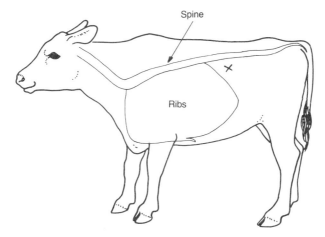

Figure 2.3 Where to insert the needle to deflate a blown calf. A trocar and cannula would be inserted at 'X' and pushed towards the elbow of the right foreleg.

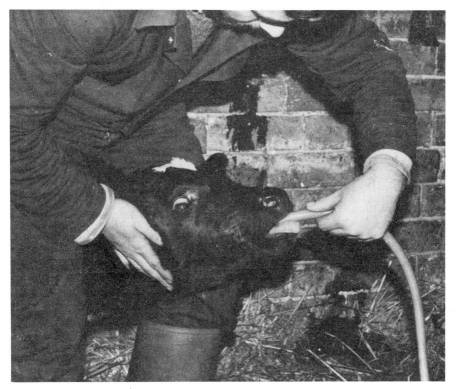

Plate 2.12 Passing a stomach tube. It would be better if the free end of the tube was resting over the operator's left shoulder.

easily. From figure 2.1 it can be seen that when the tube is inserted into the calf's mouth it must pass over the top of the larynx and trachea before it can be swallowed and fed down into the oesophagus. If you are in any doubt as to whether the tube is in the oesophagus or the trachea, simply place your ear over the end of the tube and see if you can feel or hear air moving in and out in parallel with the breathing. If the answer is yes, the tube is in the trachea and it needs to be withdrawn and reinserted.

For less severely affected calves, drenching with antibiotic by mouth (e.g. an anti-scour preparation, either as a tablet or as a liquid) will reduce the bacterial fermentation and sometimes results in a cure. This should be continued for several days and at the same time all solid food should be removed (to allow the rumen to empty and clean itself). For the first three days the calf should be fed on an electrolyte solution only (see section on calf scour), before slowly and carefully reintroducing milk. Sometimes chronic bloat occurs in calves soon after weaning, again due to 'souring' of rumen contents or inadequate rumen development. Similar treatment should be given:

• release the gas in severely affected cases;
• remove all solid food and return the calf to a liquid diet for seven to ten days minimum;
• dose with antibiotics by mouth.

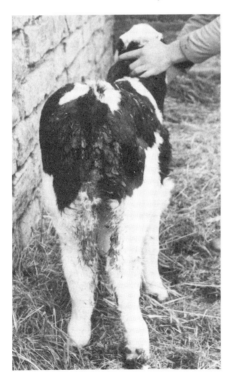

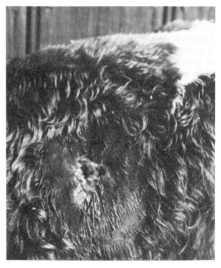

Plate 2.13   A blown calf. The soiled tail is typical of the digestive upset associated with a sour rumen.

Plate 2.14   Relief of bloat: the rumen has been sutured to the skin to provide a permanent route for the escape of gas.

Occasionally bloat becomes a repetitive problem and the calf shown in plate 2.13 was a typical example of this. He had been weaned for two weeks and was unthrifty with periodic bouts of bloat and scouring. His soiled tail is a good indication of the digestive upset associated with a sour rumen. A permanent hole was made by suturing the rumen wall to the skin as shown in plate 2.14, and this is also the point where the trocar and cannula would be inserted. Rumen contents spilled down over its side but this did not worry the calf as much as its owner! It improved almost immediately after the operation and certainly grew better than when it was bloated. It is not a difficult operation and the success rate should be almost one hundred per cent. With any of the other measures there is always the risk that bloat will unexpectedly form again, causing death before any treatment can be given. Sometimes the hole will slowly close itself, although more often it is necessary to have it sutured at twelve months old or more. Beef animals could be left with the hole open.

THE SCOURING CALF

Scouring is the commonest disease in young calves and it is without doubt the greatest single cause of death. I find it extremely frustrating to examine a

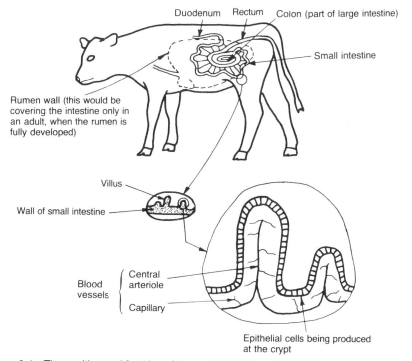

Figure 2.4   The position and function of the small intestine and its villi.

collapsed scouring calf and to realise that it is 'too far gone', especially when you know that correct treatment a few days or even hours earlier, could have saved the animal. In order to understand fully what goes wrong, we need to spend a few minutes discussing the normal calf. The small intestine is responsible for absorption of nutrients and water. To increase its surface area and hence its functional capacity, the inner surface consists of a mat of small, finger-like projections called villi. These are shown in detail in figure 2.4. Each villus is covered with a lining of epithelial cells. These are produced at the base of the villus (the crypt) and slowly pass up towards the tip. A small blood vessel (an arteriole) runs down the centre of the villus, with small branches (capillaries) radiating out towards the epithelial lining cells. The epithelial cells at the tip of the villus pump water into the central arteriole, making the blood at this point more dilute. Salts (e.g. sodium, bicarbonate or potassium) and other nutrients (e.g. glucose and amino acids) are now drawn in from the intestine by diffusion. This flow of material is shown in figure 2.5. There is also a flow of water from the blood into the intestine, in fact the total amount of water passing into and out of the normal intestine is approximately 100 litres per day each way. Water therefore enters the small intestine firstly from drinking and secondly from the blood.

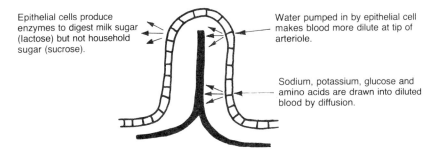

Figure 2.5   Flow of water and nutrients in a normal calf.

This flow of water into and out of the intestine is shown diagrammatically in figure 2.6. Let us assume for this particular length of intestine that 1.1. litres/day are drunk and 4 litres/day passes into the intestine from the blood supply. In the normal calf, 5 litres/day would be reabsorbed, to produce semi-solid faeces, containing only 0.1 litres water per day, i.e.

1.1 litres + 4.0 litres *in* → 5.0 litres + 0.1 litres *out* in faeces.

So what happens with diarrhoea? There are a variety of different causes and these will be dealt with individually later, e.g.

- bacterial infections
- viral infections
- digestive upsets.

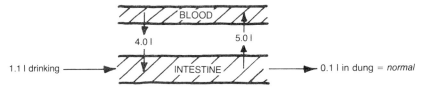

Figure 2.6   Water flow in a normal calf. The quantities are arbitrary, but in the correct proportions to one another.

In each case the overall effect is the same. Scouring means that more fluid is lost via the faeces and if this is not replaced by additional intakes by mouth, *dehydration* occurs: the blood becomes 'thicker' and more difficult for the heart to pump, poor circulation develops, body temperature drops and the calf goes into a state of shock.

Bacteria have adhesive properties. They stick to the epithelial cells of the villi and produce toxins which stimulate an increased flow of fluid *into* the intestine—this is the intestine's defence to try to flush the bacteria away. The flow of fluid from the blood into the intestine increases from 4.0 litres to 6.0 litres, and so our overall fluid balance equation becomes:

1.1 litres + 6.0 litres *in* → 5.0 litres + 2.1 litres *out* (figure 2.7).

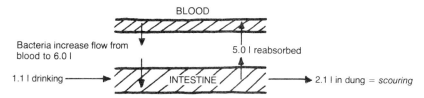

Figure 2.7   Bacteria cause scouring by sticking to the villi and causing an increased flow of fluid from the blood into the intestine.

Reabsorption of fluid remains the same, so excess is voided with the faeces producing scouring.

Viruses on the other hand destroy the villi and reduce the rate of reabsorption of water. The rate of flow of water into the intestine remains normal (4.0 litres), but because the villi are damaged let us say that only 3.0 litres are reabsorbed. The fluid balance equation now becomes:

1.1 litres + 4.0 litres *in* → 3.0 litres + 2.1 litres *out* (figure 2.8).

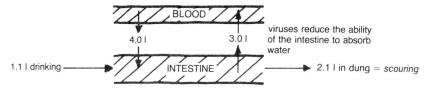

Figure 2.8   Viruses cause scouring by destroying the villi and preventing water absorption from the intestine.

Far more fluid is therefore voided in the faeces and scouring again occurs.

In both types of scouring the excess water in the faeces carries with it salts and other nutrients which would have been absorbed by the villi had they not been damaged. The capacity of the villi to produce digestive enzymes will also be reduced and hence whole milk, including lactose, may pass straight through into the large bowel, ferment and cause further diarrhoea. Treatment of the scouring calf should therefore consist of:

1. Withholding milk—because the intestine may no longer possess the enzyme capacity to digest it.
2. Providing fluids—to try to counteract the massive loss in the faeces. Remember that a scouring calf has a much higher fluid requirement and may need to be offered small quantities four or even six times a day.
3. Replenishing the salts and nutrients. Several commercial preparations exist (e.g. Beechams Scour Formula, Lectade, Ion-Aid) formulated to correct the balance of water, salts and nutrients, and these can produce excellent results in terms of recovery. There is also a plastic dispensing bag

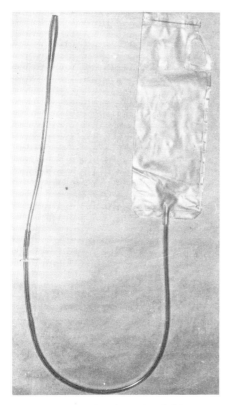

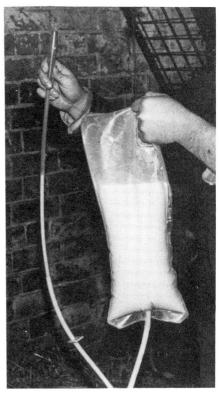

Plate 2.15   Bag for dispensing fluids to sick calves.

Plate 2.16   Dispensing bag filled with colostrum. The stomach tube part is held in the operator's right hand.

combined with a stomach tube (plate 2.15) available for calves which will not drink. This is much safer than drenching them. Plate 2.16 shows the same bag filled with colostrum ready to dose a newly-born calf too weak to suckle.

4. Administering antibiotics. They may be given by mouth, and/or by injection if there is a risk of septicaemia, and your veterinary surgeon will advise you on the most suitable preparation. There is considerable evidence that prolonged overdosing with oral antibiotics can in fact *induce* scouring, so care must be taken to ensure that a lengthy treatment is not making the situation worse.

Establishing the exact cause of scouring is often not an easy task and it is certainly an area where veterinary assistance will be required. For the stockman, treatment must be the first priority, and the guidelines given above apply to all types of scouring. At the same time, and especially if several calves have been affected, some thought ought to be given to prevention and the following points apply, irrespective of the cause of the scour:

- Separate scouring calves from the remainder of the group, thus reducing the 'challenge dose' of infection to otherwise healthy calves.
- Pay strict attention to cleaning buckets after each feed, or ensure that each calf has its own individual bucket. Salmonella, for example, can be spread via the saliva.
- Ensure that the milk substitute is fed at the correct strength and temperature and that feeding times are regular each day. This promotes both oesophageal groove closure and subsequent abomasal clot formation and digestion.
- If it is necessary to enter calf pens, consider providing a disinfectant foot dip to prevent infection being carried from one pen to another.
- As soon as possible, depopulate the calf house for cleaning as described on page 17. Start introducing new calves into a different building with clean pens and make sure that these calves are fed and attended each day before the scouring group.
- Ensure beds are dry and warm and that calves are not exposed to draughts. Sick animals may have a fever or a subnormal temperature from dehydration and shock. In both cases a heat lamp will be beneficial.

Prevention
The majority of strong, healthy and well-managed calves can withstand a substantial challenge of infection and the most important preventive measures are to provide suitable housing, ensure adequate colostrum intake and avoid digestive upsets. These factors were all discussed in detail in the early part of this chapter. Vaccination against E. coli is used but as the calf is being exposed to E. coli from birth onwards and therefore creating its own active immunity and as the vaccines may not contain the correct serotype or stimulate high levels of immunity, it would be unwise to place too much emphasis on their rôle in the overall control of scouring.

Let us now examine some of the specific causes of scour in more detail.

White Scour

The majority of calves pass yellowish dung when they are scouring and often the very fluid nature of the dung is simply a reflection of an excessive milk intake, or possibly a digestive upset. If the faeces turn to a white or off-white colour however this is strongly indicative of scouring caused by *Escherichia coli*, more commonly known as E. coli, a bacterium that will be mentioned on several occasions in this book. The dung may not be particularly loose, but affected calves become dull and listless, and in the early stages they will have a high temperature. This is due to *septicaemia*, which means that some of the E. coli have left the intestine and are multiplying in the bloodstream and tissues throughout the calf. Sometimes this is called *colibacillosis*, or coli septicaemia. Typically only calves in the first week of life are affected, and the majority will have received insufficient colostrum. At this stage treatment with antibiotics by injection is necessary and careful nursing, with warmth and a dry bed, is important, in addition to the fluid replacement measures which were discussed earlier.

White scour can spread rapidly through a group of animals, so individual cases should be isolated as quickly as possible. A variety of measures are available for prevention and the steps most suited to your unit will depend on when the problem occurs, the layout of the pens and the feeding system. Careful hygiene is always essential. In addition, calves can be given *antiserum* at birth to boost their immunity. Antiserum contains preformed antibodies against E. coli, but as there are over a hundred different strains of E. coli its effectiveness will depend on whether the commercial antiserum you are using contains antibodies to the E. coli causing the scouring on your farm. In other words, does the antiserum have the correct specificity? The same considerations apply to *vaccination*. If scouring has been occurring at two to four weeks old or more, then a killed E. coli vaccine can be given as two doses two weeks apart, thus providing the calf with the means to boost its own antibody levels before exposure to the heavy challenge dose of infection. Sometimes the problem can be correlated with a particular stage of management and in such cases the use of antibiotics, administered during the period of risk, may be a justifiable short-term preventive method of reducing the bacterial challenge while management is being improved. However, if there is a very heavy environmental challenge, infection may be ingested within hours of birth.

Rotavirus, Coronavirus and BVD Infection

Although it is not possible to identify the cause of scouring with any certainty, virus infections generally affect calves during their first week of life and cause a watery diarrhoea. This is because the virus destroys the cells lining the intestinal villi and water reabsorption is prevented (see page 33 and figure 2.8). The main clinical feature is therefore *dehydration*—the calf is dull, its eyes are sunken and the coat feels cold. The temperature may be slightly increased in the early stages, but it soon falls. Fluid therapy is vital and although antibiotics have no effect against the primary virus infection (see page 14), they may be of value in preventing a secondary bacterial attack on the damaged intestinal wall.

Rotavirus and coronavirus scouring may be seen in herds where heifers are reared separately from infected cows. If the heifer herd is not infected, the calves born to the heifers will not be provided with anti-virus antibodies from the colostrum. As soon as these calves are mixed with calves from the main herd, therefore, they succumb to disease. Calves from cows may not be affected because they have been given sufficient colostral antibody to counteract the virus. However, with the heifers' calves shedding vast quantities of virus, the overall level of infection on the unit may become so high that even the colostral antibody levels will not be sufficient protection, in which case both heifers' and cows' calves may succumb to disease.

The virus of bovine viral diarrhoea, BVD, can also cause problems, especially if the dam herself is infected in mid-pregnancy. BVD virus can pass the placenta and if it attacks the foetus during a specific stage of the development of its immune system, then the cells which would produce BVD antibodies later in life are destroyed and the calf is known as *immune tolerant*: it can no longer recognise BVD virus as an antigen. Such animals do not produce antibodies to BVD and contact of animal with virus later in life can lead to a severe disease and possibly the death of the calf. This could occur at any age and would not necessarily be a problem of the young calf. It can be a cause of chronic scouring and weight loss in one or two cattle in a group, not uncommonly leading to eventual death.

Salmonellosis

This is a bacterial infection which can cause a wide range of symptoms. The overall problem of salmonella in cattle is dealt with more fully in Chapter Ten and the disease in weaned calves in Chapter Three. At this stage only the disease in the young milk-fed calf will be considered. The commonest serotype found in young calves is *Salmonella typhimurium*. Disease is seen as a profuse yellow diarrhoea, with septicaemia and a high temperature, and death may occur in twenty-four hours or less. More chronic forms do occur, however, in which an affected calf simply has pasty dung and is unthrifty and, at the far end of the spectrum, some calves may carry the infection without suffering any adverse effects. In some ways it is these latter animals which cause the difficulties. They probably have good levels of antibody defences against salmonella, but are *intermittent excretors*, that is sometimes they shed salmonella in their faeces and sometimes they do not. Excretion is far more likely during period of stress and this has a considerable practical significance, for example:

- the stress of transport. Carrier calves are more likely to be infecting their pen-mates when they are in the market, or if they have recently been brought home from market.
- the stress of a digestive upset. The primary cause of scouring in a calf unit may have been a faulty milk mixture, or some other digestive upset but this

can lead to increased salmonella excretion and then a breakdown with clinical salmonellosis.

● the stress of intercurrent disease. Carrier calves may develop navel ill or calf pneumonia and this can lead to increased activity of the salmonella, either causing disease in the carrier animal itself, or spreading it to others.

Because the carrier calf may be an *intermittent excretor* of *Salmonella typhimurium*, it is not possible to take a faecal swab for culture and on the basis of one negative bacteriological result be sure that the animal is 'safe' to introduce into your calf unit. Swabbing daily for five days would be a better screening, but it would still not conclusively eliminate a hundred per cent of carrier calves and it would also be extremely costly. Anyone purchasing calves should therefore try to reduce the risk of salmonella by taking the following measures.

1. Buy from as few different sources as possible and try to ensure adequate colostrum intake at birth.

2. Avoid market calves—these have been exposed to many other possibly infected calves, all of which have been subjected to the stresses of transport, cold, lack of food etc., which would increase the salmonella excretion rate from carrier animals.

3. Buy only strong and healthy calves which could withstand a low level of salmonella challenge.

4. Treat calves very gently on arrival—separate penning, warm and dry bedding, feeding electrolytes only for the first twelve to eighteen hours, then increase milk gradually.

5. Vaccination—a live vaccine is currently available against S. typhimurium and S. dublin. This can be given at any time from one day old or from the day of purchase and it gives a very good immunity within seven days. There is a small risk of death from hypersensitivity within hours of administering the vaccine however and its use needs to be discussed with your veterinary surgeon. It may also be dangerous if administered to a calf already incubating salmonella.

It should be pointed out that *Salmonella typhimurium* can cause diarrhoea in man and even death in young children. Personal hygiene, especially washing hands, is always important after handling calves and especially scouring animals. The importance of markets and calf dealing in the spread of S. typhimurium was clearly demonstrated in 1977–8 when a chloramphicol resistant strain of the bacterium, called DT204, was responsible for a severe outbreak of disease in calves in Somerset and the South-West of England. The organism travelled with calves to cause outbreaks of disease on farms in the Yorkshire area and even up to the North-East of Scotland. Proposals have been submitted which would prohibit calves from being offered for sale at markets more than once every four to six weeks. If accepted, this would help to reduce the rate of spread of salmonella.

Cryptosporidia

This is a small protozoan parasite which affects the lower small intestine (the same area as E. coli) of calves in their first week of life to cause scouring. Affected calves may or may not develop a temperature and the symptoms are those of dehydration, loss of appetite, scouring, sometimes with mucus, and unthriftiness. Special techniques are required for diagnosis and if you have an unresponsive scour problem you should seek veterinary advice. Cryptosporidia are related to coccidia (see page 43) and similar drugs have been used for treatment, though not very successfully.

ALOPECIA (HAIR LOSS)

On occasions one or more calves in a group start to lose their hair. The animals concerned are usually being bucket-fed and the hair loss is most noticeable around the muzzle, on the neck and extending down the hind legs. Careful examination fails to reveal any lice, the skin is soft and there are no scurf or scabs which might indicate a fungal infection. A typical example, affecting the head and front legs only, is shown in plate 2.17.

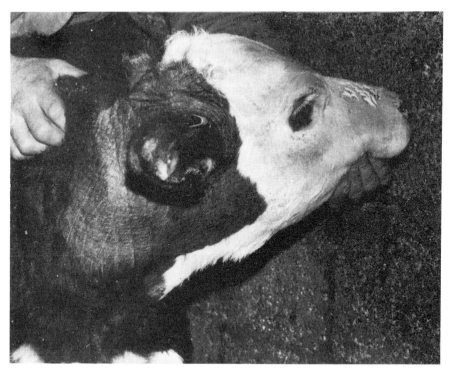

Plate 2.17 Alopecia, or hair loss, affecting the calf's head and front legs. The calf was suckling a cow when it developed only a mild fever, but then lost its hair a week later.

A previous severe attack of scour is one possible cause, or improperly mixed or cold milk leading to separation of fat globules and their accumulation on the calf's muzzle. The condition can occur spontaneously however and may be associated with high-fat diets leading to an increased vitamin E requirement. Some people have reported a good response to vitamin therapy, especially A, D and E, and others have suggested a more definite link with muscular dystrophy. Although it is probable that a proportion of these cases would recover without treatment, an injection of vitamins would be a sensible measure.

Chapter 3

THE WEANED CALF

TRADITIONALLY calves were weaned at almost eight weeks old, although in recent years this has been reduced to six weeks or even five weeks old. Calves may be weaned as soon as they are eating significant quantities of concentrate, for example 1–2 kg per day, and the concentrate being offered needs to be highly palatable to achieve these intakes. Some calves are abruptly weaned, but it is more common to reduce to once-daily feeding for a few days before totally withdrawing milk. Fresh water and palatable forage (hay or straw) should be freely available throughout. The change from a liquid to a solid diet is a critical time for the calf, and to be successful it is important that preweaning feeding has allowed the rumen to develop to its full size and that it is functioning correctly. Inadequate ruminal development before weaning can lead to many post-weaning digestive problems, with bloat and scouring being the most common. After weaning the calf needs to be given a highly nutritious diet to compensate for the loss of milk. It has probably been moved from individual pens to group housing, where it must compete with others for trough space. If the stress of this is combined with an overall reduction in nutritional status, then the calf is rendered more susceptible to disease, and this is at a time when its passive antibody levels (see page 7) are still declining. As with the young calf, many health problems are exacerbated by poor management, and one of the most important preventive measures for all the diseases of the weaned calf is to provide adequate space, good housing and a well-balanced diet.

The diseases of the weaned calf will be considered on the basis of their main symptoms. These are:

Digestive problems
> bloat
> colic
> coccidiosis
> salmonellosis

Skin conditions
> ringworm
> lice
> mange

41

Respiratory problems
  calf pneumonia

Deficiency diseases
  muscular dystrophy
  nutritional deficiencies

Nervous diseases
  lead poisoning
  cerebrocortical necrosis
  meningitis
  tetanus

DIGESTIVE PROBLEMS

It is not unusual to see scouring in calves soon after weaning. The faeces are dark, grey and pasty, and the most likely cause is simply an excessive concentrate intake. This may be because hay or straw has been restricted and the calves have consumed an excess of concentrate, although poor-quality forage making it unpalatable would have a similar effect. In both cases, concentrate intakes ought to be reduced until scouring ceases and the primary causes are found. If scouring is allowed to continue, calves become unthrifty and dirty, the intestine becomes damaged and poor growth results. Sometimes treatment is needed and a kaolin/chlorodyne mixture, 50 ml/calf/day, can be very effective as a physical anti-scour remedy, although you would be best to consult your veterinary surgeon for other possible treatments and to make sure that one of the more serious conditions mentioned later in the chapter is not involved.

Bloat

Bloat is seen most commonly immediately post-weaning and is due to cessation of ruminal movements, such that the gas produced during the normal fermentation processes cannot escape. Often ruminal contents become sour and this may lead to a pale, grey-coloured, pasty scour, which tends to stick to the calf's tail. A typical example is shown in plate 2.13. Even in an individual calf the extent of the bloat will vary, usually being at its worst one to two hours after a feed of concentrate. Some calves recover spontaneously although others, if left, develop severe bloat and can quickly die.

Treatment
It is often difficult to assess how severely affected the calf is, but because there is always a risk of fatality it is better to overtreat, rather than undertreat. The steps are similar to those discussed in the previous chapter, page 28, for preweaned calves, i.e.

- release the gas by stomach tube or a needle into the rumen;
- dose with oral antibiotics for four to six days;

- return the calf to milk feeding for seven days and withdraw concentrate;
- if these measures fail, a permanent hole, a ruminal *fistula*, can be prepared surgically (see plate 2.14).

Prevention

Make sure that the calves are eating reasonable quantities of concentrate and forage before weaning and avoid over-consumption of concentrate in the early post-weaning stage. As it is the presence of long fibre in the rumen which stimulates ruminal contractions, it is essential to ensure that good palatable hay and straw are available at all times. Bloat in the adult animal is described on page 317.

Colic

The word 'colic' simply means severe abdominal pain; it does not give any indication as to what is causing the pain. It may be due to a twisted gut or an intussusception or one of the other more serious conditions discussed in Chapter Twelve. However on occasions calves may be seen kicking at their stomachs or even rolling on the ground and bellowing with pain. They can make a rapid recovery, less than one to two hours following the administration of drugs to relax the intestine. In such cases the pain must simply be due to a spasm, that is an excessive contraction, of the intestine. A similar syndrome may be seen in calves still on liquid diets.

Coccidiosis

This is caused by a small protozoan parasite called *Eimeria zurnii*, which burrows into the wall of the lower gut. Typically, affected calves pass semi-solid faeces, usually with variable quantities of chocolate-brown blood mixed with it. Scouring is a feature and the calf's tail becomes soiled, but the faeces are not as liquid as in some cases of diarrhoea in younger calves. If the faeces are examined carefully, small lumps of a fawn-coloured gelatinous material may be seen. This is the *mucosa*, or lining, of the intestine. Probably the most characteristic clinical sign of coccidiosis is *straining*, technically known as *tenesmus*: the calf stands with its tail raised and appears to be continually trying to force out small quantities of blood, mucus and faeces. After a few days this makes them dull, they run a moderate temperature and lose weight rapidly. Death can occur in untreated cases and you will need your vet to confirm the diagnosis so that specific anticoccidiosis therapy (e.g. sulphonamides or amprolium) can be given. Affected calves should be dosed at treatment level and any in-contact animals at preventive level, because it is likely that all calves are exposed to the same source of infection and the condition can rapidly spread.

The coccidian life cycle

This is shown in figure 3.1. The coccidiosis eggs or *oocysts* are taken in by

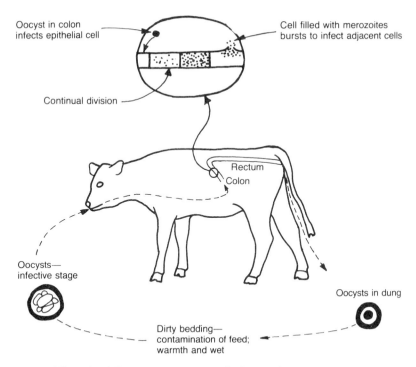

Figure 3.1   Life cycle of *Eimeria zurnii*, the coccidiosis parasite.

mouth, pass through the acid barrier of the abomasum and hatch out in the large intestine (colon, caecum and rectum—figures 2.4 and 12.4), where they invade the cells lining the gut wall. Once inside the cell the oocyst repeatedly divides, to produce thousands of vegetative forms, the *merozoites*. These rupture the cell and are liberated into the intestine to infect and destroy adjacent healthy cells. Resistant forms, the oocysts, are produced sexually at a later stage and are passed out in the faeces. The oocyst has a very thick wall and as such it can survive in the environment for many months, waiting to be eaten by another calf so that its life-cycle can start again.

The initial source of infection is most probably the cow, since many adult animals carry the infection without showing any symptoms. Affected calves can rapidly pass infection to their pen-mates, however, and this occurs especially where hygiene is poor and there is an increased risk of faecal contamination of the feed, for example when water and food troughs are dirty, or inadequate bedding is used. The oocyst is an extremely resistant form and is not affected by many of the standard disinfectants. Dirty pens should be thoroughly cleaned, washed and then soaked with an ammonia-based product or a specific proprietary anticoccidial disinfectant, before a new group of calves is introduced.

Salmonellosis

The disease in young calves, usually involving S. typhimurium, has been described in Chapter Two, and the overall problem of salmonellosis is dealt with in Chapter Ten, where the wide range of other species of salmonella, called *serotypes*, are described. A common type in weaned calves is S. dublin. Infection is contracted from symptomless carriers (see page 38), either the dam or from other calves when groups are mixed at weaning. One of the peculiar and often frustrating aspects of S. dublin is that infection may exist within the herd for several years without ever causing disease. When disease does occur, and no stock have been purchased, it is difficult to explain *why* the outbreak has occurred. In the carrier animal, infection persists in the mesenteric lymph glands, the small 'drainage' organs associated with the intestine. Excretion of infection, i.e. the passing of salmonella in the faeces of carrier calves, is likely to be very intermittent and may not occur at all for quite long periods. This means that it is difficult to identify carrier animals simply by taking faecal swabs and trying to isolate S. dublin in the laboratory. A positive result shows that infection is present and action can be taken. However, a negative result can either mean that the calf is not a carrier, or it may simply mean that the calf was not shedding infection when the swab was taken. Serial swabbing of a group of calves, e.g. at weekly intervals, would give a better chance of identifying carriers, but even then a negative result would not be conclusive proof of absence of infection.

Clinical signs

S. dublin can cause scouring, and in this respect it resembles S. typhimurium, but it can also cause other clinical signs such as septicaemia, pneumonia, or meningitis, and these may occur without any obvious change in the faeces. The affected calf will run a high temperature in the early stages and scouring may occur, but it may not be particularly severe. Sometimes scouring is profuse, however, and lumps of intestine wall, blood and mucus are passed. The calf will be dull, its coat bristling rather than smooth, its appetite reduced and there may be some coughing. On occasions a group of calves may simply appear unthrifty and sudden deaths occur, but following post-mortem examination the organism can be isolated from throughout the carcase. Salmonella in weaned calves is often an extension of the disease which has been present earlier in life. The acute phase is over and the calves remain unthrifty with pneumonia and/or arthritis.

Treatment and control

Diagnosis is difficult and your vet will need to examine the calves and take faecal samples to the laboratory for culture. Once the presence of S. dublin has been confirmed, antibiotic therapy may be administered to affected calves and, whenever possible, the calves should be isolated, to reduce the weight of challenge of infection to the remainder of the group. There is a good live vaccine available (Mellavax—Burroughs Wellcome) and other calves can be vaccinated to give them protection before entering the infected area.

Although antibiotics need to be given to avoid fatalities, there is now good evidence that they in fact *prolong* the period of excretion of the organism, and in so doing they reduce the chances of self-cure and increase the risk of an animal becoming a carrier. Treatment needs to be considered very carefully therefore, since many animals will throw off the infection themselves and achieve a full cure.

S. dublin can infect adult cows (see Chapter Ten), so careful hygiene is needed to prevent the spread of infection. When the infected group has left the building, clean out and rest as described on page 17. Ideally, soiled bedding needs to be stacked and heated to avoid pasture contamination, since it has been shown that faeces may remain infectious for several weeks even when spread onto pasture.

Skin Conditions

Ringworm

This is a fungal infection caused by *Trichophyton verrucosum*, although occasionally other species of ringworm may be involved. The fungus grows on the skin and penetrates the hair follicle (figure 3.2). Affected hairs become very brittle and they break off at the surface of the skin, producing circular bald patches. The presence of the fungus also leads to thickening and flaking of the skin and grey-brown debris can be easily picked off. The head and neck are the most commonly affected areas (plate 3.1), especially around the eyes, nose and ears, although lesions may occur over the whole body. Occasionally secondary bacterial infection occurs and the lesions become moist and discharge pus.

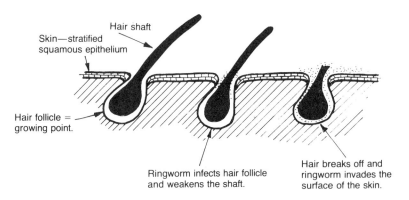

Figure 3.2   Ringworm infection. This leads to loss of hair and a crusty scaling over the skin surface.

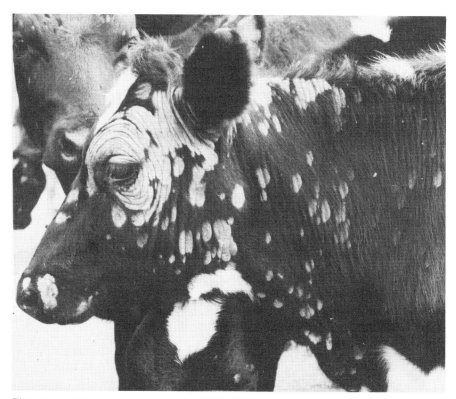

Plate 3.1 Ringworm infestation, typically on the head and neck.

Ringworm causes irritation. Affected calves rub their heads on troughs and hayracks and these act as a source of infection for other animals. Spread from one calf to another is especially common at feeding time.

Treatment
Traditionally, affected skin was painted with creosote, diesel oil, or other chemicals which would physically kill the ringworm. Aerosol cans of copper-based chemicals achieve a similar effect and are often used. While these treatments are not without merit, they can be dangerous to the calves' eyes and they have been largely superseded by more modern drugs, the two most important being:

1. Griseofulvin. This is an antibiotic-based drug which is given by mouth daily for seven days. The drug is incorporated into the growing hair and skin, so that by the end of a week's treatment the whole animal is covered by a protective layer of griseofulvin, and this persists for four to six weeks. Griseofulvin does not actually kill ringworm, it only prevents its growth. (It is fungistatic, not fungicidal—see page 12). The calf's own immune defences destroy the fungus, and this has two important practical considerations.

Firstly, healthy calves in good condition respond to treatment better than do poor and unthrifty animals, which may have concurrent pneumonia or salmonella infections. Secondly, although the lesions may start to resolve by the end of the first week, the calf remains infectious to others for a further two to three weeks.

Treatment should be given to the whole affected group. Since the incubation period of ringworm is approximately three weeks, attempts to separate and treat individual affected calves are generally unsuccessful, because further cases will probably continue to appear in the non-affected group.

2. *Natamycin*. This is administered as a spray and it is essential that all parts of the animal are thoroughly soaked, at the rate recommended by the manufacturer. It is simply not sufficient to spray across the top of the calves at random. As with griseofulvin, the whole group should be treated and it is also worthwhile applying any remaining spray to troughs and fittings, since it will also counteract infection at these sites.

Prevention
The only sure way of prevention is to avoid contact with other animals and infective material. Ringworm seems to occur even in a closed herd, however, and often it affects successive crops of calves for two or three years, then it is not seen again for a further few years. The spores produced are very resistant and may persist for up to four years if they are in a dry place. Elimination of infection from a building is therefore very difficult and is usually attempted either by a flame-gun or by painting with creosote or 4 per cent sodium carbonate. Calves in poor condition are often the worst affected and maintaining a high standard of general health and nutrition will help to reduce the effects of ringworm. Sometimes an injection of vitamins A, D and E aids recovery. Ringworm is killed by ultra-violet light and many cases resolve spontaneously when calves are turned out in the spring. This is probably a combination of the effects of the sun and improved nutrition. Ringworm can also occur in outdoor cattle however, especially in the autumn, and if they are then housed under rather cramped conditions the disease can spread rapidly.

All species of animal ringworm are infectious to man, especially younger children, and care should be taken when handling affected animals.

Lice

Although there are many cheap and effective treatments available, it never ceases to surprise me how many farms suffer reduced growth rates from heavy lice infestations. There are two separate types of lice:

Sucking lice:
  Haematopinus eurysternus
  Linognathus vituli
Biting lice
  Bovicola bovis.

Lice live on the surface of the skin and can just be seen with the naked eye. They are dark grey/brown in colour and approximately the size of a flattened pin-head. To see them, it may be necessary to look in several places, pulling aside the hair with both hands and looking for movement at the base of the hair. The other sign of infestation is the presence of lice eggs which are glued to the hair-shaft and are seen as small white dots (plate 3.2). The life-cycle is very simple: adults lay eggs which hatch after ten to fourteen days into 'nymphs' or immature lice, and these take two weeks to develop into maturity. The whole life cycle, that is from an egg being laid to a mature egg-laying female, takes four weeks.

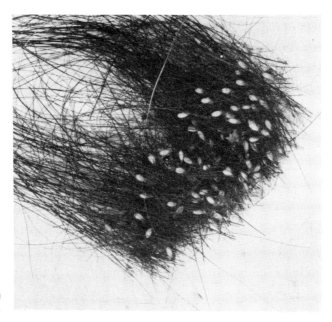

Plate 3.2   Lice eggs on
            hair shaft.

Clinical signs

The first sign of infestation is irritation. Affected animals rub their necks and backs, or there may be patches of hair loss where calves have been biting at their skin (plate 3.3). This is especially true for biting lice, which can be intensely irritating. The shoulders, neck and back are usually the worst areas, although the belly and scrotum may also be affected. On a louse-infested neck, the coat is often arranged in lines running from top to bottom (plate 3.4) and this makes diagnosis easy. Biting lice produce a crusty scurf on the surface of the skin, while sucking lice can produce a severe anaemia. I have often seen instances where calves are so badly 'run down' with a heavy louse infestation that they lose weight and are much more prone to ringworm, pneumonia and other diseases. Calves of poor nutritional status, on the other hand, are also far more susceptible to lice.

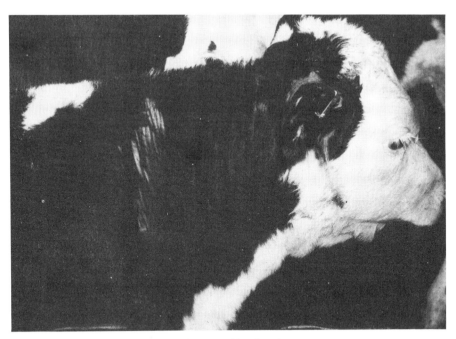

Plate 3.3 Lice—bite marks and hair loss on side of neck.

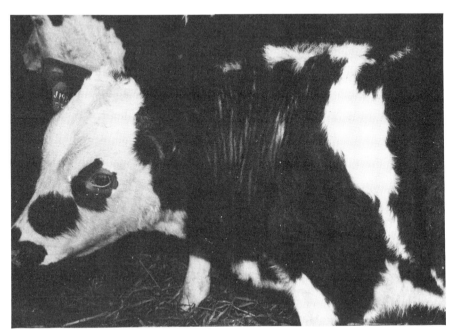

Plate 3.4 Lice—coat tends to be arranged in lines along the calf's neck.

Treatment

The traditional 'louse powder', 0.6–1.0 per cent gamma benzene hexachloride (BHC) is effective, provided that it is thoroughly worked into the coat. Organo-phosphorus compounds can also be used and these will be available in the form of fly-repellents or warble-fly treatments. There are many brands of commercial fly-repellent and provided that they are well applied, they should give a persistency of two to four weeks, although it is sometimes difficult to get the full recommended dose to stay on the animal. Warble-fly treatments are normally 'pour-on'. The chemical is applied to the animal's back, absorbed through its skin and then carried in the blood to all parts of the body to kill the lice. Sucking lice are very effectively treated in this way. Normally half the warble dose is sufficient to kill lice, and most products are not recommended for use in calves less than two to three months old, but you should always check the manufacturer's instructions before application.

Ivermectin is an anthelmintic (i.e. a drug against intestinal and lungworms) which when given by subcutaneous injection is also effective against lice, mange and warbles. Its small-volume dosage means that it is very easy to administer, although it is more expensive than some of the other treatments, and would probably be used mainly in the autumn when the whole range of its actions would be needed.

Only fly-repellents and possibly ivermectins have any persistency against lice and none of the products mentioned have any effect against their eggs. When using BHC or warble dressing therefore, a repeat treatment should be given after two weeks to kill any lice which have recently hatched from eggs which were present at the time of the first treatment.

Infestations drop to a low level in the summer. This is probably because the animals' coats are cleaner, they are less tightly confined, their nutrition is better and some lice are killed by the high temperatures of direct sunlight.

Mange

This is another skin condition of calves and adult animals, this time caused by small mites from the families sarcoptes or chorioptes. Chorioptic mange is the most common form in cattle, and both types are closely related to 'scabies' in man, 'scab' in sheep and 'canker' in dogs' ears. Whereas lice live on the top of the skin, mites, which are much smaller and cannot be seen with the naked eye, burrow under the skin surface. They cause intense irritation and a 'lifting' of the upper layers of the skin to produce thick, scabby crusts. These occur especially around the root of the tail (plate 3.5) but they may also be seen over the neck (sarcoptes), along the lower part of the abdomen or on the legs (chorioptes).

Treatment

Organo-phosphorus warble preparations or ivermectin injection are the most effective, used in the same way as for lice. A second treatment of warble dressing will be needed after ten to fourteen days to kill the young mites which have hatched from their eggs.

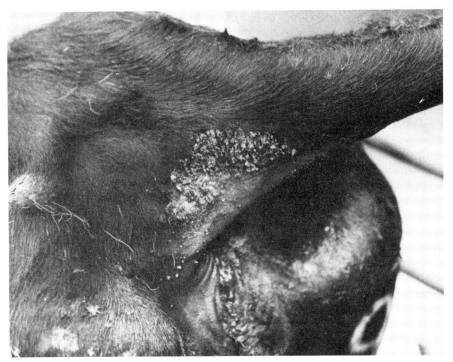

Plate 3.5 Crusty lesions of mange around the base of the tail. This can be intensely itchy.

CALF PNEUMONIA
(Virus pneumonia or enzootic pneumonia)

This must be the most common of all the diseases of the weaned calf and it undoubtedly causes the highest losses in this age group in terms of both mortality and reduced growth rates. Preweaned calves can also be affected, but generally they are protected by antibodies obtained from the colostrum. Passive colostral antibody levels (see page 7) drop significantly by two or three months old, however, and it is often at this age that pneumonia starts to be seen, although it may occur in housed animals of any age.

Clinical signs
Probably the first indication of the presence of pneumonia will be that a few calves have a slightly red eye and there is a clear discharge, making a wet mark over the calf's face (plate 3.6). This should not be confused with New Forest disease or a foreign body in the eye. Both of the latter conditions produce a discharge, but they are also painful and the calf keeps its eye tightly closed. With calf pneumonia, the eye remains open. Soon after, or maybe at the same time, coughing will be heard and the cough is generally a deep 'chesty' type, almost as if the calf is trying to cough up phlegm. Some calves

may then develop a noticeably faster breathing rate, while more severely affected animals will be standing with their heads down, backs arched and breathing very heavily, finding it difficult to get enough air. The hair on their backs often stands up with a 'spiky' ungroomed appearance, the result of sweating from a high temperature. These calves will not be eating and are likely to be standing apart from the rest of the group. Even in the early stages, affected calves may be off their food and running a high temperature (105–107°F; 40.5–42.0°C) and sometimes acute outbreaks may occur, with fatalities, before any significant coughing has been heard.

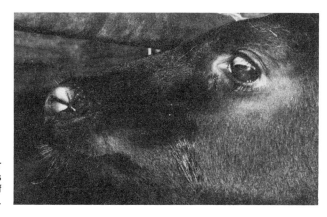

Plate 3.6 A clear discharge from the calf's eye—an early sign of pneumonia.

Causes

Calf pneumonia is known as a multiple aetiology syndrome, that is it is caused by one or more of a whole range of organisms, including bacteria, viruses and mycoplasmas.

Some of the infectious agents commonly found in outbreaks of pneumonia are:

Viruses

Respiratory syncytial virus (RSV)
Para-influenza type 3 (PI3)
Infectious bovine rhinotracheitis (IBR)
Bovine viral diarrhoea (BVD) (= mucosal disease virus)
Coronaviruses.

Bacteria

Pasteurella multocida and *P. haemolytica*
Haemophilus somnus
Corynebacterium pyogenes.

Mycoplasmas

Mycoplasma dispar, M. bovis, ureaplasmas,
Acholeplasma laidlawii.

Other causes are listed in table 1.2.

All calves, on any farm, will be carrying some of these infectious agents, but disease occurs only when levels of infection become excessively high, when immunity is low or when there are adverse environmental influences.

These factors were discussed in detail in Chapter One, as an example of the 'balance phenomenon' of disease, and pages 8 to 11 should be read in conjunction with the following. Some of the major factors which help to reduce the incidence and severity of pneumonia are worth repeating however:

1. Provide adequate ventilation: given the choice, even young calves may lie outside on a cold day. Provided that there is protection against direct draughts, high air-flows will carry away infection and reduce the challenge dose to adjacent animals.
2. Avoid overcrowding.
3. Provide a dry, warm bed. This helps to:
   - Prevent chilling, a 'stress' factor (see Chapter One).
   - Reduce the levels of ammonia and other noxious gases, which damage the normal protective mechanisms in the calf's respiratory system (page 4).
   - Lower the overall house humidity. Humid air contains a far larger number of infective particles (and therefore a higher challenge dose) than dry air.
4. Avoid mixing calves of different age-groups (as they will have different levels of antibody) and especially calves from different sources (which may be carrying a variety of infections). In this instance 'mixing' should mean avoiding using the same air-space.

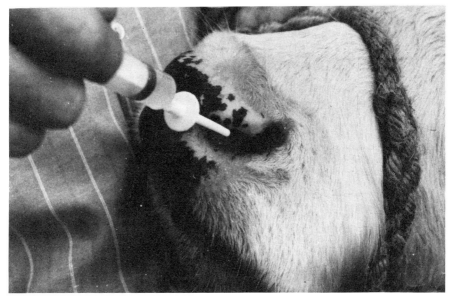

Plate 3.7 Administering an intranasal vaccine against IBR or PI$_3$ viruses. The applicator on the syringe produces a spraying effect.

5. Maintain good levels of antibody protection by:
   - Ensuring an adequate colostrum intake.
   - Vaccination. A variety of commercial preparations are available, some aimed at one specific agent (e.g. RSV, PI3 or IBR) and others at a range of infections. This is a complex area and before using any vaccines you would need to ask your vet to take blood samples to see which of the infections are commonly involved on your unit.

There are good live vaccines available against both IBR and PI3. They are temperature attenuated strains of virus, that is the virus can multiply in the lower temperatures of the nose (and this contact stimulates the calf to develop an immunity), but the normal body temperature of the calf's lungs inhibits the growth of the vaccine virus and so disease cannot occur. The vaccine is applied by spraying 2.0 ml of a liquid into the animal's nose (plate 3.7) using a special applicator.

Ventilation, stocking rates and humidity are the key environmental factors in outbreaks of pneumonia. Levels of infectious particles in the air of a calf house, sometimes called the atmospheric load, may be as high as 100,000 per cubic metre of air. Many of these organisms come from the skin of the calves and would not cause pneumonia; others however, could lead to disease. The rate of reduction of this atmospheric load is governed by several factors:

- The death-rate of organisms in the air. This is by far the most important factor and it is humidity-dependant. For example, increasing the humidity from 60 per cent to 90 per cent r.h., *decreases* the death rate and can lead to a ten-fold increase in the atmospheric load of organisms. It is one reason why pneumonia is much more common in foggy weather.
- The rate of ventilation. Surprisingly, ventilation has only a secondary rôle in reducing the atmospheric load and it is important to note that once stocking density exceeds a certain level in a calf house, no ventilation system is able to reduce the burden of infection adequately and so the risk of pneumonia then becomes very high. Reducing stocking density is thus an extremely important factor in pneumonia control.
- The rate of sedimentation, i.e. particles physically dropping out of the atmosphere.
- Respiration. The calf's air passages act as a very efficient filtering system (page 4 explains the mechanisms) and 95 per cent of the infectious particles inhaled are retained, only 5 per cent being breathed out again. Very few ever penetrate as deep as the lungs, however, and fortunately the majority of particles trapped by the filtering system do not cause disease.

Treatment
The first factor one should consider when faced with a group of coughing calves is whether any treatment is necessary. If coughing and eye discharge are the only symptoms, all the calves are eating and none have a significantly elevated temperature, I would not treat. The infection should spread and the calves should develop their own active immunity without any disease. On the other hand, if a proportion are panting, off their food and have elevated

temperatures, I would treat the whole group. Antibiotics are the primary treatments and your vet will advise you on the most suitable drug for your situation. Remember that antibiotics do not have any effect against viruses (see page 14) and hence response to treatment may be disappointing. Treating the whole group is intended to lower the overall level of bacteria and mycoplasmas in the environment to the extent that the calf's own defences will then be able to cope with the reduced challenge and develop an immunity.

Severely ill animals will need respiratory stimulants and supportive therapy, and veterinary attention should be sought for these. Others may develop chronic lung infections, leading to poor growth and intermittent bouts of pneumonia for weeks after the initial outbreak. I have found prolonged antibiotic cover to be well worthwhile in such cases; for example, giving a long-acting penicillin or tetracycline injection twice-weekly for three weeks or more.

DEFICIENCY DISEASES

Because growing animals generally have a higher requirement than adults for minerals, vitamins and trace elements, it is in this age group that nutritional deficiencies are most likely to be seen. Weaned calves are normally reared indoors on a forage and concentrate diet, and problems may occur towards the end of the winter, especially when feeding and management are poor. The mineral and vitamin requirements of the animal and the effects of the various deficiences are given in detail in Chapter Eleven, and in this section I shall be dealing only with one of the slightly unusual deficiencies, that is muscular dystrophy or white muscle disease.

Muscular Dystrophy (White Muscle Disease)

The name muscular dystrophy means 'abnormal development and function of the muscles' and it is a muscular abnormality which causes the clinical signs and the white areas seen in the muscles at post-mortem. Disease generally occurs at turn-out in the spring and can be precipitated by the stress of bad weather. Calves which have been fed rations containing inadequate levels of vitamin E and/or selenium during the winter develop muscles which are weak and have areas of degeneration. Often no clinical signs are seen indoors, where the calves are relatively inactive. A few days after turnout, however, when they have been running around, a stiffness of gait may be noticed, with the legs unusually rigid. Some animals may be so badly affected that they become recumbent, while others may be found dead from heart failure, the heart muscle having degenerated. Muscle degeneration leads to release of the pigment myoglobin and this is occasionally seen as a red discoloration in the urine. If the chest muscles are involved there will be difficulty in breathing and affected calves may appear to have pneumonia.

Occurrence
With improvements in testing procedures for selenium and vitamin E deficiency in both plants and animals, large surveys have been carried out which have shown that deficiency is very common. Deficiency does not always seem to be associated with disease, however, and the cost benefits of treatment must be carefully evaluated before embarking on any control programme. Traditionally disease occurred in beef suckler herds which had been over-wintered on a diet of straw and turnips. Many pastures have now been found to be deficient, however, and Table 3.1 gives an idea of the feedingstuffs which are good or bad sources of vitamin E.

Table 3.1 Some dietary sources of vitamin E

Good	*Average*	*Poor*
Grass and dried grass	Cereal grains	Poor hay
Grass silage	Maize silage	Straw
Kale	Good hay	Root crops
	Brewer's grains	

Total dietary selenium requirement = 0.1 ppm in dry matter.

Vitamin E and Selenium. Although they are two totally unrelated chemicals, they act on similar mechanisms (involved with the metabolism of unsaturated fatty acids) within the animal. Animals with a marginal selenium status can be precipitated into disease by vitamin E deficiency and vice versa. Selenium deficiency is closely related to soil type and hence all crops grown in certain areas may be deficient. On the other hand, vitamin E levels are more related to the type of plant, its stage of growth, or the method of conservation of the crop. For example, vitamin E levels are very low in hay which has been badly weathered in its making and in grain which has been stored using propionic acid as a preservative.

Treatment and control
This is an area where you will undoubtedly need veterinary advice, since selenium is extremely toxic. There is a wide range of possible courses of action, however. For example:

1. Inject a selenium/vitamin E preparation. This is essential in the treatment of affected animals to achieve a rapid effect. A long-acting product is also available as a control measure, although it is rather expensive.
2. Selenium bullets. These are given by mouth and slowly dissolve in the reticulum over a period of two or three years.
3. Add sodium selenite to the ration to produce a final dietary concentration of 0.1 ppm. This is an extremely low level however, only one-tenth of a gram in one ton of mix, and it is impossible to achieve an even distribution of selenium unless specialist mixing facilities are available.
4. Water-soluble preparations are available, which can be placed in the drinking water and slowly dissolve at a specified rate to provide the

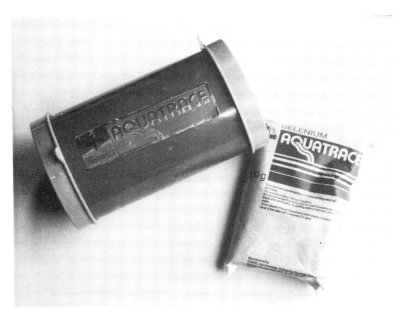

Plate 3.8   An Aquatrace dispenser used to boost selenium levels in drinking water.

animal's selenium requirement. One such system is known as Aquatrace, the canister for which is shown in plate 3.8. The pellets are formulated such that when the selenium concentration in the water reaches a level which will satisfy the animals' requirements no further selenium will dissolve. If some of the water is drunk, fresh water flows into the tank, the selenium concentration falls and this then permits more pellets to dissolve.

Nervous Diseases

There are four major disorders producing nervous symptoms in calves. These are:

Lead poisoning
CCN (cerebrocortical necrosis)
Meningitis
Tetanus.

Hypomagnesaemia (grass staggers) can occur, but it is highly unlikely other than in calves of four to six months old which are still suckling their dams and this situation would be unusual for dairy replacements. Milk is a poor source of magnesium so a rapidly growing single-suckled calf on a whole-milk diet would slowly deplete its magnesium reserves unless additional dietary supplementation (e.g. in concentrates) was given. Tetanus is the least likely of the four disorders.

Lead Poisoning

Lead is still the most common cause of poisoning in farm animals and it is usually young calves or heifers which are affected, probably because of their inquisitive nature and tendency to lick and chew at unusual objects. There are several possible sources of lead, the most common being paint, and old doors are still used in the construction of calf pens. This is extremely dangerous, since old paint invariably contains large quantities of lead and calves tend to chew at woodwork. Other possible sources of lead include:

- putty and traditional 'liniment' or 'white lotion';
- golf balls and lead shot;
- lead plates from batteries;
- pasture contamination, e.g. beside motorways (from petrol), near lead mines and from certain types of industrial workings. The latter are now very carefully controlled.

Clinical signs

The signs of the disease vary, depending on whether there has been a high intake of lead over a short period (acute poisoning), or a lower intake over a more prolonged period (chronic poisoning). Acute poisoning is more common and calves may show symptoms a few days after eating the lead. The affected animal is blind and experiences periods of extreme excitement, bellowing, frothing from the mouth and trying to run up the wall. Quiet periods may follow, when the calf stands almost motionless, often pushing its head into a corner or against the feeding trough. It stops eating, it will probably be constipated and it may run a temperature. Death may occur in as little as one to three hours after the onset of the symptoms, with the calf finally lying on its side, kicking with its legs and bellowing, as if it has severe abdominal pain.

Treatment

Lead poisoning is a serious condition and you should consult your veterinary surgeon if you suspect it. He will most probably take blood and dung samples to confirm the diagnosis and then administer calcium disodium versenate by intravenous injection. This chemical combines with the lead in the animal's blood, producing an inert form which is readily excreted from the body. The affected calf, and the others in the group, should be given 100 grams of magnesium sulphate (Epsom Salts) by mouth. This has the double action of producing insoluble lead sulphate in the gut, thus reducing the rate of lead absorption and also acting as a purgative to quickly carry ingested lead out of the intestine. All possible sources of lead should be carefully considered and removed.

Unfortunately in many calves the disease is too far advanced and treatment is not successful.

Cerebrocortical Necrosis (CCN)

The name means degeneration of the grey matter of the brain. Disease can occur in any age of calf, although it is most commonly seen at three to nine months old and especially in housed calves on a fairly high concentrate diet. The cause is a bacterium which lives in the rumen and produces an anti-metabolite to thiamine (thiamine is also known as vitamin B_1). This means that although the calf is receiving a normally adequate dietary intake of thiamine, the thiamine is unable to function because the bacterial antimetabolite (a *thiaminase*) which is very similar in shape, is sticking to the thiamine receptor sites in the brain. This produces the symptoms of thiamine deficiency.

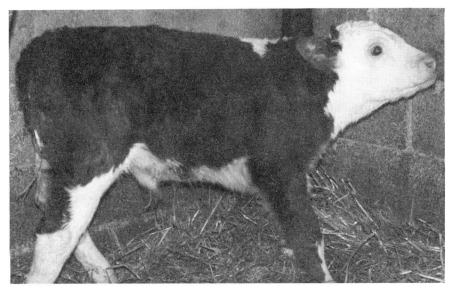

Plate 3.9   Typical 'nose up' position of calf, blind from CCN. It made a full recovery following treatment with thiamine (vitamin B_1).

Clinical signs

Blindness is a common clinical sign and the affected calf tends to wander around the pen with its head held up and nose forward, often walking into things. This rather characteristic position is shown in the calf in plate 3.9. Its temperature will probably be normal, although it may stop eating and soon develop a very hollow appearance. If the disease is allowed to progress, the calf becomes recumbent, lies on its side and may die following bouts of kicking and struggling.

Treatment

Treatment consists of giving large doses of thiamine and it is surprising how quickly quite severely affected calves recover. The first dose will most probably be administered by your veterinary surgeon as an intravenous injection, to obtain rapid action. He may use a multivitamin complex or a simple thiamine solution. If several cases have occurred in a group of calves, it may be worth supplementing their ration with thiamine-rich sources, e.g. 60 grams of brewer's yeast per calf per day.

Meningitis

The meninges are the fibrous layers which surround the brain and separate it from the skull. Meningitis simply means inflammation of the meninges, and may be caused by a range of bacteria including streptococci, *Salmonella dublin* and E. coli.

Although meningitis occurs in calves, it is a difficult disease to define, since the clinical signs depend on the nature of the infection invading the meninges and on the part of the brain affected. The calf may or may not be blind, but often the pupils are dilated and the eyes move from side to side in a jerking movement known as *nystagmus*. The calf may appear to have an intense headache, in that it stands apart from the others with its head down, possibly pushing it against a feeding trough or into the corner. In this respect it resembles lead poisoning. More severe cases tremble and eventually fall to the ground. There is usually a raised temperature.

Treatment

Your veterinary surgeon will prescribe a suitable antibiotic. It needs to be the correct drug and at a high dosage, because there is a physiological barrier preventing many drugs from entering the brain. Nursing is very important. The affected calf should be penned on its own and, if it has stopped eating, drenched with milk to maintain its strength.

Tetanus

Tetanus is quite rare in calves. Its clinical signs are similar to those seen in adult animals and these are described in the section on clostridial diseases in Chapter Four (page 90).

Chapter 4

REARING DAIRY HEIFERS

FOR PROFITABLE heifer rearing, the age of calving needs to be decided well in advance. It is now common practice to calve heifers in batches and if at all possible growth rates should be adjusted to ensure that the animals in a batch are all approximately the same weight at calving. Generally the faster-growing animal is more efficient, because a smaller proportion of its food is used for maintenance and a greater proportion for growth. It is for this reason that the two-year-old calving heifer is now very common. The age of puberty is also affected by growth rate, with well-fed animals showing their first oestrus as early as 9–12 months old. Approximate targets for growth are given in table 4.1:

Table 4.1 Growth targets for heifers to be calved at two years old

Age	Bodyweight	
	kgs	(lbs)
5 weeks	55	(121)
3 months	85	(187)
6 months	145	(319)
Turnout	175	(385)
12 months	275	(605)
Service	330	(726)
18 months	385	(847)
Precalving	510	(1122)
Postcalving	455	(1001)

The bodyweight of heifers at calving affects subsequent milk yield: those which are too small give disappointing production. However, heifers calving at less than two years old will give reduced yields, irrespective of their bodyweight and condition. There are many different types of management and feeding systems for rearing. The most important factor is to decide on a policy and then adhere to it. As general guidelines however, the following points are important:

1. Calves which become overfat during the first six months of life may have reduced yields.

2. High liveweight gains during their second winter can be wasteful because this prevents full utilisation of cheaper summer grazing and the 'compensatory growth' effect.

3. For optimum conception rates, heifers need to be above a certain minimum size (table 4.1) and *gaining weight* at around 0.7 kg/day at the time of service. To achieve this, supplementary feeding with 1.8 kgs cereals will probably be necessary, particularly if conserved forage is being fed. Further details of service regimes and the advantages of batch calving heifers are given on page 226.

4. Weight gains in late pregnancy (that is, in the last two to three months) should be moderate only. Since the majority of the bodyweight of the calf is produced in late pregnancy, high-level feeding can lead to oversize calves. In addition excessive fat may be deposited around the wall of the vagina in the pelvis, and a combination of the two factors can lead to serious calving problems, a point which is referred to again on page 119.

5. When a heifer has calved at two years old she is then both a growing and lactating animal, and feeding levels should be adjusted accordingly. If she does not reach her full mature size, total lifetime production will suffer and many disadvantages of the two-year calving will be lost.

The achievement of reasonable growth rates depends on adequate feeding, full utilisation of the feed and minimising the effects of disease. Disease contracted during rearing can have great carry-over effects on longevity and total lifetime production. Problems of the young calf and the post-weaning animal have been described in Chapters Two and Three. Now we can turn our attention to the diseases which are encountered in the first grazing season, the second winter indoors and miscellaneous conditions of the second grazing season leading up to calving.

Many of the diseases affecting the growing heifer cause few symptoms apart from reduced growth rates and failure to thrive, and this means that it is even more important to be aware of the weight targets for specific ages of animal. The growing heifer is often a grazing animal, and if she receives little or no concentrate supplements she will be particularly susceptible to deficiency diseases. This is especially true during her second grazing season when she will have the requirements of pregnancy added to her needs for growth. Some of the more common causes of failure to thrive are listed on the next page, and for easy reference I have added the page number where each condition is discussed.

Some of these conditions have already been dealt with, and others (for example liver fluke and deficiency diseases) are included in later sections. In this chapter I shall be discussing ostertagia and lungworm, the three viral conditions, eye problems, photosensitisation and the clostridial diseases.

Common Causes of Failure to Thrive

Inadequate feed levels
A very common cause of poor growth, but not discussed in this book.

Parasites
- Ostertagia = stomach worm (66)
- Dictyocaulus = lungworm (71)
- *Fasciola hepatica* = liver fluke (329)
- Ticks and tick-borne disease (redwater and tick fever) (335)

Trace element deficiencies
- copper (300)
- cobalt (302)
- selenium/vitamin E (56, 304)

Virus infections
- IBR, infectious bovine rhinotracheitis (78)
- BVD, bovine viral diarrhoea (80)
- MCF, malignant catarrhal fever (82)

Eye problems
- New Forest Eye (83)
- Other causes of damage (86).

There will, of course, be many other diseases affecting heifers where failure to thrive is not the main symptom. Examples include:

Clostridial diseases
- tetanus (90)
- blackleg (91)
- black discase and botulism (91, 92)

Skin conditions
- ringworm (46)
- mange (51)
- lice (48)
- photosensitisation (88)

Udder problems
- summer mastitis (189)
- teat warts (195)

Conditions of the mouth
- tooth abscesses (312)
- lumpy jaw (313)
- wooden tongue (313)

STOMACH AND INTESTINAL WORMS

Ostertagia

Although there are some eighteen different species of stomach and intestinal worms of cattle known in Great Britain, very few cause disease and those which do follow a similar life-cycle. One possible exception to this is the worm nematodirus, which is sometimes found in early spring and late autumn. Although nematodirus infection of cattle does occur, as it is uncertain whether or not it causes any adverse effects, I have not included a description in this book. By far the most important is the stomach worm *Ostertagia ostertagi* which will be dealt with in detail. The adult worm lives in the abomasum, or fourth stomach and lays eggs which pass out in the faeces (see figure 4.1). The eggs have small larvae developing inside them and after a period of time they hatch, releasing the third-stage larvae, L3. Under suitable conditions the L3 swim up blades of grass in a film of moisture and remain there ready to be eaten by grazing animals. This migration from the dung pat to grass occurs best in warm, wet conditions. Once eaten, the L3 burrows into one of the gastric glands lining the wall of the abomasum and here it feeds and grows (figure 4.2) and develops into an adult. As an adult it emerges into the abomasum and begins to lay eggs. The period between eating the L3 on pasture and eggs appearing again in the faeces is three weeks.

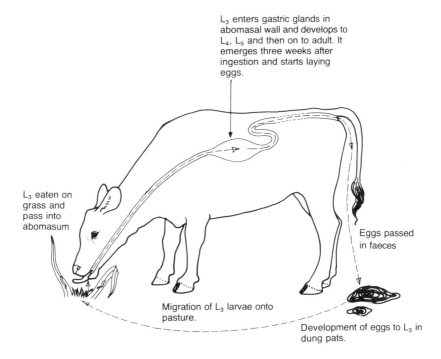

L₃ enters gastric glands in abomasal wall and develops to L₄, L₅ and then on to adult. It emerges three weeks after ingestion and starts laying eggs.

L₃ eaten on grass and pass into abomasum

Eggs passed in faeces

Migration of L₃ larvae onto pasture.

Development of eggs to L₃ in dung pats.

Figure 4.1   Life cycle of the stomach worm, *Ostertagia ostertagi*.

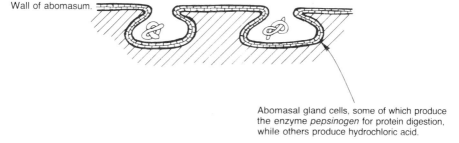

Wall of abomasum.

Abomasal gland cells, some of which produce the enzyme *pepsinogen* for protein digestion, while others produce hydrochloric acid.

Figure 4.2   Ostertagia larvae developing L₃ to L₄ in gastric gland in the abomasum.

Clinical signs

Disease is the result of the damage caused by the developing worms in the gastric glands of the abomasum. The gastric glands produce hydrochloric acid and the enzyme pepsinogen, both of which are essential for protein digestion. Following ostertagia infestation there is less acid produced, the pH of the abomasum rises, protein digestion is impaired and this is seen clinically as *scouring*. Mildly affected calves may have only semi-solid dung and this may be difficult to detect in animals on lush grazing. As the condition progresses, however, the scouring becomes profuse, watery and bright green, and calves lose weight rapidly. Severely affected animals may show a fluid swelling under the chin ('bottle-jaw'), which is in fact oedema ('dropsy') caused by the protein lost in the scour. Death is not common, the main symptoms being massive weight loss and subsequent growth retardation.

Disease is generally seen from mid-July until October, and to understand why this occurs and how to control outbreaks we must look carefully at the life-cycle. Start with calves turned out in mid-April onto a pasture which is contaminated with L3 (see figure 4.1). The infective L3 are eaten with the grass, they develop into adults and begin to lay eggs some three weeks later, that is in early May. The rate of development and hatching of these eggs depends on temperature, so that eggs deposited on the pasture in April and May take several weeks to develop, while those passed in the warmer midsummer months complete the transition to infective L3 in only two weeks. Consequently all the eggs passed in the dung from May onwards develop at approximately the same time, namely mid-July, and this can produce a massive increase in the level of herbage L3 infestation. The calves are now eating the L3 which developed from the eggs which they themselves passed earlier in the summer and this massive increase in the challenge dose may be sufficient to produce disease. Even where clinical symptoms are not seen, the worm burden may be sufficient to reduce weight gains (see figure 4.3). Towards the end of the grazing season an immunity develops. This has the effect of restricting the life of the adult worm to approximately one month and hence only moderate worm burdens are then likely to be carried. This feature has two important consequences. Firstly if calves are moved to and maintained on pastures free of infestation in September, their worm burdens will quite quickly decrease, because the adult worms die in four weeks. Secondly, anthelmintic treatment *without* moving onto a clean pasture will give only a very temporary relief, because the worms killed by the anthelmintic would soon have died anyway and new infections are rapidly established from fresh larval intakes.

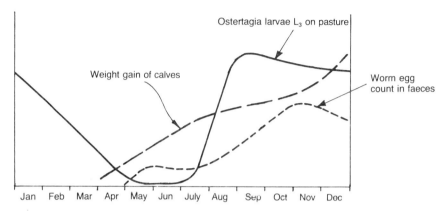

Figure 4.3   The pattern of summer ostertagia infection. Overwintered L_3 are the primary source of infection, and these are present on pasture until mid June. Disease is caused by the secondary wave of L_3 produced in July.

Even if no further worm eggs are passed from July onwards, herbage larval infestations (that is the number of L3 present on the grass) will persist at a high level over the winter and will only start to decline during the spring of the following year. If there are no calves grazing this pasture, i.e. no way in which the larvae can be multiplied, then the pasture should be virtually free of worms by mid-June of the following year. These points are illustrated graphically in figure 4.3. If calves are left until late June before being turned out and they are then put onto pasture which has not been grazed that year, then larval intakes would be very low and hence the risk of disease would be minimal. The incidence and severity of disease will therefore be affected by a variety of factors, namely:

1. The level of pasture larval infestation produced during the previous grazing season.
2. The time of year chosen for turnout.
3. Stocking density. Heavily stocked fields lead to tighter grazing, greater larval intakes and more extensive faecal contamination of pasture. All these factors could lead to a high larval challenge in mid/late July.
4. Rainfall. Heavy rain physically scatters dung pats and hence spreads larvae over the pasture. In addition, high moisture levels make it easier for L3 to swim up blades of grass, whereas larvae are killed by direct sunlight and very dry weather.

5. Intercurrent diseases, especially debilitating conditions such as copper or cobalt deficiency, reduce the calf's ability to develop an immune response and hence increase the severity of the ostertagiasis.

Control of ostertagia
There are a variety of control measures available and each farmer must choose the system most suited to his own farm. The following are the most common:

1. Dose calves with anthelmintic at intervals of three weeks after turn-out. The length of time from ingestion of larvae to their development into egg-laying adult females is three weeks. Hence anthelmintic dosing of the calves at regular three-weekly intervals from turn-out kills the females just before they reach the egg-laying stage. The pasture does not become contaminated with worm eggs and there is no massive increase in pasture larvae from mid-July onwards. This situation is shown in figure 4.4, which should be compared with the undosed calves shown in figure 4.3. Calves turned out in late March/early April should be dosed three times at three-weekly intervals, while for those turned out in late April, two dosings will be sufficient. The calves can then be left on this pasture for the remainder of the year. An inexpensive levamisole drug can be used, either by drench, injection or pour-on, whichever is most convenient.
2. Use a slow-release anthelmintic. There is a very large and heavy tablet (= a bolus) of the anthelmintic *morantel* available (Paratect; Pfizer Ltd.) in a slow-release form. It is given to calves at turn-out and its weight keeps it in the bottom of the reticulum. A continual low level of morantel is released for ninety days following its administration, and this ensures that no egg-laying worms become established in the abomasum. One dosing

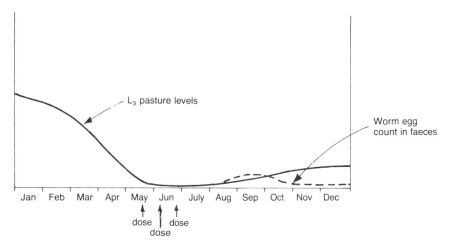

Figure 4.4 Dosing calves at three-week intervals after turn-out in late April reduces the level of ostertagia larval infection on the pasture.

therefore produces a situation identical to the three three-weekly treatments shown in figure 4.4. It is more convenient than repeatedly handling the calves, but it is considerably more expensive.

3. Dose and move in mid-July. The secondary wave of pasture larvae reach a peak in mid-July. Calves can be given anthelmintic just before this date to eliminate their burden of egg-laying adults and then moved onto larvae-free pasture, for example, silage aftermaths which have not been grazed by calves earlier that year. The disadvantages of this system are:
   - any delay in the 'dose and move' may allow an outbreak of clinical disease
   - the pasture that the calves grazed during the early summer will remain highly infested until May/June of the following year, and should not be used for grazing during the remainder of the season.

4. Ensure that calves are turned out onto pastures which have a very low level of larval herbage infestation; for example, those which were used only for conservation and/or sheep in the previous year, or new seeds planted after an arable crop. Alternatively, delay turn-out until after early June. However, recent research has shown that larvae may pass down into the soil and maintain pasture infestation for two years, so no pasture can be considered completely 'safe'.

5. Rotational grazing of cattle and calves, or sheep and calves. Two-year grazing plans can be devised whereby calves are turned out onto pastures with low larval herbage infestations and moved again before any significant worm burdens are established. Such procedures require careful planning and I would recommend that anyone considering such systems seek veterinary advice well in advance.

It is important to realise that anthelmintic treatment of clinically affected calves *without* moving them to a clean pasture will give relatively little relief, because new infestations are rapidly established. There is also a tendency for some people to treat at cattle turn-out. This is *never* necessary for calves which have not previously been grazing, and it could only be justified in second-season cattle if they had been inadequately treated the previous year.

Winter ostertagiasis

Earlier in this section we discussed the way in which ingested L3 larvae completed their development in the gastric glands of the abomasum (figure 4.2) before emerging as adults. From September onwards, however, many of the ingested L3 undergo *arrested development*, that is, they remain dormant as L4 in the abomasal gastric glands. This is the fate of a large proportion of the larvae eaten in the autumn and, by the time of housing, a calf may have a burden of some eighty thousand ostertagia, forty thousand of which are adults in the abomasum and forty thousand are L4 larvae in the gastric glands. The latter may remain as dormant L4 until March to May of the following year, when a sudden development into adults and emergence from the gastric glands can produce an outbreak of profuse, watery diarrhoea. The 'calves' will be twelve to eighteen months old at this stage and may be housed or out-wintered. Diarrhoea is the most prominent clinical sign, although 'bottle-jaw', rapid weight loss and anaemia are also seen. Calves may die if treatment is not given quickly, which is in contrast to the summer (type 1) disease, when deaths are relatively rare.

Prevention of winter (type II), ostertagiasis is achieved simply by dosing with a suitable anthelmintic at housing (or in December for stock which are to be out-wintered); 'suitable' meaning an anthelmintic which is effective against inhibited L4 larvae. For summer treatments, almost any anthelmintic can be used, e.g. levamisole, morantel or thiabendazole, but at housing the choice is restricted to the benzimidazole derivatives (e.g. fenbendazole, oxfendazole) or the ivermectins. The range of activity of the various anthelmintics is given in table 1.3, but if you are in any doubt you should seek veterinary advice before dosing.

Worms in older stock
After the first year, cattle develop an immunity to ostertagia, although it may take a complete grazing season for this immunity to fully develop and worm burdens may still be high (e.g. eighty thousand) in the first October following turnout. Heifers in their second grazing season will carry much lower burdens however (perhaps five thousand worms) and at least half of these may be present as arrested L4 larvae. Adult cows will be carrying even fewer worms and although the risk of clinical disease in cows is virtually zero, you may still see improvements in growth rates and milk yields following treatment. For example, one large trial involving nine thousand dairy cows in the UK showed a 42 litre improvement in the milk yield of treated cows compared with untreated controls in the same herds and this would more than cover the cost of treatment. As one might expect, the response varied enormously from herd to herd, with some herds showing a dramatic improvement and others none. As any animal under 'stress' is more susceptible to disease, it would seem sensible to at least give two-year-old heifers a precalving treatment even if you do not treat all the milking herd. I would also recommend dosing beef cattle at housing after their second grazing season, in both cases ensuring that the anthelmintic used was effective against arrested L4 larvae (table 1.3). In lactating animals, consideration may have to be given to milk-withholding periods following treatment.

Lungworm (Husk)

Lungworm, 'husk', 'hoose', or parasitic bronchitis, is caused by the small worm *Dictyocaulus viviparus*, whose life-cycle is depicted in figure 4.5. The adult lungworms live in the trachea and bronchi (the air-passages to the lungs), laying eggs which rapidly hatch into first-stage larvae, L1. These larvae cause irritation and are coughed up into the throat. They are then swallowed, passing through the intestine and out onto the pasture in the faeces. Maturation of the larvae from L1 to L3 (i.e. the growth from the first- to the third-stage larvae) is dependent on temperature, but takes a minimum

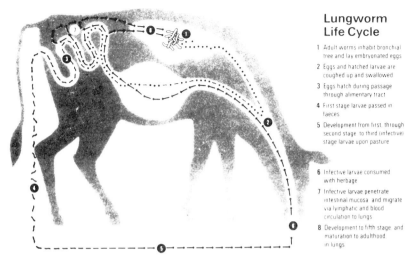

Lungworm Life Cycle

1 Adult worms inhabit bronchial tree and lay embryonated eggs

2 Eggs and hatched larvae are coughed up and swallowed

3 Eggs hatch during passage through alimentary tract

4 First stage larvae passed in faeces

5 Development from first, through second stage, to third (infective) stage larvae upon pasture

6 Infective larvae consumed with herbage

7 Infective larvae penetrate intestinal mucosa and migrate via lymphatic and blood circulation to lungs

8 Development to fifth stage and maturation to adulthood, in lungs

Figure 4.5   Life cycle of the lungworm.

of seven days even under ideal conditions of warmth and humidity. When mature, the L3 move up the blades of grass in a film of moisture, are eaten by the calf and pass into the intestine. They then burrow through the intestinal wall and travel via the bloodstream to the lungs. Up to this stage no clinical signs would be observable. However, as the larvae penetrate the air-sacs of the lungs (figure 4.6) and the young adults begin their climb up the air-passage to start egg laying, clinical signs of coughing and panting will be seen.

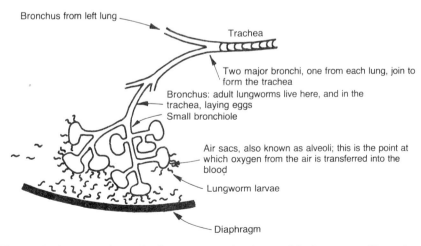

Bronchus from left lung

Trachea

Two major bronchi, one from each lung, join to form the trachea

Bronchus: adult lungworms live here, and in the trachea, laying eggs

Small bronchiole

Air sacs, also known as alveoli; this is the point at which oxygen from the air is transferred into the blood

Lungworm larvae

Diaphragm

Figure 4.6   Lungworm larvae begin to penetrate the airsacs of the lungs ten to fifteen days after being eaten. Symptoms are first seen at this stage.

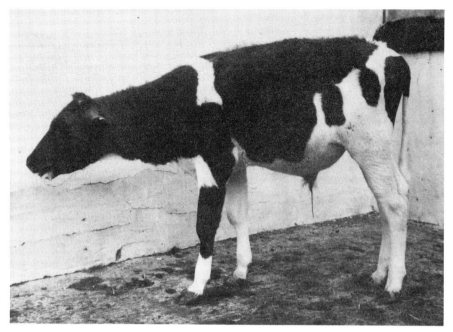

Plate 4.1   Calf with severe lungworm infestation. Note its open mouth and laboured breathing.

Clinical signs

Usually disease is seen in calves during their first season at grass, although occasionally second-year heifers or even adult cows can be affected following a heavy larval challenge. Outbreaks occur from late July until September and are most common in the milder and wetter parts of the country. No symptoms are seen immediately following the ingestion of large numbers of larvae, but ten to fifteen days later, as the larvae penetrate the lungs, rapid breathing and grunting will be noticed, especially when the calves are moved. Heavily infested animals will have an increased temperature, they may be reluctant to move, they stand with their backs arched and their mouths open, and are often fighting to obtain enough air. A typical case is shown in plate 4.1. Because they are not eating there will be a rapid weight loss. Deaths may occur in as little as fifteen to twenty days after exposure to heavily infected pasture. As the worms move up the air-ways to become adults and begin egg laying, coughing becomes more pronounced, a deep abdominal cough, as the calf is trying to clear the worms from its trachea and throat. Plate 4.2 gives an idea of how many worms may be present in the trachea. By this stage (twenty-five to fifty days after infection), larvae will be present in the faeces and your veterinary surgeon can take a dung sample to confirm the diagnosis. A word of caution, however. Severe panting and deaths may occur at fifteen to twenty days after infestation, as the larvae are penetrating the lungs and, at this stage, L1 larvae will not be present in the faeces. This is known as a *prepatent* husk infection.

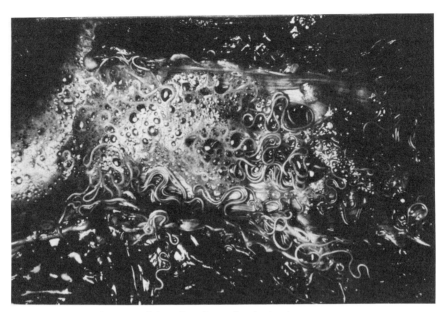

Plate 4.2   Heavy lungworm infestation obstructing the trachea.

Treatment

Remove the calves from the infested pasture, possibly by bringing them indoors, and dose with a suitable anthelmintic (table 1.3). Injectable preparations (e.g. levamisole or ivermectin) probably provide a more rapid effect. Unfortunately anthelmintic treatment causes death or paralysis of the lungworms and this allows many of them to fall back into the air-sacs, so the treatment itself may lead to a fatal pneumonia in some calves. A severe outbreak of husk can be a crippling condition and many of the calves which do survive may be so severely affected that they never reach mature bodyweight. Antibiotics and general supportive therapy may be prescribed by your vet for animals which develop a secondary bacterial pneumonia.

Reservoirs of infection

Contaminated pasture, leading to a clinical outbreak of husk, may arise from a variety of sources, for example:

1. Overwintered L3 larvae, passed by calves infected in the previous summer, are the most likely source of infection. These larvae will certainly persist on pastures until April or May. Lungworm larvae have also been found deeper in the soil, even in earthworms, and both may remain potential sources of infection for a year or more.
2. Carrier animals. Six to eight weeks after exposure to infection an immunity develops which has the effect of restricting the number of adult lungworms living in the air passages at any one time. Even after treatment there will be a few worms remaining, however, and this produces carrier animals

which can infect pastures the following spring. Young calves should not be turned out with second-season cattle therefore, or to areas where they have been grazing.

3. A somewhat more unusual method of spreading infection is provided by a fungus called Pilobolus. This grows on dung pats and produces a seed head which explodes when it is ripe (figure 4.7). Lungworm larvae can climb onto the seed head and they are then carried away from the dung pat with the explosion. This takes them beyond the foul area around the dung, which cattle are normally reluctant to graze, and is a very effective way of increasing the larva's chance of finding a new calf to infect.

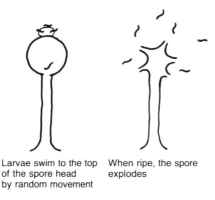

Larvae swim to the top   When ripe, the spore
of the spore head   explodes
by random movement

Figure 4.7   Lungworm larvae are dispersed by the explosion of the spore of the pilobolus fungus. There may be as many as fifty larvae on one seed head, and they are thrown well clear of the foul area around the dung pat by the explosion.

4. Other methods of transmission of infection from one field to another, or even from farm to farm, include infected dung on boots and tractor wheels, or even the spreading of slurry. Worm larvae are surprisingly resistant and transmission of infection in this way is often overlooked.

Occurrence of disease

Young calves turned out in the spring may be exposed to only low levels of L3 infection. However, these rapidly multiply. For example, each L3 eaten and established as an egg-laying female can be producing over three thousand new larvae per day in the faeces. This means that in one month a single female could shed approximately a hundred thousand larvae onto the pasture and, should weather conditions become favourable for their simultaneous development, calves could be exposed to a very high challenge of infection. With ostertagia it is possible to predict when outbreaks of disease are likely to appear. High intakes of lungworm larvae occur far more randomly however and hence control of husk by strategic anthelmintic treatment during the summer is *not reliable*.

Prevention

The only reliable way of preventing lungworm is by vaccination. The vaccine consists of larvae which are alive but have been rendered harmless by irradiation. It is a 'prescription only' medicine which you order through your vet, but it is posted direct to you from the manufacturer. Each dose is in an individual bottle (plate 4.3) to be administered as a drench. It must be stored

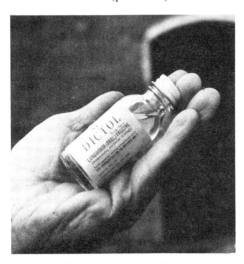

Plate 4.3   A single dose of an oral vaccine against husk.

in the fridge and used within one to two weeks of arrival, so carefully check the expiry date given by the manufacturers. Two doses, each of a thousand larvae, are given at six weeks and two weeks before turn-out, and calves should ideally be eight weeks old before receiving their first dose. Other dosage regimes are possible, however, and if you have a late-born group of calves or have simply forgotten to order the vaccine, reasonable levels of immunity are produced by dosing at intervals of less than four weeks. There is also no reason why calves should not be given vaccine after turn-out, except of course they will not have adequate protection until two weeks after the second dose, and that no anthelmintics can be given over this period. This could interfere with the ostertagia control programme (see page 69). Once turned out, calves may be exposed to low levels of natural infection and this will boost their immunity. Vaccinated calves can still become carriers and can infect pastures the following year, however, so vaccination cannot be discontinued after a few years simply because no outbreaks of disease have been seen. It takes only a very small number of larvae, under favourable conditions, to build up to significant disease levels if susceptible calves are available. The morantel slow-release bolus (see page 69) can be used two weeks after the second vaccine dose has been given since by this stage the vaccine will have stimulated an immunity in the calf. Although morantel kills the majority of L3 lungworm, it is not effective against adults, and even in the presence of the drug sufficient numbers of L3 become established as adults to allow the maintenance of a good level of immunity.

THE VIRAL DISEASES

Husk is likely to be the most common condition affecting the respiratory system of grazing cattle, although as herd sizes have increased and cattle have tended to be kept in progressively larger groups, there are three viral conditions which have increased in prevalence. These are IBR (infectious bovine rhinotracheitis), BVD (bovine viral diarrhoea, also known as mucosal disease) and MCF, malignant catarrhal fever. All three conditions affect organs other than the respiratory system, and all three may also cause problems in adult dairy cows. Although they occur in grazing cattle, they are perhaps a greater problem in housed animals, when nutrition is generally poorer and where crowding increases the risk of animal-to-animal transmission. All three diseases may also play a part in the enzootic pneumonia complex of calves described in Chapter Three, when they would not necessarily be recognisable as a single clinical condition.

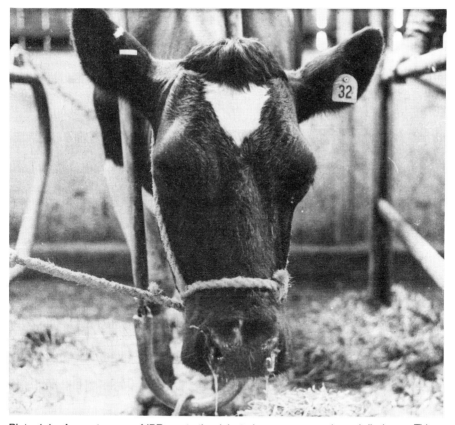

Plate 4.4   An acute case of IBR—note the dejected appearance and nasal discharge. This cow died within 24 hours despite treatment.

IBR (Infectious Bovine Rhinotracheitis)

This is a virus disease of cattle and, as its name indicates, it affects primarily the nose (rhino-) and windpipe (-tracheitis), although there are other manifestations. The condition was first reported in Scotland in 1968, but is now widespread throughout Great Britain. Disease is seen in a variety of forms, depending on the age of the animal and on its previous level of immunity. All ages of animals can be affected, from the young calf to the adult cow. The three main groups of clinical signs are:

1. Acute respiratory form—this is the classic type of disease. Affected animals run a very high temperature, are dull, off their food and a discharge is likely to be seen from the nose and sometimes from the eyes. The cow in plate 4.4 was so badly affected that she died twenty-four hours later, despite treatment. Panting and coughing do occur, but may be fairly late clinical signs. Deaths can start within a few days of clinical signs first being noticed, although at the other extreme, disease may be quite mild, for example simply as an additional agent in the calf pneumonia complex, while still other animals may contact the infection and develop an immunity but never even produce clinical signs.
2. Eye lesions may be seen on their own or in association with respiratory symptoms. The conjunctiva lining the eye becomes very reddened and swollen and, if examined carefully, small ulcers caused by the IBR virus

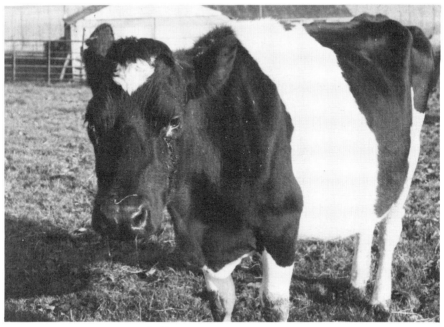

Plate 4.5   A cow drooling and with an eye discharge typical of IBR. She recovered within a few days.

can be seen. A white discharge appears and this may be so severe that the eye closes, with a thick layer of pus between the lids. Although it looks unpleasant, it does not seem to be very painful and generally growth rates are not seriously affected. Plate 4.5 shows a typical example. This cow was drooling and had an eye discharge and a high temperature, but made a good recovery.

3. Abortion or foetal death caused by IBR can occur at any stage of pregnancy and may be quite difficult to diagnose. It is thought that the virus multiplies in the placenta and this may well occur without any other clinical signs of generalised illness being seen in the cow. Abortion occurs some weeks or months after the initial infection, by which time the virus has disappeared from the placenta. Diagnosis is usually based on blood-sampling the cow to look for high antibody titres and on presumptive evidence, for example, eye lesions having occurred in these or other cows in the herd a few weeks or months before the abortions.

Treatment

With the disease showing such a variety of symptoms, treatment depends on the type of IBR present. For the acute disease, your veterinary surgeon will prescribe a suitable antibiotic to prevent secondary bacterial pneumonia, but there is no specific treatment against the virus (see page 14). Drugs to reduce the temperature and aid recovery may also be used. If there is a purulent eye discharge, then topical antibiotic ointment or a subconjunctival 'depot' injection (see page 85) is indicated. There is no treatment for the abortions.

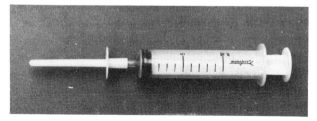

Plate 4.6 IBR vaccine applicator, designed to spray the vaccine into the animal's nose.

Prevention

The best method of control is by vaccination. The vaccine is a live, *temperature-attenuated* strain of IBR, which means that it can only live at the lower temperatures found in the nose. It would be killed by the normal body temperature in the lungs. The vaccinal virus multiplies in the nose to produce immunity, but it cannot spread to cause disease. It is administered using a syringe which has a special applicator (plate 4.6) to produce an aerosol into the animal's nose. This procedure was also described in Chapter Three (see plate 3.7 and page 55). One dose is sufficient to provide immunity for a year, although in some herds annual boosters are necessary. These would be required if herd replacements were normally purchased from the open market, although even in this case it may be decided that vaccination of only incoming animals provided sufficient protection.

As IBR is quite widespread in the national herd, one of the problems is deciding whether or not vaccination is necessary. This is especially so if animals from different sources have been mixed and only one animal in the group is showing symptoms of IBR. In such a case it is impossible to know how many of the group have been previously exposed and are therefore already solidly immune. For these immune animals vaccination would clearly be a waste of money. To be safe, however, you should always vaccinate the whole group as soon as a single case has been confirmed. On occasions I have done this and when no more cases have occurred I have felt that perhaps vaccination had not been necessary. On the other hand I have also delayed vaccination on a 'wait and see' basis and this has led to a serious outbreak of disease!

BVD (Bovine Viral Diarrhoea [and Mucosal Disease])

At one time it was thought that these were two separate diseases, Mucosal Disease in the young animal and Bovine Viral Diarrhoea in the adult. They are now known to be caused by the same virus. The virus attacks all the mucosal surfaces in the body, causing inflammation and ulceration and it is the results of this which cause the symptoms seen. As with IBR, the clinical signs can vary enormously from one animal to another, depending on which of the mucosal surfaces is the worse affected, and on the severity of the attack. The latter will be a reflection of the balance between the size of the challenge dose of infection and the immunity of the animal (see page 8). The mucosal surfaces which may be affected are:

- The mouth and throat: here the ulcers can be seen with the naked eye as small red spots. Affected animals are reluctant to eat, especially if the hay or straw is very coarse, and there will be drooling or even frothing from the mouth.
- The nose and trachea: small ulcers may be seen around the muzzle. Those in the nose undergo secondary bacterial infection and this causes thick white nasal discharge. If the lungs are also affected, the animal will take very short, shallow breaths because of the pain of breathing.
- The intestines: scouring is then the most prominent feature, sometimes a black scour, the dark colour being blood from bleeding intestinal ulcers. Very often whole lumps of intestinal lining are shed and these are seen as gelatinous tissue mixed with the dung. The other characteristic feature is the severity of the scour. The dung may be almost 100 per cent water, with so little solid material that the tail is not soiled and you are not even aware that the cow is scouring. The cow shown in plate 4.7 was feeling so ill with BVD and her mouth was so sore, that she stopped licking herself and maggots were growing in the ulcers at the angle of her lips. Note the nasal discharge, which would also normally be removed by licking.

Treatment

As with all other viral infections, there is no specific therapy and treatment is based on alleviating the symptoms and providing antibiotic cover to prevent

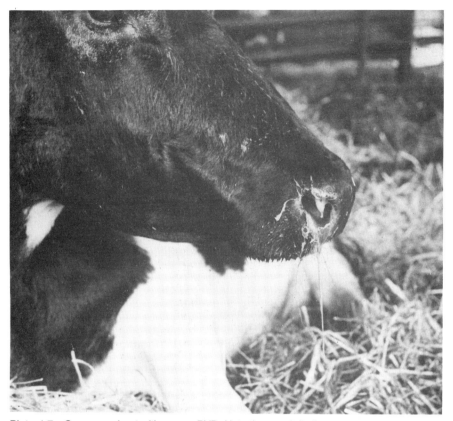

Plate 4.7　Cow recumbent with severe BVD. Note the nasal discharge.

secondary bacterial infection. Affected animals run a moderate temperature, they are off their food and they usually stop cudding, so appetite stimulants may be indicated. Vitamins, especially A and D will help in the repair of the mucosal membranes and B vitamins will act as a general tonic. Animals with very sore mouths may have to be given liquid gruel and those which are scouring should be given kaolin or kaolin and chlorodyne. I find 250 g kaolin twice daily to be useful symptomatic treatment for scouring cows and your veterinary surgeon may prescribe a suitable antibacterial, e.g. 33 per cent sulphamezathine, to mix with this. Copper sulphate is another useful astringent drench.

Prevention and Control
There is no licensed vaccine currently available in Great Britain against BVD, but fortunately the disease does not usually affect large numbers of heifers in a group. Although all animals will be exposed to infection, only occasional ones develop severe clinical disease. This is now thought to be associated with a syndrome known as *immune tolerance*. There are two separate strains of

BVD virus, called cytopathic and non-cytopathic because of their effects on tissue culture preparations. The developing calf is unable to produce its own antibodies until after 180 days of gestation, known as its age of immunological competence. If the cow is infected with the non-cytopathic strain of BVD virus at a stage of pregnancy earlier than this, the virus enters the developing foetus and destroys the memory line cells (see page 37) which would have produced anti-BVD antibodies later in life. Such calves are born with non-cytopathic virus still circulating in their blood but no antibodies. Unfortunately they are also unable to produce antibodies to the more virulent (i.e. more severe) cytopathic BVD, so if exposed to this infection later in life, the animal has very little protection.

Disease can be very severe, and if not fatal it leads to such a severe growth retardation that full mature size may never be attained. A similar syndrome of immune tolerance exists with border disease in sheep and rubella (measles) in man. On occasions it is possible to identify a period when dairy cows are exposed to BVD, then by looking at the performances of the calves which were in early to mid gestation at this time it may be found that many of them develop bouts of scouring or are generally unthrifty later in life.

Waves of infection may pass through dairy herds, especially during the winter housing when the risk of faecal contamination is much greater. Some authorities consider that BVD is the primary agent of the so called 'winter dysentery' of dairy cows, although others consider that a separate bacterial infection called *campylobacter* is involved. In the first year that disease is seen, up to 80 per cent of cows may be affected by this condition over a two to three month period, each animal running a temperature for a few days, scouring, off its food and with a sharp drop in milk production. Mouth and nose lesions are less common in adults. Occasional cases develop a very severe scour and die within a few days. However, the majority recover, although yield may be affected for the remainder of the lactation. During the second winter, further cases may be seen, but far fewer in number, and thereafter the disease becomes 'endemic' in the herd, producing occasional cases each winter, especially in heifers or purchased cows. Although BVD/MD is not too serious in these herds, it does cause a considerable nuisance and loss of milk.

Malignant Catarrhal Fever

This is the third in the group of virus infections which cause respiratory disease in older cattle. It is not as common as either IBR or BVD, although infection generally results in a more severe illness, luckily affecting only one or two animals in a group. The clinical signs are very similar to those of the acute respiratory forms of IBR described on page 78. In the acute disease, affected animals run a very high temperature and are extremely ill in themselves, standing motionless with a dejected appearance. There is a purulent discharge from the eyes, nose and mouth and the animal stops eating. Diarrhoea is often present, arising from ulcers which may occur throughout the intestinal tract, and this can sometimes develop into a bloody dysentery.

There may be skin changes in other parts of the body and some animals show nervous signs, although many have died before reaching this stage. One feature which is almost diagnostic but unfortunately does not necessarily develop in every animal, is an accumulation of a white flocculent material in the anterior chamber of the eye, and at the same time the cornea may become blue/grey in colour and opaque. This obscures the colour of the iris and leads to blindness. It is often associated with the development of nervous signs.

MCF is an interesting condition because, although it is thought to be caused by a virus, the virus itself has still not been isolated. The most widely held theory is that the causal virus, or at least part of its genetic material, becomes incorporated into the genetic material of one of the strains of the animal's lymphocytes. (A similar situation exists with EBL.) The class of lymphocyte affected is called the 'large granular lymphocyte'. This cell line has two functions. Firstly it regulates the growth and activity of T-lymphocytes, and secondly it destroys animal cells which have become infected with virus. When MCF virus becomes incorporated into the large granular lymphocyte, the cell loses its ability to control the growth of T-lymphocytes, and so these cells continue to multiply. This is seen in the clinical disease as enlargement of the lymph nodes. At the same time the large granular lymphocytes themselves get out of control and begin to destroy normal healthy tissue cells, rather than just those infected with virus. This produces ulcers in the nose, mouth and intestine, and in so doing leads to the drooling and scouring seen in clinical MCF.

Treatment
Symptomatic only, as for IBR and BVD. There is no vaccine available.

Eye and Skin Disorders

New Forest Eye

Sometimes known as 'pink eye' and, scientifically, as infectious bovine keratoconjunctivitis (IBK), this is an extremely painful condition affecting all ages of stock, and particularly calves of up to one year old during their first summer grazing. Winter infections are becoming much more common, however, especially in tightly housed calves. Disease is caused by the bacterium *Moraxella bovis*. When it lands on the cornea (the surface of the eye) Moraxella starts to burrow inwards, forming a pit or ulcer and this is seen as a small white spot or a white ring on the surface of the eye (plate 4.8 and colour plate 1). The reaction of the eye to the infection is a fascinating series of events. Firstly, with only mild infections, tears are produced. This has the effect of washing away the bacteria and the tears also carry antibodies to counteract the infection. The animal in colour plate 1 shows these early changes. At a slightly later stage the eyelids may close to reduce pain and protect the eyeball. This is especially true in bright sunlight, which acts as an irritant. In fact ultra-violet light itself can damage the corneal surface of the eye and this reduces healing. As the ulcer becomes deeper an alarm signal is

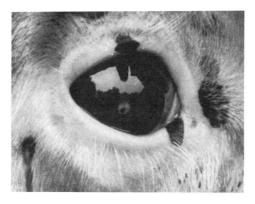

Plate 4.8   White spot on eye, typical of the corneal ulcer caused by New Forest infection.

sent out and blood vessels start to race across the front of the eye, carrying antibacterial cells and antibodies to kill the infection, as well as 'building materials' to repair the ulcer. The blood vessels appear as a red ring progressing inwards from the rim of the cornea (see colour plate 1) and this is known as *pannus* formation. The eye may become totally red and sight has now been temporarily lost but there is still a chance of recovery. When the bacteria burrow completely through the cornea, however, and the ulcer perforates, the fluid (the aqueous humour) in the anterior chamber of the eye

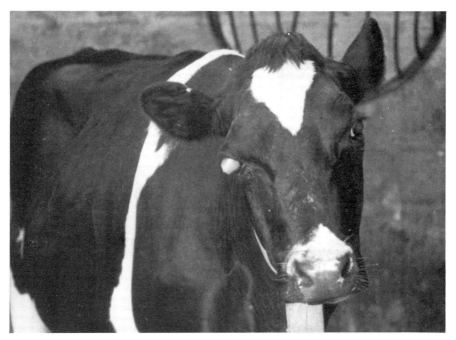

Plate 4.9   Total loss of sight due to bacterial infection of the whole eye. The rough edges of the original ulcer are still visible three years later.

starts to leak out. The iris, the coloured part of the eye which we can see, is then sucked forward from behind to block the hole. This maintains the remaining fluid pressure in the eye, but vision has been permanently destroyed. Provided that the cornea has not ruptured in this way, once the pannus blood vessels have finished their repair work they eventually withdraw and sight is restored, with the only blemish being a small white dot in the centre of the eye. However, sometimes other bacteria get into the eyeball, producing pus, so that the eye becomes totally white and sight is permanently lost. The cow in plate 4.9 had lost her sight three years before the photograph was taken. The rough edges of the perforated corneal ulcer can still be seen.

Treatment
Antibacterial ointment applied to the surface of the eye is very effective in killing the infection and your veterinary surgeon will recommend a suitable preparation to use. Most products need to be applied for at least four days, however, and preferably twice daily, although there is one longer-acting topical preparation which should persist for forty-eight hours. I do not like using antibiotic powders. They may be easier to apply, but tears very quickly wash away the antibiotic and the powder itself may be an irritant.

An alternative is to have an injection of antibiotic deposited behind the conjunctiva, that is, the membrane lining the eye. This is released slowly over three or four days and provides continual antibiotic cover against the bacteria. There are several techniques for giving the injection. One method is shown in plate 4.10. In all cases the animal must be held very still, otherwise

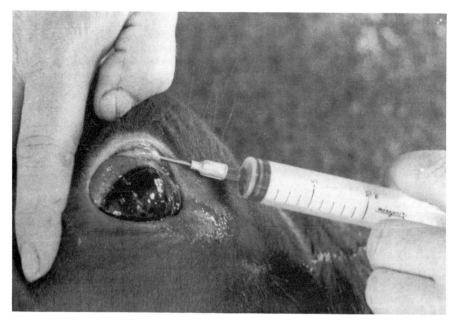

Plate 4.10   Injecting antibiotic behind the conjunctiva of the eye.

severe eye damage could result. Sulphonamide injections given into the muscle are excreted in quite high concentrations in the tears and this is another useful treatment for severe cases. Whatever is used, treatment *must* be applied *early*, before the eye is severely damaged. The speed of healing is almost entirely dependent upon the severity of the initial eye damage which in turn depends on the dose of bacteria received and the length of time before treatment is applied. Prompt treatment also reduces the risk of spreading the infection to other animals. Ideally, infected calves should be removed from the remainder of the group and placed in a dark box (for their own comfort), but this is often impractical.

Prevention and control

New Forest infection is thought to be spread by flies and hence fly control, by spraying or ear-tagging, should be helpful in reducing the condition. Fly control is dealt with in more detail in the section on summer mastitis (page 190). If several animals in a group are affected, and especially if disease is spreading rapidly, it is well worth while asking your veterinary surgeon to inject both eyes of every animal in the group. This sharply reduces the reservoir of infection and it therefore decreases the challenge dose to other animals. Often no further cases are seen. Anything leading to irritation of the eye may be important in the spread of disease and factors such as dust, grass-seeds, ringworm and overhead feeding racks are important.

Inadequate trough space and overcrowding will increase the likelihood of contact spread and if calves are grazing areas with a heavy fly burden (e.g. near water or trees), they are likely to group together in a bunch and this in itself increases the risk of disease. There is also a small nematode worm called *Thelazia* which lives in the eyes and tear ducts of cattle and this may be a further contributory factor. Immunity develops after recovery from infection, although the other eye could still develop disease. So far no effective vaccines have been produced, possibly because there are many different strains of Moraxella which can occur.

Other Causes of Eye Damage

There are a number of conditions which may be confused with New Forest disease, in that they also lead to painful eyes and the production of tears.

1. *Grass seeds, barley awns or other foreign bodies.* These often become wedged in the corner of the eye and may cause damage to the cornea, thus resembling New Forest. The ulcer produced is usually at the side of the cornea however (thus differing from New Forest where it is invariably towards the centre), and there is usually more haemorrhage present, with blood vessels growing in from one side of the eye only. Before treating for New Forest, the eyes should be carefully checked for such objects and if they have penetrated deep into the conjunctival sac at the corner of the eye they are easily missed. Forceps are needed to remove them.

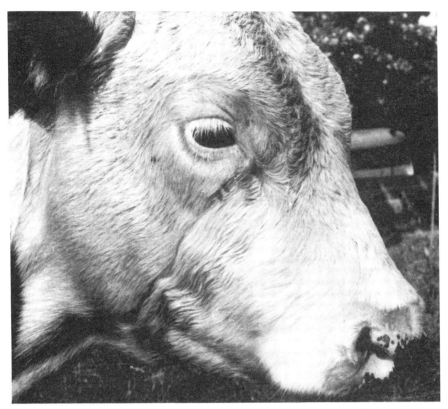

Plate 4.11　A clear eye discharge, commonly seen in the summer and probably caused by fly irritation or ultra-violet from sunlight.

2. *IBR, Infectious Bovine Rhinotracheitis.* This is covered in detail on page 78. Although it leads to a red and painful eye, often with the eyelids closed, the discharge is more of a white, creamy pus (plate 4.5) rather than clear tears and it is the conjunctiva, the membrane lining the eye, which is inflamed. The cornea is normal, and there is no white ulcer present.

3. *Irritation caused by flies or ultra-violet sunlight* can lead to calves rubbing their faces and this can produce runny eyes during the summer, particularly in white-faced animals. A typical example is shown in plate 4.11. Even if the eyes are examined very carefully it is sometimes difficult to tell whether New Forest disease is present or not. New Forest infection *may* cause nothing more than a mild eye discharge, when no ulcer is visible. This would be impossible to differentiate from fly or ultra-violet irritation.

4. *Tumours of the third eyelid* are seen as a red, fleshy lump protruding from the inner corner of the eye and attached to a white fibrous membrane. A typical example is shown in plate 4.12. They occur in older animals at

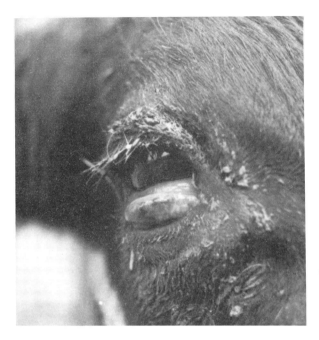

Plate 4.12 Tumour of the third eyelid. This was removed surgically, allowing the cow to continue her normal lactation.

any time of the year and only one case is likely to be seen in a group, so confusion with New Forest is unlikely.

Photosensitisation

This is a condition seen in grazing animals but it is equally as common in adult cows as in young stock. It is caused by an accumulation of light-reactive pigment in the skin. When the skin is exposed to sunlight the pigment absorbs radiant energy and this triggers off a chemical reaction which eventually leads to the release of histamine and causes extensive skin damage. Photosensitisation can be either primary or secondary:

Primary—this is caused by the animal actually eating the photosensitising compound, for example the chemicals contained in the plants St. John's Wort or buckweed.

Secondary—in this instance there is a dysfunction in the liver and chemicals which are normally detoxified at this site accumulate in the body. Alternatively a bile duct may be obstructed, and this can also lead to the accumulation of toxic products in the circulation which are eventually deposited under the skin. The most common of these is phylloerythrin, a breakdown product of chlorophyll, the green pigment found in plants.

Clinical signs

In the very early stages of the acute case the animal may simply be showing signs of liver failure, e.g. depression, off food and inco-ordination. Skin lesions are first detected as a thickening of the white skin and, if you run your hand from black to white pigmented areas, the division can be easily felt. The skin over the back and sides is the worst affected, these being the areas most directly exposed to sunlight, although sometimes in severe cases the teats are so badly inflamed that the cow is impossible to milk. The thickened skin is very painful to touch and after a few days it forms a dry, leathery crust. This eventually drops off, leaving red, raw tissue exposed underneath. The animal shown in colour plate 2 had reached this healing phase before she was noticed and this was probably one to two weeks or more after the initial histamine release and skin damage. In time new skin forms, but this may take several months. If the liver was badly damaged in the initial stages, poor growth and severe laminitis may develop as secondary features.

Treatment
In the early stages the aim is to minimise the effects of the photoreactive chemical. If you suspect the condition, take the animal away from direct sunlight as soon as possible and shut it in a loose-box. After your veterinary surgeon has examined it, he will probably prescribe antihistamines and/or cortisone to counteract the effects of the histamine and reduce any further skin damage. Antibiotic cover may be given to prevent skin infection and vitamins (especially A and D) to promote healing. While the skin is very raw, that is immediately after the initial 'peeling', fly repellents are useful to reduce irritation and to prevent 'strike' and subsequent maggot infestation. Keeping the skin supple with a bland emollient cream also helps healing.

It can easily take a whole summer for the skin to completely heal and during this time the animal should be allowed out to graze at night only. There is no reason why photosensitisation should recur the following year, although the skin may be permanently damaged, similar to the scarring left after severe burns.

THE CLOSTRIDIAL DISEASES

There is a group of infections in cattle all caused by one family of bacteria, the *Clostridia*. The clostridia are also responsible for some of the major diseases of sheep, that is pulpy kidney, lamb dysentery, enterotoxaemia, braxy etc., and they are the cause of gas gangrene in man. In cattle there are four major syndromes, namely:

Tetanus	—caused by *Clostridium tetani*
Blackleg	—caused by *Clostridium chauvoei*
Black Disease	—caused by *Clostridium oedematiens*
Botulism	—caused by *Clostridium botulinum*

Anthrax, caused by *Bacillus anthracis* is a very closely related organism and will be dealt with in the chapter on notifiable diseases.

All four diseases are similar, in that infection can persist in the soil in a very resistant spore form (see page 2) and the bacteria grow best in the absence of air, that is, they are *anaerobic*.

Tetanus

Tetanus can occur in cattle of any age and should always be considered as a possibility if an animal is showing nervous symptoms. It is generally associated with a deep and dirty wound, although in cattle the original wound may no longer be detectable by the time the symptoms of tetanus have developed. Wounds caused by an object originally coated with soil, for example penetration by a muddy nail, are especially dangerous because they take infection deep into the tissues and away from air, and anaerobic conditions such as this are exactly what the clostridia prefer. Improper application of castration rings, for example to calves which are too old, can also lead to a festering wound and tetanus. Traditionally wounds were flushed out with a solution of hydrogen peroxide. This not only kills the tetanus bacteria, but it also supplies a large quantity of oxygen to prevent their growth by destroying their anaerobic environment. Modern antiseptics have a similar effect but it is important that wounds are always cleaned first to remove dirt and soil contamination. The use of an antibiotic and gentian violet aerosol after cleaning is also beneficial.

Clinical signs

When infection has gained entry to the body the bacteria start to multiply and produce *neurotoxins*. The neurotoxins pass via the bloodstream to affect the nerve cells in the brain, and this causes either spasms or loss of function of the muscles. It is this effect which produces the clinical signs of tetanus. Initially the affected animal is dull, shows a small trembling of the muscles and is disinclined to move. A slight bloat may be noticed on the left flank because the rumen muscles have stopped working and the paralysed third eyelid passes part way across the front of the eye. Problems with swallowing may lead to drooling and later it becomes very difficult to open the animal's mouth, the classic 'lock-jaw' syndrome. This can be very helpful in making a specific diagnosis. As the disease progresses, stiffness becomes more apparent, then waves of muscle tremors occur, especially if the animal is excited, and its whole body may shiver uncontrollably. Eventually it is unable to stand and death follows periods of more severe muscle spasm, when all four legs and the neck become completely rigid. It is a most distressing condition to witness and as in the final stages treatment would be hopeless, such animals should be humanely slaughtered.

Treatment

Your veterinary surgeon would undoubtedly be advising you on this, since treatment is extremely complex. The clostridial bacteria are easily killed by penicillin and this should prevent any further toxin from being produced, but only time and the natural defences of the animal can remove the toxins which are already present. Antiserum, containing specific antibodies to tetanus toxin, may be used and muscle relaxants and sedatives will help to overcome the muscle spasms. Animals which are not drinking should be *carefully* drenched (the swallowing reflex may not be functioning correctly either) and in severe cases fluids may be given intravenously.

Prevention
There are two important aspects in the prevention of tetanus. The first is to ensure that all deep wounds are thoroughly cleaned and dressed, especially if soil contamination is a possibility.

Secondly, *vaccination* is highly effective and comparatively inexpensive. If animals are to be grazing areas of known tetanus risk, then they should be given two doses of vaccine at ten weeks and four weeks prior to turnout, plus an annual booster where there is a high risk. On occasions, hard swellings may develop in the skin at the site of vaccination. These are not significant and will slowly disappear without treatment.

Blackleg

Blackleg affects cattle approximately six to eighteen months old and it is almost always a disease of grazing animals. It is caused by the bacterium *Clostridium chauvoei*, which is present in the soil and may be eaten during grazing. Although the disease has been recognised for many years, we still do not know the factors which lead to its appearance, since it is possible to dose calves with *Cl. chauvoei* spores and produce no effect.

Clinical signs
It is unlikely that you will see anything but a dead animal, because the disease is so acute. However, on occasions you may witness an animal which is very dull, standing apart from the others and perhaps panting. Characteristically there will be a swelling somewhere in the muscles where the bacteria are growing, and this is seen in both the live and the dead animal as an enlargement under the skin, often along the back or in the hind legs. If squeezed, a cracking sound is heard, due to the massive accumulation of gas produced by the bacteria. After death the affected muscles have a butyric or rancid smell and are much darker in colour—hence the name 'blackleg'.

Treatment and control
Treatment is rarely possible, although if a live, affected animal is seen, massive doses of penicillin may be effective. Vaccination is the only means of prevention and a combined blackleg and tetanus vaccine is commonly used.

Black Disease

This is certainly not a common disorder, but may occasionally be seen in grazing calves. The organism, *Cl. oedematiens*, is ingested with soil-contaminated food and multiplies in the liver, where it causes a type of 'gas gangrene' similar to blackleg, and, again, very rapid death. If a live affected animal is seen, then penicillin would be the drug of choice for treatment. Control is by vaccination and this is highly effective. Combined tetanus, blackleg and black disease vaccines are available and cost little more than the tetanus vaccine alone.

Botulism

This is a rare disease of cattle in the British Isles, although it does occur overseas, and it is mentioned here only for the sake of completeness. Botulism is an intoxication, not an infection. The bacteria, *Clostridium botulinum*, may be present in the gut of normal healthy animals and cause no problems. After death, however, the bacteria may multiply rapidly and produce a toxin. If other cattle then consume (probably inadvertently via contaminated feed or water) part of the dead carcase containing the toxin, they will develop a progressive paralysis, eventually causing death from loss of function of the respiratory muscles. The toxin of *Clostridium botulinum* is one of the most deadly substances known to man, with minute quantities being fatal.

Chapter 5

THE COW AT CALVING

Gestation Length

THE AVERAGE gestation period for a Friesian cow is approximately nine months, usually quoted as 281 days, although male calves tend to be carried for one day longer and Holsteins one day more than Friesians.

There is considerable variation between the other breeds. For example table 5.1 shows the effect of varying breeds of bull on subsequent gestation length when used to serve Friesian cows.

Table 5.1   The influence of the breed of the bull used on Friesian cows and its effect on gestation length, calf birth weight, calving problems (in cows and heifers) and calf mortality

| | Gestation length Friesians (days) | Calf birth wt. rating | % Dystocia | | | Heifers | Calf Mortality % |
| | | | Cows | | Mean | | |
Breed of Sire			Male Calf	Female Calf	—		
Aberdeen Angus	278.8*	—	—	—	—	1.4	5.3*
British Friesian	281.0	1	—	—	2.7	5.7	2.4
Hereford	282.1	2	1.3	0.4	1.2	2.7	2.3
Charolais	284.2	7	7.9	2.2	3.4	6.7	4.7
Simmental	284.3	6	—	—	1.0	8.8	3.8
South Devon	284.9	4	3.3	1.4	2.7	—	5.6
Chianina	286.1	8	9.6	2.2	6.1	—	6.5
Blonde D'Aquitaine	287.3	5	—	—	2.0	—	3.6
Limousin	287.4	3	3.0	1.7	2.4	3.2	3.3

*Aberdeen Angus bull on Friesian maiden heifers, not cows).
(From: J. W. Stables, *Bovine Practitioner* (1980) *15* 26).

It is interesting to note that although the Limousin bull gives the longest gestation length when used on Friesian cows, its calves are not the heaviest at birth. There is a certain amount of compensatory growth however, and the Limousin cross steer reaches a final slaughter weight approaching (but not equal to) the Charolais cross. The heaviest calves are sired by the Chianina and Charolais, and these are the two breeds which lead to the highest number of births requiring assistance. This is known as the incidence of *dystocia*, and is usually expressed as a percentage. As one might expect there is a higher dystocia rate in heifers than in cows (table 5.1) even if the same bull is used. The number of calving problems also increase when there is a male calf born rather than a female and in the data used to construct table 5.1 the highest incidence of dystocia was given by the Chianina bull producing male calves, although the figures would undoubtedly have been worse had the bull been used on heifers and not cows. Calf mortality, possibly better called the full-term stillbirth rate, is the percentage of calves born dead, and this increases with the relative birth weight of the calf, with the Charolais and Chianina giving the heaviest calves and two of the highest mortality figures. In addition to the interbreed variations, individual bulls *within* a breed will also vary in gestation length and in the ease of calving of their offspring. Provided that heifers are not overfed for the six weeks prior to calving, there is no reason why an 'easy-calving' Friesian bull should not be selected to give an additional crop of Friesian heifer calves. (This is considered in more detail on page 226). Although the average incidence of dystocia using a Friesian bull on Friesian heifers is given as 5.7 per cent, this could be reduced considerably by careful bull selection. It is not advisable to routinely use the Chianina, Charolais or South Devon breeds on Friesian heifers, however.

It is the developing calf which determines exactly when birth will occur. Increased activity of its adrenal gland immediately prior to calving triggers off a reaction in the cow to produce a rise in her oestrogen levels and a fall in progesterone, and this in turn leads to the sequence of events which induces birth.

The Birth Process

To understand the mechanisms of the birth process, it is necessary to appreciate the basic anatomy of the reproductive tract and the structure of the calf in the uterus. Figure 5.1 and plate 5.1 show the reproductive organs viewed as if you were standing above the cow and looking directly down onto her back. The opening to the outside is known as the *vulva* and the fleshy folds of skin surrounding it are the *vulval lips*. The passage leading forwards from the vulva into the cow is known as the *vagina* and this goes as far as the *cervix*, a thick fibrous structure which seals off the inner tract, thus preventing the entry of infection and protecting the calf during pregnancy. The *uterus* is the womb, the part of the tract which enlarges during pregnancy to accommodate the calf. It consists of a main *body* which divides into two *horns*. From the tip of each horn a very narrow and convoluted tube, the *oviduct* or *fallopian tube* runs forward to the *ovary*, the organ which produces the eggs to initiate pregnancy.

These structures will be referred to later in the chapter on fertility control and for the moment we will return to the cow at calving.

Figure 5.2 shows the position of the calf in the cow's uterus towards the end of pregnancy. The calf is floating in fluid which acts as a 'shock absorber',

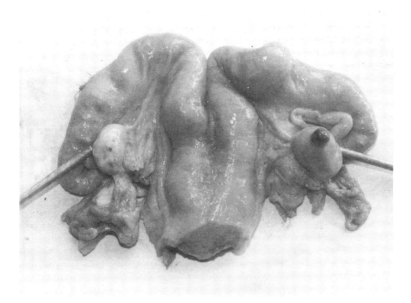

Plate 5.1 The reproductive tract of the cow, amputated at the end of the cervix. The right ovary shows a large corpus luteum and the oviduct can be seen behind the ovary as a convoluted tube running to join the tip of the uterine horn.

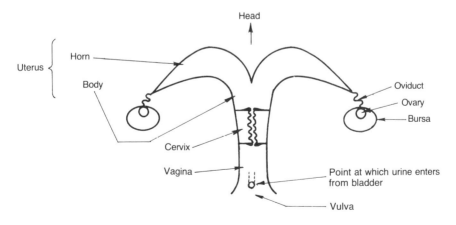

Figure 5.1 The reproductive tract of a cow (as shown in plate 5.1).

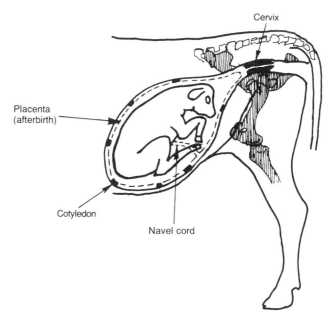

Figure 5.2   Position of the calf in the uterus towards the end of pregnancy but before the first stage of labour.

protecting it from the cow's movements. This fluid is contained in a membranous bag formed by the *placenta*, sometimes called the *afterbirth* and it provides lubrication at the time of birth. The placenta is attached to the wall of the uterus only at certain points, known as *cotyledons*, where there is a very delicate interchange of materials across the maternal and foetal blood vessels (figure 5.3). The cow and the calf each have completely separate blood supplies; there is no direct flow of blood from one to another. Instead, their blood vessels grow *very* closely together at the cotyledon so that food and oxygen can diffuse from the cow's blood supply into the placenta, while urea and other waste materials flow from the calf to the placenta and back into the cow. All the nutrients which have passed from the cow into the placenta at the cotyledons are collected together by a series of blood vessels and eventually these join as one and enter the calf via the *umbilical* or navel cord. The blood vessels of the cord pass directly to the calf's liver, which is the organ where many of the nutrients are utilised.

The point of placental interchange at the cotyledon also acts as a filter, allowing only small molecules of nutrients and waste products to pass. Bacteria, moulds, large viruses and certain drugs are unable to gain access into the normal calf, and if bacteria cause abortion they do so by destroying the placenta and 'starving' the developing foetus. Although the placental filter is a useful protective mechanism, it means that the calf is not exposed to the majority of the infectious organisms and other antigens in the cow's environment, and so it cannot produce its own antibodies before birth. (The

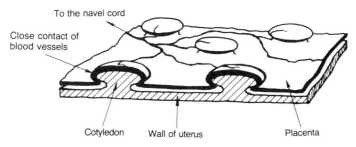

To the navel cord

Close contact of
blood vessels

Cotyledon   Wall of uterus   Placenta

Figure 5.3   The cotyledons of the uterus. There is no direct flow of blood from mother to foetus. Nutrients must diffuse across the blood vessels at the cotyledon area.

mechanisms of antibody production are explained on page 7.) In addition, antibodies from the cow are such large molecules that they cannot pass the placenta either. The newborn calf is almost totally devoid of immunity therefore, and this is why the antibodies it receives in its colostrum are of such vital importance to its survival. There are a few very small viruses, for example BVD (page 80) which can cross the placenta. These may result in either the loss of the developing calf or the phenomenon of immune tolerance (see page 82), or, if the calf is old enough, antibody production.

Freemartin Calves

The twinning rate for Friesians varies from approximately 1.5 per cent in heifers to 5 per cent in older cows. Unless they are identical twins, the sexes of the calves will be randomly distributed, that is 25 per cent of the twins will be male–male, 25 per cent female–female and 50 per cent male–female. In the latter combination, over 80 per cent of the female calves are infertile due to incomplete development of their reproductive tract, and they are known as *freemartins*.

The cause of this occurs in very early pregnancy. In all but a small proportion of twin calves, the placentae fuse together and have a common blood supply. Because male hormones are produced at an earlier stage than those of the female, the heifer calf starts its development as a male. Later, its own female hormones take over, so the calf is born with almost normal external reproductive organs (the vulva etc.), but parts or all of the cervix, uterus and ovaries are missing. Often the freemartin vagina ends just in front of the point where the urethra enters from the bladder which would be the equivalent position of the hymen (see figure 5.1). By measuring the vaginal length of your female twin calf and comparing it to a normal calf, your vet may be able to decide whether your heifer, born twin to a bull, has an abnormally short vagina and is therefore one of the unfortunate 80 per cent which will be unable to breed. Another useful sign of a freemartin is the presence of an enlarged clitoris and a tuft of hair between the lower lips of the vulva.

However, the only accurate tests are either to take a blood-sample from the calf and perform a chromosome analysis, or wait until the young heifer is mature when your vet will be able to carry out a rectal examination. A chromosome analysis consists of culturing certain blood cells (the lymphocytes) and then examining the chromosomes (that is the genes) in their nucleus. True female calves will have only XX chromosomes, true males XY, whilst the freemartin will have a mixture of XX and XY because of the interchange of blood in the early stages of pregnancy.

There is one final point of interest. A very small proportion of single heifer calves were also originally twin to a bull, but because the male calf died early in pregnancy (early foetal death—see page 227) there is no way that you could know that it had been a twin. These heifers may also be freemartins. It is worth noting that the *hippomane*, the small irregular-shaped rubbery mass approximately the size of a 50-pence piece and often seen in the foetal fluids at calving is *not* the remains of an original twin. It is simply an accumulation of fibrin and placental cells.

Calving Facilities

Calving is the most critical time of a cow's life. A smooth calving will help to ensure a successful and profitable lactation, and so it is important to provide adequate facilities. Ideally there should be sufficient loose boxes to allow each cow to calve on its own (plate 5.2), and the boxes ought to be positioned within easy access of the dry-cow yard so that the herdsman doing his late evening rounds can easily separate an individual cow for the night. They need

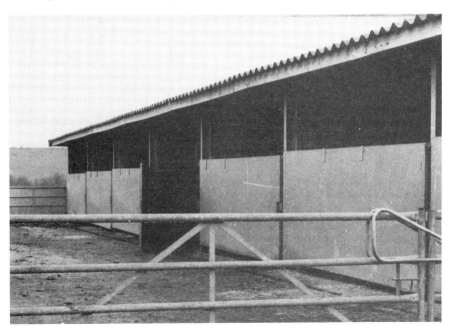

Plate 5.2   A row of calving boxes with wide doors and easy access.

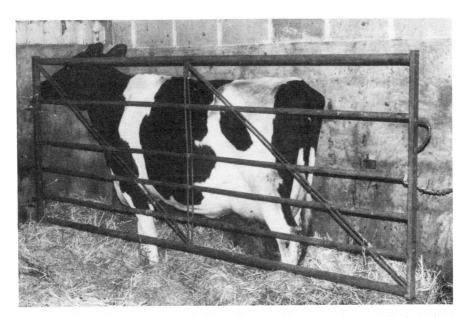

Plate 5.3 Each of the seven boxes is fitted with a set of hinges, and one gate is always kept available to be taken into a box whenever it is needed.

to be large enough for several attendants to enter should assistance be required, and I strongly favour an internal handling gate, as shown in the boxes in plate 5.3. If it is easy for one person to restrain and examine a cow, there is far less risk of problem cases being overlooked or neglected. The cow should remain with her calf for the first twenty-four hours when every effort must be made to ensure an adequate colostrum intake (see page 17). This period of isolation also allows a regular check for milk fever, mastitis and the other post-calving complications described at the end of this chapter. There must be facilities for food and water and there must also be good lighting. Boxes ought to be regularly cleaned to decrease the risk of mastitis and uterine infections, although this means there would then never be more than a shallow bed of straw present, and this may not be sufficient to provide an adequate grip for cows with nerve damage. The door should therefore be large enough to carry a cow out on a gate, and also to remove the unfortunate fatalities that are bound to occur.

Signs of Calving

During late pregnancy the cow's abdomen enlarges, especially the lower part, and her udder progressively fills. There is no set time-scale for these changes to occur, however, and they seem to vary with the individual animal. The secretion in the udder changes from a tacky, clear, honey-coloured fluid in the dry cow, to a much cloudier, off-white liquid, the start of the colostrum. At forty-eight hours or so before calving, the ligaments of the pelvis relax to

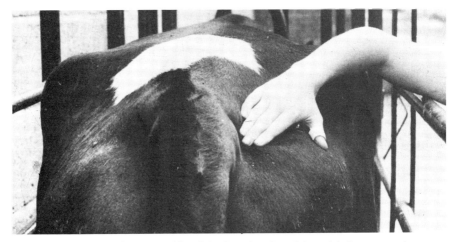

Plate 5.4 The point where cows 'drop in'—the relaxation of the pelvic ligaments prior to calving.

allow additional room for the calf to pass through and this can be seen as a depression in the skin on each side of the tail at its base, that is, where it joins the main body. This point is shown in plate 5.4 and the cow is said to be 'dropping in'. There is also enlargement of the lips of the vulva and the cow shows increasing discomfort.

Stages of Labour

Traditionally, the process of giving birth has been divided into three parts, known as the three stages of *labour*.

First stage labour
This is the opening of the cervix. Waves of contraction pass through the muscles of the wall of the uterus leading to discomfort but the cow is not seen straining. A thick, cloudy, slimy discharge may occur and this is the plug which was originally blocking the cervix. The calf alters from the position shown in figure 5.2 bringing its front feet up, so that they are extended forward ready to lead the way through the cervix, and its nose also comes upwards.

Second stage labour
This is the actual delivery of the calf. Externally it is seen as the start of the contractions of the abdominal muscles, that is the cow begins to strain. The contraction of the muscles of the uterus forces the calf and the fluid-filled placenta through the cervix and into the vagina and it is the presence of these large objects, dilating the vagina, which stimulates the cow to contract her abdominal muscles, thus giving further help to the expulsion of the calf. The hormone *oxytocin* is involved in these reflex actions.

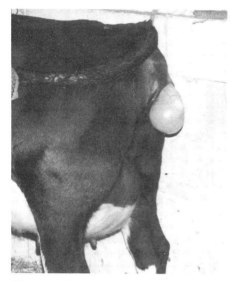

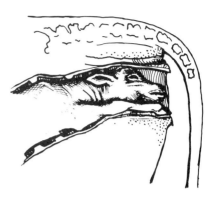

Figure 5.4 Calf at the second stage of labour.

Plate 5.5 Second stage labour. The calf's feet can be seen at the vulva still covered by the inner placental membrane (the amnion).

After a period of forceful straining, the outer placenta ruptures and liberates a large quantity of straw-coloured allantoic fluid. This is known as the bursting of the *waterbag* or allantoic sac. The calf is still enclosed in an inner placental bag, however, and this inner bag (the amniotic sac) contains the thicker and more lubricant amniotic fluid which will assist the birth process. As the contractions increase in strength and frequency, the feet of the calf may be seen appearing at the vulva, usually covered by the inner placental membrane. This is seen in plate 5.5 and figures 5.4 and 5.6.

When the calf's head reaches the vagina, the cow often lies flat on her side as the abdominal muscles contract to push the calf's head through the vulva. After this stage has been passed, the cow may rest for a few minutes before making the final effort to expel the calf's chest and then its hips. If the inner placenta has not broken during birth, the calf's own movements should be sufficient to clear it from its face and nose, thus allowing breathing to start. If you happen to be present at the time of birth, however, it is always worth checking that the airways are clear and that the calf cannot suffocate. The navel cord breaks very quickly, either when the calf moves or by the cow standing up, and the blood vessels, which have elastic walls, spring back into the calf's umbilicus to prevent bleeding.

Third stage labour
During birth there has been a slow separation of the placenta from the uterine cotyledons (see figure 5.3) and the third stage of labour is the expulsion of the placenta. Under normal circumstances this should occur within one to six hours after the birth of the calf and the cow will eat its afterbirth if given the opportunity. In the natural state there is some evidence to suggest that the

placenta even supplies hormones required for mothering and early lactation. Although it is not a great danger to her, others have associated eating the placenta with digestive problems and would say that if it is possible to take it away, this is best done. Usually the calf is standing and suckling some thirty minutes after birth and the suckling itself leads to the release of oxytocin, which in turn stimulates uterine contractions and helps with the expulsion of the placenta.

Time sequence

One of the great questions with regard to calving is 'how long should I wait?' Unfortunately no specific time sequence can be given. Heifers, especially, can show discomfort some two or three days before calving and this may be due entirely to distension and tightness in the udder. The first stage of labour, leading to the opening of the cervix, involves only uterine contractions: the cow is not seen to be straining. Straining is the second stage of labour and a vaginal examination at this time should show that the cervix is open. If the calf is still covered in the inner placental membrane, as shown in plate 5.5, there is usually no hurry. As a very rough guide I would suggest the following:

First stage: allow nine hours.
Second stage: allow three hours.

This assumes that the birth is proceeding normally. If any abnormality is suspected, the cow should be examined immediately so that any necessary help can be given.

Manual Examination

You can learn a great deal from examining the cow yourself and it is unlikely that any harm will occur, provided that you follow these simple instructions.

1. Restrain the cow, preferably by standing her behind a gate, rather than using a halter which may cause her stress. I think all calving boxes should be fitted with gate hinges slightly offset from one corner, so that a gate can be brought in and the cow easily and calmly restrained by one person, as shown in plate 5.3.
2. Ask an assistant to hold the tail to one side, and wash the vulva with warm soapy water, possibly containing a mild antiseptic.
3. Thoroughly wash your hand and arm, then, with your sleeve rolled well back and using ample lubrication, insert your hand through the vulva and into the vagina. At the time of insertion your fingers and thumb should be together and pointing forwards, with the thumb uppermost. This will cause least discomfort to the cow.
4. Once in the vagina, push your hand slowly forward towards the cervix. If the vagina ends in a hard protruding button, and in the centre of that button there is a hole into which only one finger can be inserted, then the cervix is fully closed and the cow should be left (figure 5.5) as calving has not started.

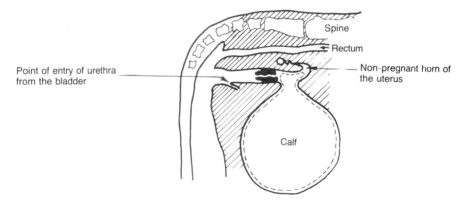

Spine

Rectum

Point of entry of urethra
from the bladder

Non-pregnant horn of
the uterus

Calf

Figure 5.5 The cervix is still tightly closed: you may be able to insert one finger but nothing more.

5. If the cervix is open, you will be able to push your hand into the uterus. Now it should be possible to feel the calf's head and two front legs, although they will most probably be covered by a placental membrane, probably the amnion. Do not break this membrane. Withdraw your hand into the cervix. If the rim of the cervix can easily be felt as a ring or a thick fibrous band running around the inside of the vagina (figure 5.6), then the cervix is not fully dilated and the cow should be left for a little longer. Sometimes you need to wait until the cow is straining and forcing the calf into the vagina to be able to feel this incompletely dilated cervical ring.

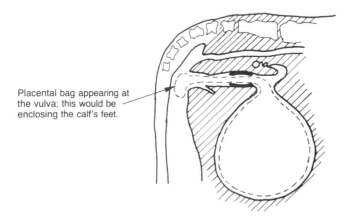

Placental bag appearing at
the vulva; this would be
enclosing the calf's feet.

Figure 5.6 Although the calf's feet covered by placenta may be appearing at the vulva careful examination would reveal that the cervix was detectable as a thick ring running around the vaginal wall. The cow is still not ready to calve.

Births Needing Assistance

The majority of cows calve quite easily without assistance and one of the great features of stockmanship is knowing precisely when additional help is necessary. If the calf's feet are appearing at the vulva, then clearly the cervix must be open and, at this stage, I would not leave a cow for much longer than an hour or so, especially if she is straining fairly violently. The most important step is to confirm that you have two front legs and a head in the vagina and that they all belong to the same calf. The latter point is easily checked by sliding your hand along each leg until you can confirm that they both join the same body and that the head in the vagina also comes from that body (plate 5.6). If there is any doubt, check that you have two front legs and not two back legs. This is done by bending the legs: starting from the foot, if the first two joints bend the same way it is a front leg. If the first joint moves the foot up and the second joint moves the leg down, then you are dealing with a hind leg. These differences are shown in more detail in figure 5.7. It is most important to check for these features when the calf's head cannot be felt. The commonest cause of two feet with soles uppermost in the vagina is a calf coming backwards, although the possibility of it being a forward delivery, but with the hcad back and the calf upside down must not be overlooked, and this can also be checked by bending the leg.

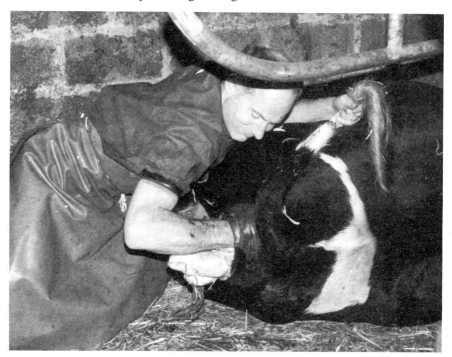

Plate 5.6   Before pulling, make sure that both legs belong to the same calf, and decide whether they are front or back legs.

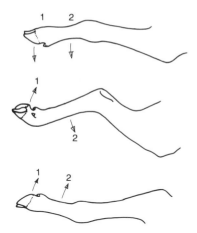

Front leg: joints 1 + 2 (fetlock + knee) would both move the foot downwards.

Hind leg, calf coming backwards: the fetlock joint (1) would move the foot upwards but the hock (2) moves it downwards.

Front leg, but the calf is upside down and its head is not detectable. Joints 1 + 2 still both move in the same direction, but upwards and not down.

Figure 5.7   Distinguishing the presentations of the calf in the uterus by examining its leg.

Having satisfied yourself that the calf is positioned correctly, next attach the ropes. I would strongly recommend that you purchase a special set of calving ropes, that these are used *only* for calvings and that they are washed and stored in the same place after each occasion. Calvings seem to occur at the most inconvenient times and there is nothing worse than not having the equipment to hand when it is needed. The rope should be looped *above* the calf's fetlock as shown in figure 5.8 and plate 5.7 and you must make sure that there is no placenta between the rope and the calf's skin (this has in fact happened on the left leg in plate 5.7) otherwise there is a risk of it slipping off when you start to pull. The rope could also slip if it is attached just above the hoof and below the fetlock (figure 5.8a).

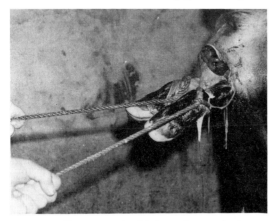

Plate 5.7   The ropes should always be attached *above* the fetlock joint. There is placenta between the rope and the skin on the left leg, which could lead to the rope slipping off.

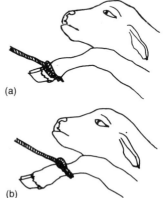

Figure 5.8   Rope should be attached above the fetlock (as in b), *not* below the fetlock (a).

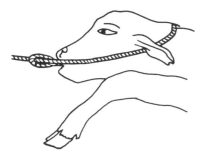

Figure 5.9   The head rope must go behind both ears of the calf, and passing it through its mouth will help to lift the nose when traction is applied.

Next tie short bars to the ropes (sawn-off axe handles are ideal), ready for the pull. A steady but continual pressure can be applied with one man on each rope, but as the cow strains the pull should be increased, so that the increased forces of man and cow coincide. In the early stages of the pull it is vital that two factors are checked. First that the head is coming with the feet. If not, a third rope may have to be attached to the head as shown in figure 5.9. Second, check that there is enough room for the calf's head to enter the bony pelvis of the cow. If not, then you are dealing with an impossible case and a Caesarian section will be necessary.

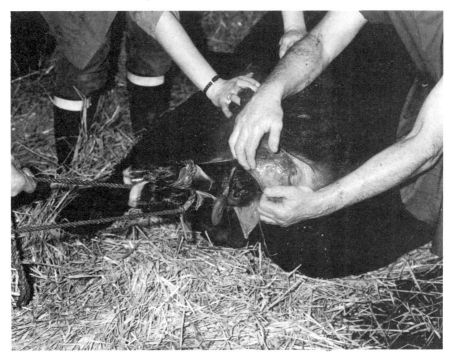

Plate 5.8   One of the most difficult parts of the birth is drawing the head through the vulva. Stretching the vulval lips with your hands helps a great deal.

With a pull, the feet should pass through the vulva fairly easily. However, as the head approaches there may be some difficulty, especially in heifers, and an additional operator can provide very useful assistance by standing beside the animal and manually stretching the vulva with both hands as shown in plate 5.8. It is much better to dilate a tight vulva with your hands, since excessive pulling will reduce the calf's chances of survival, and there is also a risk of tearing the vaginal wall. Sometimes it is simply not possible to stretch the vagina and vulva enough to allow the calf to pass, and in this case your vet could cut through the constriction, cutting along the line of the operator's first finger (right hand) in plate 5.8. This is known as an *episiotomy*. The incision has to be sutured afterwards, but a controlled cut through soft tissues is far better than a tear which might rupture blood vessels and lead to fatal haemorrhage. Adequate lubrication is vital at all stages of the birth, but especially when the head is stretching the vulva. If there is any dryness, the friction between the skin of the calf and the wall of the vagina can easily lead to tearing and even severe bleeding. Proprietary lubricants are available, but personally I find that soapflakes are the easiest to use, while others recommend lard. Choose a moment when the cow is not straining, allow the ropes to slacken and, taking a handful of dry soapflakes, briefly immerse your hand in a bucket of water and then push the now pasty soap into the vagina. The top of the calf's head is especially important, but put soap all around the head and shoulders if you are at all doubtful. Failure to provide adequate lubrication is a mistake commonly made by farmers.

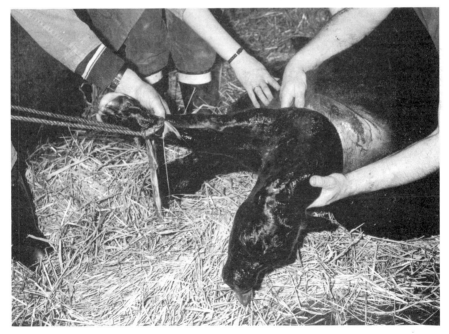

Plate 5.9 The calf's legs should be pulled obliquely downwards and not straight back.

When the head is passing through the vulva, the calf's ribs will be passing through its mother's pelvis and if the birth is tight the umbilical cord may be constricted. Time is now more important. Continue to pull, co-ordinated with the cow's straining, ensuring that the calf's legs are pulled obliquely down towards the cow's feet as shown in plate 5.9, rather than straight backwards. This enables the calf to pass in an arc through the mother's pelvis and facilitates the passage of the calf's hips. Additional pressure may be required to get the calf's hips through and a slight rotation of the calf may also help, so that the calf's hips pass obliquely through the mother's pelvis. The idea is shown in plate 5.10 and diagrammatically in figure 5.10. In a more difficult birth it may be necessary to pull the head of the calf under its front legs and over its body (from the position shown in plate 5.10) to achieve a more forceful rotation while traction is being applied.

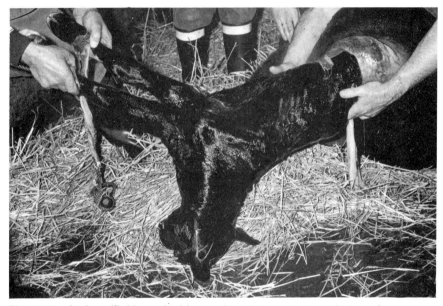

Plate 5.10   As the calf's hips and pelvis pass through the mother's pelvis, it may be necessary to slightly rotate the calf to facilitate delivery.

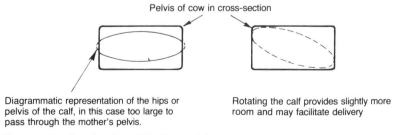

Pelvis of cow in cross-section

Diagrammatic representation of the hips or pelvis of the calf, in this case too large to pass through the mother's pelvis.

Rotating the calf provides slightly more room and may facilitate delivery

Figure 5.10   Rotating the calf facilitates delivery of its hips and pelvis.

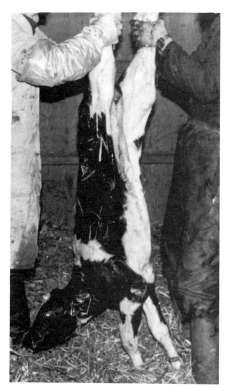

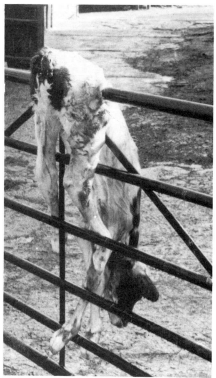

Plate 5.11 Hold the calf by the hocks with its head downwards to drain fluid from its mouth and trachea *before* breathing starts. Swinging it from side to side will also help to expel any fluid.

Plate 5.12 Calf suspended by crooking its hind legs into a gate. This allows any inhaled fluid to run out.

As the calf reaches the ground, immediately clear any placenta from its nose and mucus from its mouth. If the birth has been protracted and you feel there has been a possibility that placental fluids have been inhaled, immediately lift the calf by its hocks, and swing it with its head downwards as shown in plate 5.11. This allows the fluid to drain out. An alternative is to crook the calf's legs into a gate, as shown in plate 5.12. Breathing should start very soon after birth and the idea is to suspend the calf and drain the fluid from it *before* its first breath, so that the fluid is not drawn into the lungs. If breathing does not start, place your hand flat on its chest underneath the left front leg to check for a heart beat. Breathing may be stimulated by throwing cold water into the calf's ear, or over its whole head, or by tickling the end of its nostril with a piece of hay or straw. The latter method is especially good because it makes the calf sneeze, and the sudden breathing-out movement helps to expel any inhaled fluid. Slapping the side of its chest with the flat of your hand will also help to stimulate breathing. Stimulation of breathing is technically known as *resuscitation*.

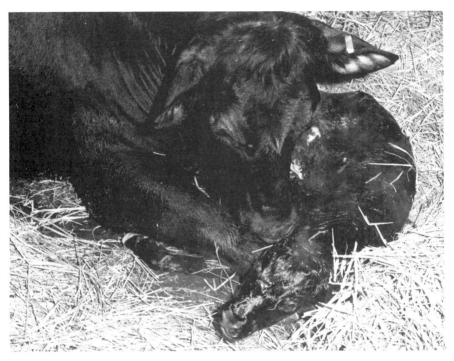

Plate 5.13   The cow licking her calf after birth dries it and thus prevents chilling. Licking also stimulates breathing and may remove any placenta from over the calf's nose or mouth which could obstruct its airways.

With the cow still restrained wash your arm then reinsert it into the uterus to check for a second calf. Check all four quarters of the udder for mastitis and check for vaginal tears and excessive bleeding. The technique for this is described in detail on page 119. Then release her, putting the calf in front of her head to encourage her to lick it dry (plate 5.13). This stimulates the calf's breathing and prevents it from getting too cold. As soon as the licking has stopped, spray the wet cord with an antibiotic aerosol to prevent navel ill (page 22), and when it can stand, guide it to the teat for a good feed of colostrum. If it does not stand within six hours, it is very important that it is kept warm and that colostrum is given by bottle or stomach tube. The importance of colostrum is described on page 17.

Calving Aids

The most common calving aid is the calving jack (plate 5.14). It can exert considerable additional force when pulling a calf and so it is vital that you are *absolutely* sure that the calf is positioned correctly for delivery before operating it. Restrain the cow, check the posture of the calf and apply the

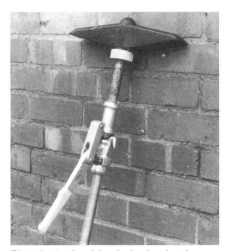

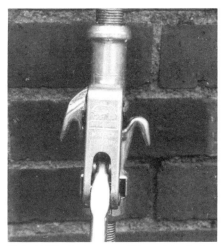

Plate 5.14 A calving jack, showing the black buffer bar which fits against the cow's hind legs.

Plate 5.15 A close-up of the calving jack showing the hooks where the ropes are to be attached.

calving ropes as described on page 105. Next slide the ratchet down to the bottom of the jack, attach the ropes to the hooks (plate 5.15) and place the transverse buffer bar of the jack (the black crosspiece seen in plate 5.14) on to the thick muscle of the cow's hind legs, as shown in plate 5.16. You are now in

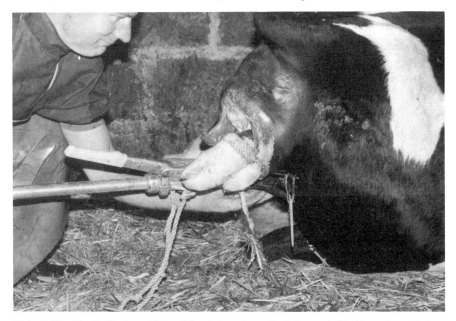

Plate 5.16 The buffer bar of the calving jack rests against the cow's hind legs, beneath the vulva and above the udder.

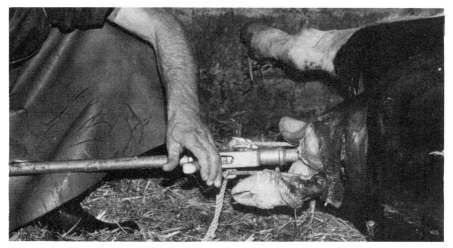

Plate 5.17 Using the ratchet handle of the calving jack. Note that the calf's tongue is quite swollen, so delivery cannot now be delayed. The calving rope is also starting to slip from the calf's left leg. The operator's right hand can push the bar downwards to give a little additional traction as the cow strains.

a position to start pulling. Slowly work the ratchet handle and start to draw the calf (plate 5.17). As the cow strains, extra pressure can be applied by pulling the free end of the calving jack downwards in a lever action; when the contraction ceases, ease the handle back up to the horizontal position and take up any additional slack rope using the ratchet. In this way the calf can be slowly delivered.

The calving jack is particularly useful for the single-handed stockman, and for assisting calvings in a field. However, in inexperienced hands or if used incorrectly, it can also be very dangerous. The main danger is that it is used in the wrong circumstances, for example before the cervix or vagina have fully opened, or before the calf has been correctly positioned for delivery, or simply when the calf is too large and veterinary assistance should have been sought. Another misuse is that the calf is drawn far too quickly. If the tissues of the vulva and vagina are not allowed to dilate naturally as the calf's head is being delivered (this critical stage is shown in plate 5.17), tearing of the vagina may occur. This in turn could lead to severe infections or even fatal blood loss.

The final disadvantage of the jack is that it is not easy to rotate a calf stuck at the hips to facilitate its passage through the maternal pelvis. Rotation may be a critical part of delivery at this stage. Great care therefore needs to be taken with its use. If in doubt, call for veterinary assistance. The possibility of losing a cow from vaginal infection, blood loss or nerve damage following an excessively tight delivery is never worth the risk. Once the calf becomes locked in the birth canal, it may be too late for the vet to carry out an embryotomy, episiotomy or Caesarian section to effect a safe delivery.*

* *Embryotomy*—cutting up the calf inside the cow and delivering it piecemeal.
Episiotomy—cutting through the vulva and posterior vagina to increase the space available for the calf.
Caesarian—cutting through the flank and into the uterus so that the calf does not have to be drawn through the pelvis.

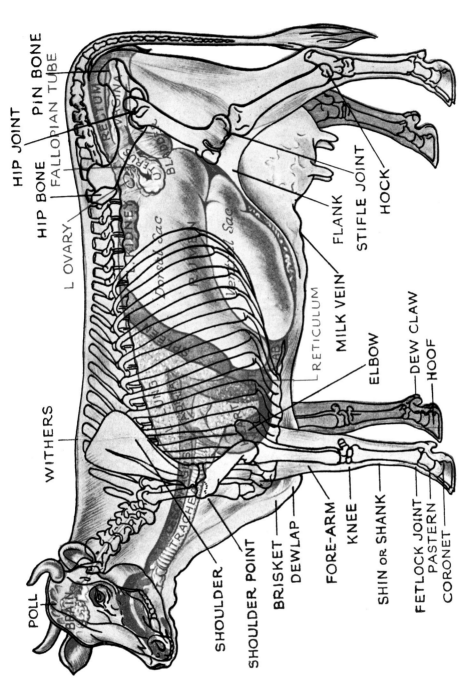

The skeleton and internal organs of the cow as seen from the left side.

Labels on figure: POLL, BRAINS, WITHERS, HIP JOINT, PIN BONE, HIP BONE, FALLOPIAN TUBE, L OVARY, RECTUM, VAGINA, KIDNEY, BLADDER, Dorsal Sac, Ventral Sac, RETICULUM, MILK VEIN, FLANK, STIFLE JOINT, HOCK, ELBOW, DEW CLAW, HOOF, SHOULDER, SHOULDER POINT, BRISKET, DEWLAP, TRACHEA, FORE-ARM, KNEE, SHIN OR SHANK, FETLOCK JOINT, PASTERN, CORONET, LUNG, HEART, DIAPHRAGM

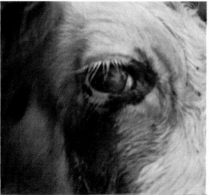

Colour plate 1   New Forest: the red ring around the eye is caused by blood vessels moving in to heal the ulcer. This is known as pannus formation.

Colour plate 2 (*below*) Photosensitisation: although photoreactive chemical is present throughout the body, only the white areas allow entry of sufficient sunlight to cause skin damage.

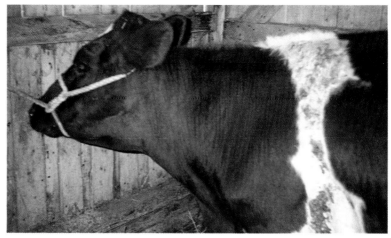

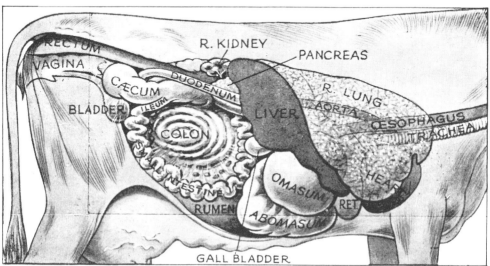

The internal organs of the cow from the right side.

Abnormalities Requiring Correction

There are some abnormalities which can be easily corrected and others which need to be recognised so that veterinary assistance can be sought. The following gives a few ideas on when a manual vaginal examination should be carried out and what may be felt:

1. Any cow due to calve which has been 'in discomfort' for more than twenty-four hours without any positive signs of the birth process starting should be examined.
2. If a piece of cleansing (placenta) is hanging from the vulva, and especially if deep red/purple cotyledons are visible on it. This is an indication that placental separation is already occurring and intervention is needed.
3. The shape of a normal closed cervix has been described as a protruding button (page 102 and figure 5.5). If this bulging structure cannot be felt, but it is still not possible to pass your hand through the cervix, you may be dealing with a twist, or *torsion of the uterus*. This would feel similar to the effect of trying to push your hand along the sleeve of a jacket which has been rotated through 180° or 360° at the elbow. If uterine torsion is suspected, veterinary attention should be sought. The condition is thought to be caused by the calf making excessively violent movements within the uterus at the start of calving and in almost every case there is a very large calf involved. Although it is possible to roll the cow and correct the torsion, in many cases the cervix still fails to dilate adequately and delivery by Caesarian section is necessary.
4. Sometimes even though the vagina and cervix are fully dilated and the calf is lying normally, the cow simply refuses to push to effect its delivery. This is the condition of *uterine inertia*. The calf will have to be delivered by traction. It is probably worth giving the cow a bottle of calcium in case milk fever is a predisposing factor.
5. We come now to the abnormal positions of the calf which have to be corrected before birth can occur. Earlier in the chapter we said that towards the end of pregnancy the calf straightens its nose and forelegs so that these are the first parts to enter the 'birth canal' (the name given to the opened cervix and vagina leading through the pelvis). However, on occasions this does not occur and abnormalities of posture result.

Leg backwards
The bend may be at the calf's knee (figure 5.11), when the point of the knee will be felt by pushing your hand along the calf's neck, through the bony canal formed by the cow's pelvis and into the uterus. It may be possible to cup the calf's hoof in the palm of your hand and draw it forwards (figure 5.12). This is especially so if the abnormality has been detected at an early stage and the head and normal leg of the calf are not already tightly locked in the pelvis. At the other extreme you may need to ask for veterinary help to inject into the spine of the cow (an epidural anaesthetic), to stop her straining, so that the calf can be pushed back into the uterus and the leg brought forwards.

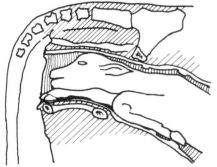

Figure 5.11   Abnormalities of posture: leg flexed at knee.

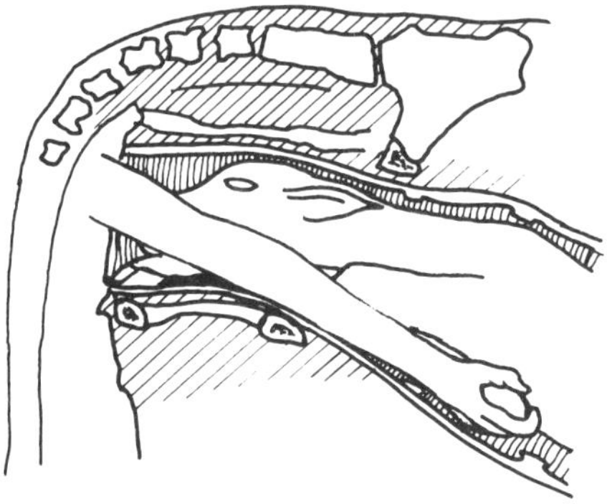

Figure 5.12   Correction of simple leg flexed (leg back) presentation. Cup the calf's foot in your hand and draw it forward.

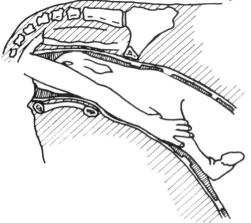

Figure 5.13   Full leg flexion from the shoulder, showing an attempt to draw it forward to the simple knee flexion position.

On occasions the whole leg may be turned backwards from the shoulder (figure 5.13) and your first impression when examining the cow is that you are about to witness the birth of a three-legged calf! With a good long reach, however, it should be possible to pull the leg forwards into the 'knee flexed' position (figure 5.11), either pulling it with your hand or by attaching a rope. It is very rare that it is not possible to push a rope around the leg, even if it is fully extended backwards. The cases which pose problems are those in which the head and one leg have passed through the vulva, as shown in plate 5.18. The cow was found like this early one morning and the calf's head had become dry and swollen. Note the protruding swollen tongue. I was unable to repel the calf even after an epidural, and the cow had to be suspended by her hind legs to give sufficient room to correct the posture and deliver the calf.

Head back
In this posture two legs will be presented in the birth canal and it is vital that you confirm that they are front and not back legs, using the method described

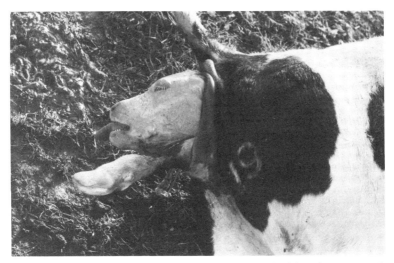

Plate 5.18   A difficult presentation. The calf had to be pushed back into the uterus so that the missing leg could be found and straightened.

on page 104. Once you are sure that they are front legs, try to locate the top of the calf's neck and follow the direction of its curve. This will tell you if the head is on the right or the left. If possible, gently cup the calf's nose in the palm of your hand (figure 5.14) and draw it forward so that it will enter the vagina. Sometimes it may be necessary to apply a rope as shown in figure 5.9. If the posture cannot be corrected easily, call for veterinary assistance. Pulling the head round with excessive force can rupture the wall of the uterus and there will be occasions when correction is not possible and delivery will have to be by embryotomy (that is after cutting off the calf's head and neck), or by Caesarian section.

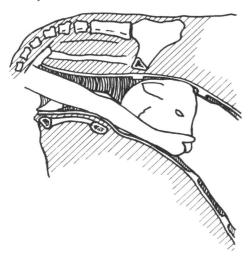

Figure 5.14   It may be possible to correct a 'head back' simply by drawing the nose around with your hand. On other occasions a rope is needed.

Backwards delivery

A proportion of calves are born hind legs first without any trouble. There are a few additional complicating factors, however. Firstly the presence of only the feet in the vagina (that is without the head) does not dilate the vagina to the same degree, so there is thus a reduced release of the hormone oxytocin (page 100) and reduced abdominal contractions. Secondly, when the calf's hips are passing through the vulva, its chest is entering the cow's pelvis and so the umbilical cord is constricted well before the calf is able to breathe. The danger of it inhaling uterine fluids is therefore much greater and calves born backwards should definitely be suspended in the manner described on page 109 (plates 5.11 and 5.12) to allow excess fluid to drain from the air passages. The situation is sometimes exacerbated by the fact that the umbilical cord is passing back between the hind legs of the calf and over its hock, as shown in figure 5.15. In this instance the cord would rupture as soon as delivery commenced, and the chances of obtaining a live calf are even more seriously impaired. If you detect this abnormality of the cord I suggest you call for immediate veterinary assistance to reposition it before delivery commences. The final danger with backward deliveries is that the tail may be pushed towards the calf's head (figure 5.16). If this is not corrected it can cause serious damage to the roof of the vagina.

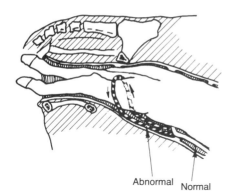

Abnormal   Normal

Figure 5.15   Backwards presentation showing normal and abnormal positions of the umbilical cord. With the latter, veterinary assistance is needed.

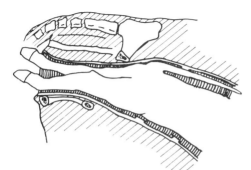

Figure 5.16   Backwards presentation: always check that the tail is not being forced into the roof of the vagina as it is in this diagram. It should be lying between the hind legs during the birth.

Breech presentation

This is probably the most difficult of all the abnormalities to correct and I would suggest that you call for veterinary assistance. In this posture the calf is coming backwards, but with its hind legs pointing forwards (figure 5.17), so that only the tail enters the birth canal. The absence of any object dilating the vagina means that the cow does not strain, nor is any part of the calf or placenta seen at the vulva. As a consequence, cows with breech births tend to be left too long and in the majority of cases the calf is already dead before assistance is thought necessary. Decomposition may have set in, and the calf may even have to be delivered piecemeal by embryotomy. Correction involves pulling the calf's foot backwards at the same time as its hock is pushed upwards and forwards, and there is thus a great danger of rupturing the wall of the uterus with the calf's leg.

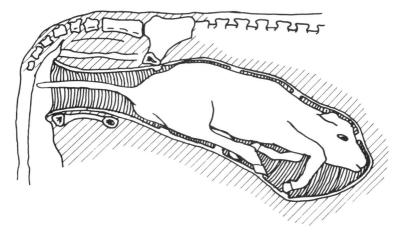

Figure 5.17 Breech presentation: the calf is coming backwards but with both legs forward so that only the tail is felt in the vagina. Because there is nothing dilating the vagina the cow often does not strain, and consequently many breech births may go unnoticed for several hours and produce a dead calf.

'Monster' calves

These are relative rarities and are mentioned only for the sake of completeness. Some have massively enlarged heads, some have two heads, and some may have the hind legs totally fused with the pelvis so that they cannot bend. This fusion of joints is known as *ankylosis*. Probably the most bizarre abnormality, although one of the most common, is the condition of *schistoma reflexus*, in which the four legs and the head of the calf are pointing one way and its open abdomen, exposing the intestine and rumen, is pointing the other. Colour plate 3 shows a schistosome calf which also had leg abnormalities. It was aborted with a normal twin at six months of gestation. Achondroplasic calves ('dwarfs' or 'bull-dogs') may also occur, and although the majority are born dead, the calf in plate 5.19 lived for several days. It also had a cleft palate.

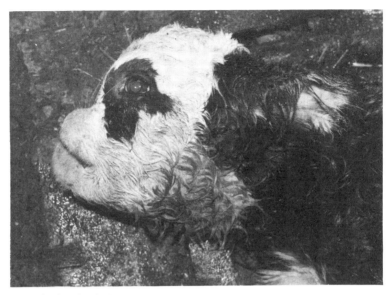

Plate 5.19   Anchondroplasia, or 'bull-dog' calf. This one was unusual in that it was born alive.

Many foetal monsters (including ankylosis and achondroplasia) are genetic defects, and as such they should be reported to the AI centre. Their incidence has decreased considerably during the past twelve years as a result of culling.

Any abnormality could lead to difficulties at calving, often requiring Caesarian section, and I would recommend that you request veterinary assistance as soon as the problem is suspected.

THE 'DOWNER' COW

Causes of the 'Downer' Cow

Cows which do not get up after calving, or, having been standing for a few hours, sit down and will not rise, are sometimes known as 'down' or 'downer' cows although some authorities reserve this term for cows which fail to respond to milk fever treatments. The expression simply describes the symptoms of the animal, that is, their inability or disinclination to rise, and the cows are said to be recumbent. There are a whole range of possible causes and considering that the life of both the cow and calf may be in danger, I would strongly recommend that veterinary advice is requested. Some of the possible causes of the downer cow are given below:

1. Blood loss
After the birth of the calf there will always be a certain amount of free blood released, due to the breaking of the umbilical cord. If large quantities of bright red blood continue to run from the vulva following a difficult birth, this is an *extreme emergency*, as it most probably indicates rupture of a major

blood vessel in the vaginal wall. First telephone for immediate veterinary help. Next insert your hand into the vagina as far as wrist depth, then hold your fingers against any tears which may be present. The blood vessels in a normal cow can be felt as pulsating tubes, approximately the size of a pencil, covered by a relatively thin membrane which is the wall of the vagina. You should get used to feeling these in a normal cow. A rupture is felt as a tear in the membrane and almost always occurs at the four or eight position of a clock face, that is, just below half-way down the vaginal wall on either side, and a broken blood-vessel will be felt as a pulsating jet of fluid on the fingertips. If possible, catch hold of this blood vessel to stop the bleeding until veterinary assistance arrives. If this cannot be done, push a small towel into the wound with as much pressure as possible, to try to stop the bleeding. I have known heifers bleed to death in less than an hour, so anything which can be done must be an advantage.

Post-calving haemorrhage is especially common in very fat heifers. Fat laid down in the space between the wall of the vagina and the cow's pelvis tends to reduce the overall size of the birth canal and it also reduces the strength of the attachments of the vaginal wall to the bony pelvis. If force now has to be applied to draw the calf, and especially if there is inadequate lubrication, the wall of the vagina tends to fold over on itself and tearing can occur. Small globular lumps of off-white fat which have been passed with the calf are indicative of vaginal damage and if these are seen in conjunction with profuse bleeding, you know that time may be limited. Even in the absence of bleeding, it may be worth seeking veterinary assistance to suture the vaginal wall to prevent severe and possibly fatal infections or peritonitis a few days after calving. Correct precalving feeding of heifers (see page 64) will help to prevent vaginal tearing.

2. Milk fever
This is the commonest cause of 'down' cows and is dealt with in Chapter Six.

3. Nerve, muscle or bone damage
The cow may have been injured during calving, especially if excessive force was applied to an oversized calf. Injuries can also be the result of the cow falling on slippery concrete, either accidentally or because she is unsteady on her feet from milk fever, or the nerve damage may be simply the result of the cow having had milk fever and having been left in an incorrect posture on a hard surface for too long. Whatever the cause of its recumbency, the cow should always be positioned so that she is sitting correctly, that is with one hind leg flexed in front of its udder and sitting on the other leg with it also in a flexed position. This is shown in plate 5.20. It should not be possible to see the lower leg in front of the udder. If you can see the lower leg up to its hock or even its fetlock (plate 5.21) then the leg is almost fully extended and research has shown that a cow left in this position on a hard surface for as little as six hours, may suffer irreversible nerve damage. In fact, the heifer shown in the plates had been trying to deliver an oversized calf, and she was found with her calf half out and locked at its hips. It was necessary to carry out an

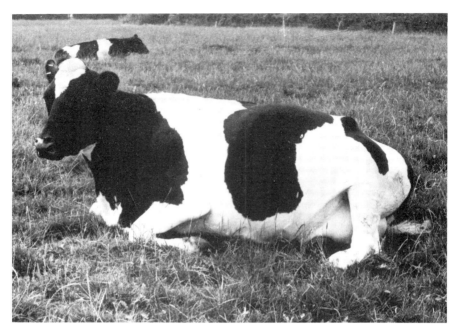

Plate 5.20   Normal sitting position for a cow. The right hind (lower) foot cannot be seen under the udder.

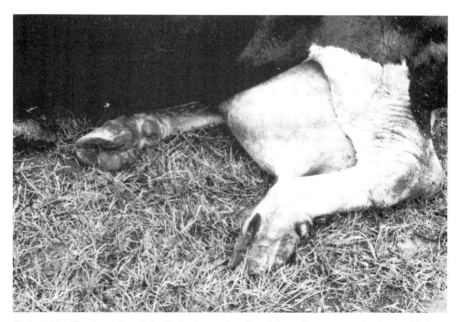

Plate 5.21   The lower leg of the heifer is paralysed, and it can be seen running forward in front of her udder.

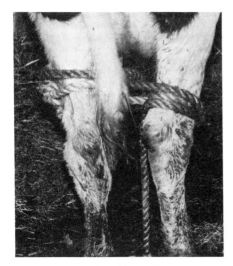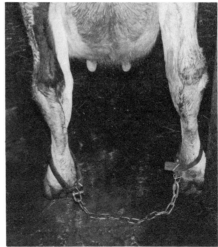

Plate 5.22(a)   Rope tied at hocks to prevent a cow 'splay-legging' following obturator nerve paralysis. Chains may also be used (plate 5.22(b)).

embryotomy, that is to cut the calf in half across its abdomen, repel its remaining hind-quarters then feed a wire between its hind legs to cut the pelvis in half and deliver the legs separately. It was several days before the heifer stood up but she did eventually recover.

The classic problem following a tight calving is that of obturator paralysis. The obturator nerve passes through the pelvis on its way down to the muscles on the inside of the cow's leg and can easily be damaged by pressure. The nerve supplies the muscles responsible for pulling the hind legs together, so that when it is damaged the cow literally 'does the splits'. She may attempt to stand, but one or both legs start to slide outwards. If obturator paralysis is suspected, the cow should immediately be moved off concrete and either onto soft pasture or into a straw yard containing a good depth of rotted straw bedding, where she can get a grip with her feet. A rope or belt can be tied just above the hocks, as shown in plate 5.22a, to prevent her legs splaying out, or a chain can be used (plate 5.22b). If left unattended, and she 'does the splits' on slippery concrete, this could result in either severe muscle tearing or in a fracture of the top of the femur, or a dislocation of the hip, or a fracture of the pelvis (see page 243). All four conditions are likely to be irreversible and would probably mean that the cow would have to be sent off as a casualty.

The other very common injury at calving is damage to the peroneal nerve, which runs from the spinal cord through the pelvis and then down over the outside of the hock towards the foot. Loss of function of the nerve results in the cow being unable to straighten the fetlock and, when she tries to walk, she knuckles forward, as shown in plate 5.23. In more severe cases the hock is also dropped, so that the cow walks with the stifle extended and the hock is almost on the ground (the normal position of these joints is given in figure 9.1). It is surprising how well cows manage to compensate for these injuries

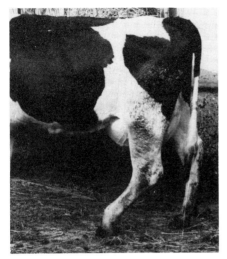

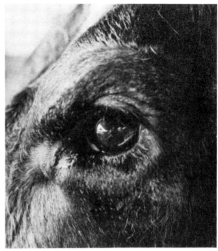

Plate 5.23   Cow with peroneal nerve
paralysis producing knuckling of the fetlock.
These cases usually recover on their own
but it may take several months.

Plate 5.24   Cow with sunken eye and a
pathetic depressed stare, typical of acute
E. coll mastitis.

and provided they get up and start walking the majority of them slowly
recover, although recovery may take anything from a few days to two or three
months. It is doubtful if anti-inflammatory drugs (e.g. cortisone or phenylbutazone) produce any significant benefit other than during the first few days
after the injury, when they may prevent the condition from deteriorating.

4. Acute mastitis

A high proportion of acute cases of mastitis occur around calving or soon
after and should always be suspected as a cause of the downer cow. In all the
cases mentioned so far, the cows generally looks quite bright and alert (except
of course in the terminal stages of blood loss). A cow with mastitis has a very
dull appearance, however, often with its eyes sinking, and it may have
developed a profuse scour. In this respect it is very different from a milk fever
cow which is always constipated. The pathetic depressed gaze of the cow in
plate 5.24 is typical of this. Its temperature is usually raised, but not always. It
may even be below normal. The udder of a downer cow should *always be
checked* before arriving at any final conclusions, although when colostrum is
present it may be very difficult to detect the early changes associated with, for
example, *E. coli* mastitis.

5. Liver failure

This generally occurs as a consequence of some other condition; for example,
an unresponsive case of milk fever, which has led to recumbency and
depression of appetite for a few days. It is especially common in overfat,
high-producing animals and will be dealt with in more detail in Chapter Six.

Care of the Down Cow

The two most critical aspects of care have already been mentioned. They are moving the cow to a field or some other suitable non-slip surface, and secondly making sure that her legs are in the correct sitting position (plates 5.20 and 5.21). It is not difficult to move a recumbent cow on a gate, a wooden pallet or a door. If she is sitting with her legs pointing to the left (plate 5.25), place the gate (in this case covered with two old doors) on the ground on her left and lift her left front and back legs onto it, getting the gate as far under her body as possible. Next push her over until she is sitting facing the right. She will now be well onto the gate (plate 5.26). Finally, lie her flat

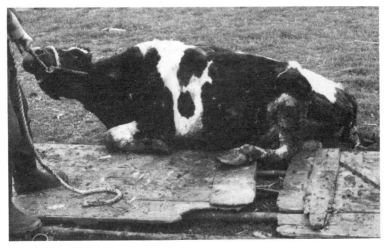

Plate 5.25   Moving a cow on a gate (1). Lift the left front and back legs onto the gate.

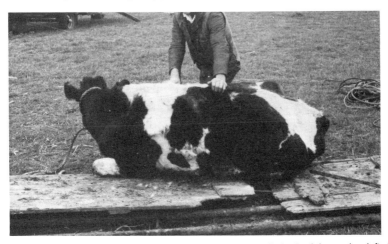

Plate 5.26   Moving a cow on a gate (2). Push the cow over until she is sitting on her left side on the gate.

onto her side, so that her legs are partly supported by the gate (plate 5.27). Her head can be tied to the gate as shown in plate 5.27, although if there was no protective door present, it would be better to pull her head back over her body. Attach the gate to a tractor by a short length of chain or a strong rope, ideally via the linkage arms, so that when it is being dragged the front end of the gate and the cow are both lifted off the ground. Ideally an assistant needs to lift the left hind leg (the lower leg) to keep the udder off the ground (plate 5.28).

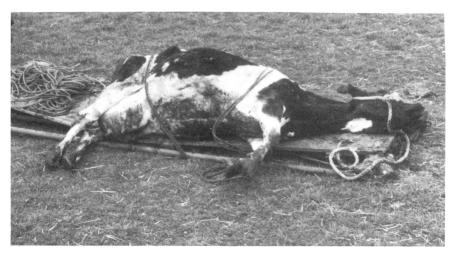

Plate 5.27 Moving a cow on a gate (3). Lie the cow flat and secure her head before transporting her. It is not normal practice to tie the whole body in the manner shown in the photograph.

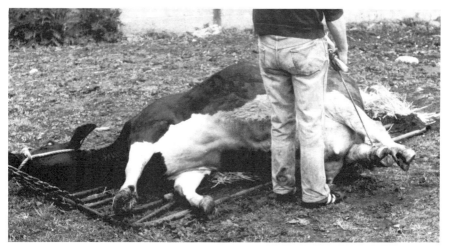

Plate 5.28 The front end of the gate should be lifted by the tractor to reduce the risk of damage to her head, and an assistant lifting the lower hind leg helps protect the udder.

Once onto the new firm surface and away from slippery concrete, it is easy to roll the cow off the gate, and with added confidence many cows will simply stand up and walk away. Those which do not, need to be positioned correctly, as described on page 119, and given food and water. If she is outside in the winter, a large carpet draped over her provides excellent protection and, if it is large enough, it will not fall off when she moves. Unless they are moving themselves, recumbent cows need to be rolled from side to side at least four times each day, and they must be given continual access to food and water. You will want your vet to check her periodically for illness, fractures and other irreversible injuries, and then much of her chances of recovery must depend on how long you are prepared to persist with nursing.

With some cows lifting aids are very valuable. The Bagshawe hoist (plate 5.29) fits over the wings of the cow's pelvis (the 'pin-bones': figure 9.1). The screw must be turned up very tight, such that the vertical part of the hoist is pressing against the edges of the bones of the lumbar spine, the point shown by the operator's fingers in plate 5.29. If the cow moved and fell from the hoist during lifting, considerable damage could occur, e.g. fracture of the pelvis. Once onto their front legs, some cows will walk forwards, and the advantage of the hoist is that the tractor can be driven along behind her, supporting her walking. For other cows the hoist appears totally ineffective, however, because the cow simply hangs, without making any effort to stand.

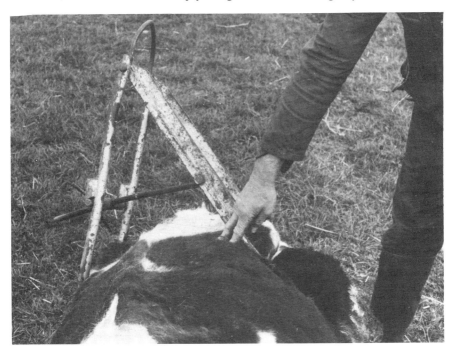

Plate 5.29   A Bagshawe hoist. The screw must be very tight, so that the vertical part of the hoist is pressing against the cow's spine. The cow is lifted via the loop on the top of the hoist.

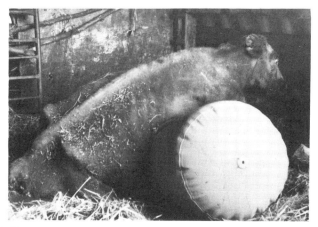

Plate 5.30 A lifting bag. The bag was fed under the cow's chest and then inflated to this position. By pushing her forwards from behind she took her weight on her front legs while the bag was supporting her under her udder.

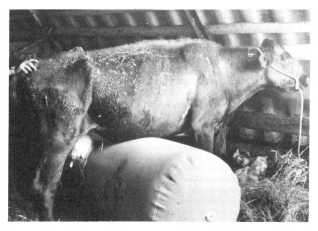

Plate 5.31 She was then taking all of her own weight and the bag could be slowly deflated.

An alternative device is a lifting bag, which is positioned under the cow's chest and then inflated (plate 5.30) using a small pump operated from a 12 volt battery. If the cow is then gently pushed forward so that the bag rolls back towards her udder, the forward lunging movement she feels is often sufficient to get her to stand on her front legs, with the bag supporting her hindquarters as shown in plate 5.31. When she takes her own weight the air can be slowly released and the bag removed. The procedure was very effective on Polly, the 27-year-old Shorthorn shown in the plates, but some cows try to rush forward as soon as they are lifted and trip over the bag before it can be removed. Much larger bags are available, but I find that because they support the whole cow, like an enormous cushion, they make no effort to stand on their own.

Dealing with any recumbent cow can be a most frustrating and time-consuming experience, and when physical injuries and metabolic problems have been eliminated, it cannot be overstressed that time and careful nursing are the two most important factors determining recovery. Unfortunately many farms simply do not have the facilities to lift a cow and turn her several times each day, but for anyone prepared to spend the time, their efforts can be amply rewarded. I have known at least two cows get up and lead a useful productive life after being 'down' for three weeks or more.

Other Post-Calving Complications

Blood loss and nerve damage are normally apparent immediately after calving, although occasionally cows suffer a severe haemorrhage two to three days later. Acute mastitis can also occur at any time during the first few weeks, and may be the cause of severe illness without necessarily leading to recumbency. The other important post-calving conditions are retained placenta, metritis, vaginal infections, prolapsed uterus, and vaginal prolapse. Failure of milk let-down, blocked teats and blind quarters would also be evident during this period and will therefore be mentioned at the end.

Retained Placenta

Earlier in the chapter we said that expulsion of the placenta (the afterbirth or cleansing) was the third stage of labour and should occur within approximately six hours of the birth of the calf. A proportion of cows will pass the placenta within twenty-four hours, but after this, uterine contractions become very weak or non-existent, and then several days will have to elapse before the attachments to the cotyledons (figure 5.3) eventually putrefy and decompose, and the placenta is dropped. Surveys of incidence have given very varying results, but if the condition exists in your herd at greater than the 10 per cent level then this undoubtedly represents a problem. The condition is easily recognised by the fact that part of the placenta is seen hanging from the vulva, although in a proportion of cases all of the placenta remains inside the uterus and the stockman may be unaware of its existence. The effects of a retained placenta on the overall health and well-being of the cow seem to vary enormously. Some cows are sick within two or three days, while at the other extreme a cow may pass her whole placenta ten or fourteen days later with no one knowing that retention had occurred and without any signs of ill-health. This is relatively uncommon however.

Treatment
This is necessary for four main reasons. First some cows may develop a bacterial infection in the uterus which can lead to illness, reduced yield and even death. Second, under the Dairy Regulations milk from affected cows is not to be sold for human consumption. Third there could be a reduced conception rate in cows which have not been adequately treated. (Retention

of the placenta in itself probably does not affect subsequent fertility, whereas retention plus infection almost certainly does.) Finally, it is unpleasant milking a cow which has a putrefying placenta hanging around its udder.

Veterinary surgeons vary in their approach to treatment, but as a general rule cows are left for three or four days without treatment, provided that they are not sick. Illness occurs either because of bacterial infection, or simply because the placenta is degenerating naturally but the cow is absorbing toxic waste products. Even on the third or fourth day the attachment of the placenta at the cotyledons is sometimes so strong that separation is not possible and your vet will have to try again two to four days later, depending on how sick the cow is. It is *essential* not to tear the placenta and it is far better to get your veterinary surgeon to have a second attempt rather than run the risk of leaving pieces in the uterus. Pessaries will be inserted through the cervix and into the uterus. These usually contain an antibiotic to kill the infection and possibly also oestrogens to help the natural uterine defence mechanisms and to stimulate its contraction. Some authorities question the wisdom of using pessaries in an otherwise healthy cow. They would say that bacterial action should be allowed to continue as it is a normal feature of placental degeneration and separation, and anyway there is a risk that the increased blood flow caused by oestrogen in the pessaries may increase the absorption of toxins. Whilst this may be sound theory, the change from a healthy to sick cow may be so sudden that in practice the use of pessaries would seem to be a commonsense safeguard.

Injections of oxytocin can be used, but they are only likely to have any effect in the first twenty-four hours after calving. Injections of oestrogens have also been suggested, but these may possibly lead to an increased incidence of cystic ovaries. If there is a large volume of stinking fluid present and the cow is very sick, your veterinary surgeon may attempt to wash out and drain the uterus using a length of tubing and a bucket of warm saline.

Causes and control

If the main causes of a high incidence of retained placenta can be identified then the control and preventive measures would be obvious. Anything which interferes with the normal third stage of labour is likely to lead to placental retention. Such factors include:

1. Abortions and premature calvings (including those induced by prosta-glandin, cortisone and other drugs). Although birth may occur normally, the processes of placental separation may not. Injection of oestrogen on the day of calving is said to aid placental expulsion in artificially induced cows.
2. Twins. Retention probably occurs because the uterus is weak after pushing out two calves, and also because a high proportion of twins are born early.
3. Milk fever is a condition of lack of muscle power and in this instance the uterus simply lacks the necessary 'push' to expel the placenta.
4. Difficult calvings. Again the uterus may be 'tired' after the calf has eventually been delivered.

5. Dirty calving boxes or unnecessary manual interference at calving. It has been shown that inflammation and infection of the placenta at the very early stages does in fact, *reduce* the chances of a normal placental separation and expulsion. On some farms there is definitely a tendency to provide assistance with calvings before it is really necessary. As well as the risk of infection and vaginal tearing, delivering a calf before the birth canal is fully opened may lead to weakness of the uterus and hence failure to expel the placenta.
6. Vitamin E and/or selenium deficiency leading to reduced muscle power in the uterus has been associated with an increased incidence of placental retention.
7. Any condition which leads to debility in the cow, for example liver fluke, copper deficiency or simple under-nutrition.

If you are faced with a herd with a high incidence of retention—and on occasions this may be up to 50 per cent of calvings—the first step towards control is a careful recording of all the calvings, with the following questions in mind. Were they on time; were there twins; was assistance or manual examination necessary; where did the cow calve; did she have milk fever; how old was she?

It is very easy to read through such a list and assume that the overall answer is known. Careful recording often leads to a different conclusion, however, and possibly more than one factor is involved. Your veterinary surgeon will probably want to take blood samples from dry cows and from cows immediately after calving, to make sure that selenium deficiency or a subclinical level of milk fever is not involved.

Metritis

Metritis simply means inflammation of the uterus. The inflammation is most commonly associated with a bacterial infection, and we can therefore say that the majority of cows with retained placenta also have a degree of metritis. Metritis often occurs in the absence of retained placenta, however. It may be an *acute* condition, that is, severe and sudden in onset and is making the cow ill. A foul-smelling brown watery discharge would be passing from the uterus through the vulva, the cow would be running a high temperature and she would probably be off her food. Treatment consists of administering pessaries into the uterus and giving antibiotic by injection, although if the cow is very sick your vet may give intravenous fluids and other anti-shock therapy.

A proportion of cases are so badly affected that they die. These are relatively rare however, and as the cow recovers the uterine discharge slowly becomes thicker, taking on a gelatinous consistency, and its colour becomes progressively lighter until you are left with white globules of pus, possibly mixed in with clear mucus. This is now at the *chronic*, or long-standing and less severe stage, and the condition is referred to as *endometritis* (that is, affecting the inner wall—'endo'—of the uterus), often known as 'the whites'. The causes of endometritis are dealt with in detail on page 231. Acute metritis can be caused by unnecessary or unhygienic assistance at calving; by dirty calving boxes; by difficult or rough calvings leading to uterine tearing, or following a retained placenta which has been improperly removed so that small pieces of tissue have been left attached to the uterine cotyledons.

Vaginal Infections

These are the result of a tear in the vaginal wall at calving which was not adequately dealt with, either by suturing and/or by antibiotic treatment. The first signs are normally seen five to seven days after calving, and it is often heifers which are affected. They become very dull, they may have a swollen

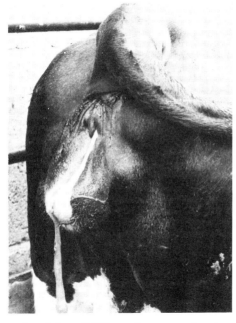

Plate 5.32   An infected vaginal tear from calving leading to an enlarged vulva.

vulva (plate 5.32) or they may simply stand with their tail raised. There may or may not be a foul-smelling uterine discharge, but they will always have a very high temperature. At this stage it is too late to suture the vaginal wall, but immediate and high-level antibiotic treatment is necessary to prevent peritonitis.

Prolapsed Uterus

Uterine prolapse occurs immediately after calving, sometimes as the calf is expelled, but almost always within twelve hours of parturition. It is thought to be associated with slackness of the ligaments holding the reproductive tract in position, and as such it is much more common in older cows. Figure 5.18 shows that the uterus turns itself inside out and passes through the cervix and

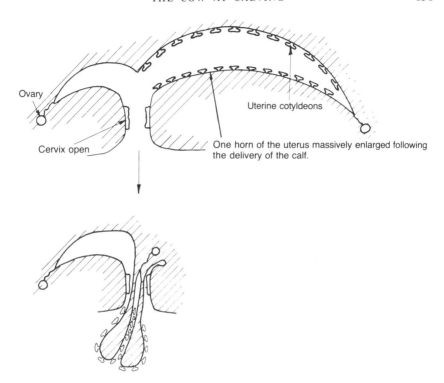

Ovary

Cervix open

Uterine cotyledons

One horn of the uterus massively enlarged following
the delivery of the calf.

Figure 5.18   Prolapse of the uterus. The cervix and vagina remain in their correct positions.

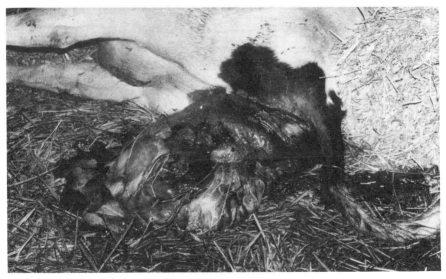

Plate 5.33   A prolapsed uterus. It is a very large organ, and the structure of the placenta and
cotyledons can be clearly seen.

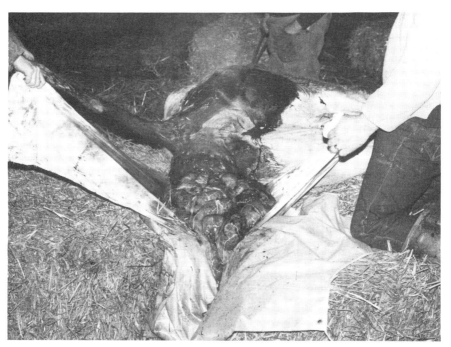

Plate 5.34 Replacing a prolapsed uterus. Two assistants lift the prolapsed uterus with a sheet ready for it to be pushed back through the vulva and vagina. They are kneeling on the platform of bales which have been used to raise the cow's hind quarters.

vagina. If the cow is standing, the prolapsed uterus will be hanging down as far as her hocks or teats, in other words it is a very large structure. The other characteristic feature is that the uterine cotyledons are clearly visible, and the placenta may still be attached. This is shown in plate 5.33, which should be compared with plate 5.35 showing the much less serious condition of vaginal prolapse.

The mass of exposed internal organ leads to a large heat loss for the cow, and a state of shock soon sets in. It is therefore a serious condition, and you should call for immediate veterinary attention to have it replaced. In the meantime it is important to keep the cow quiet and if possible cover the prolapse with a clean sheet. If she damages her prolapsed uterus by standing on it or catching it on a fence or similar object, the condition becomes far more serious. I find that the best way of dealing with a prolapse is to give an epidural anaesthetic and then either suspend the cow by her hocks from a tractor foreloader or, if this is not possible, roll her hind quarters onto some bales to give extra height. In addition to the epidural, a rope tied tightly around her abdomen, immediately in front of her udder, also helps to stop her straining, and this makes replacement easier. It is not an easy task however. Two assistants support the uterus in a sheet, lifting it up to the vulva (plate 5.34) and my task is to try to force the uterus back through the vagina and cervix. Often two people are needed to push because the uterus is so large that as you repel one part of it, another part slides back out. When back in place, oxytocin and calcium are given to contract the uterus, and antibiotic injections and pessaries to prevent infection. There is no reason why the cow should not be served again. Most cows conceive normally and the chances of a prolapse at the next calving are not significantly increased.

Vaginal Prolapse

This is a much less serious condition than a uterine prolapse, and although it is often seen during the few days after calving, it can occur at any stage of pregnancy. As figure 5.19 indicates, only the vagina and cervix are everted, the uterus remains in its normal position. You will need veterinary assistance to replace the prolapse under epidural anaesthesia and suture it into position, but make sure your vet knows that it is a vaginal and not a uterine prolapse that he is being called to. Only the latter needs to be dealt with as a matter of urgency. A vaginal prolapse is shown in plate 5.35 and this should be carefully compared with the uterine prolapse shown in plate 5.33.

Occasionally a vaginal prolapse may be accompanied by a rectal prolapse,

Plate 5.35   A vaginal prolapse. The smooth tissue is the wall of the vagina, the convoluted tissue the first part of the cervix.

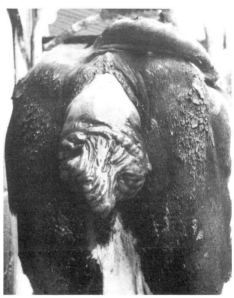

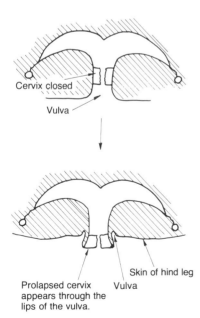

Figure 5.19   Prolapse of the vagina and cervix.

although a rectal prolapse can also occur as a separate condition. Replacement and surgical fixation is needed in both cases.

Milk Let-Down Failure

Milk let-down, that is the expulsion of milk from the glands where it is produced (see figure 7.1), down into the teat, is stimulated by the hormone oxytocin. In some cows the normal activities of entering the parlour, feeding and udder preparation do not seem sufficient to stimulate oxytocin release, and virtually no milk is given. This can be particularly true with heifers which are apprehensive or nervous, because the hormone adrenalin acts as an antagonist to oxytocin. The problem can be approached in two ways. First careful and gentle handling may overcome the heifer's fears and, second, injections of oxytocin can be given two to three minutes before the milking machine is applied. In practice you would probably use both methods. When you have established the dose of oxytocin required to produce let-down, try slowly decreasing it over a few days until the heifer's own behavioural reactions take over. This subject is discussed in more detail on page 161.

Blind Quarters

This is a condition seen primarily in heifers, and would not be noticed until the first milking. The udder appears normal, but no milk can be drawn from the teat. I have experienced three separate categories of this condition. The first, and by far the most common, is the presence of a membrane across the top of the teat, producing a permanent barrier between the teat cistern and the gland cistern (see figure 7.1, page 160). The teat feels normal but it never fills with milk during let-down. If the teat is anaesthetised and a long cannula (often called a teat siphon) is inserted through the teat sphincter it can often be forced through the membrane to allow milk to flow. Making a series of holes in this way can occasionally resolve the blockage, but many eventually heal over again. The second cause of a blind quarter is a blockage at the teat sphincter. The teat feels full of milk, but it cannot be drawn out. This is the easiest condition to deal with. With the teat anaesthetised, a small knife (called McClean's Knife) with a disc blade just below the guide tip is forced up through the sphincter as shown in plate 5.36. It is then rotated through 180° and pulled back out again. This produces two transverse cuts, and once milk starts to flow, it usually continues very successfully, although it may be best to infuse intramammary antibiotic into the teat end after each milking for the first few days as a mastitis preventive. The same procedure can also be used to dilate the teats of cows or heifers which are very slow milkers, provided the sphincter is normal. If the slow milking arises from a crushed teat or some other abnormality however, I have not found the knife particularly successful.

The third cause of a blind quarter is summer mastitis, and this is described in detail on page 189. The heifer will already have had the infection, quite possibly unnoticed, and may well have recovered without treatment, but the

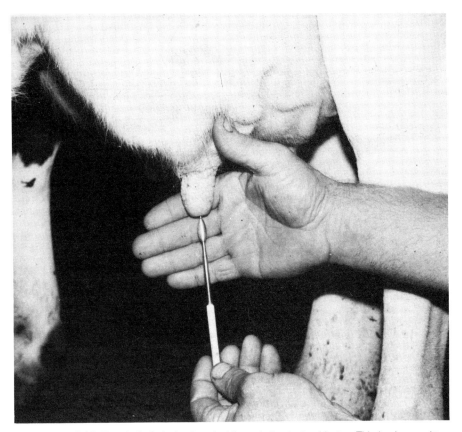

Plate 5.36   A McClean's knife being inserted through the teat sphincter. This is also used to dilate the teat of a very slow milker.

teat is left permanently damaged. It feels as if there is a thick fibrous core running up through the teat cistern. There is no treatment.

Blood in Milk

It is not uncommon for cows to calve down with blood in their milk, and I have always felt that it is more common in animals which have had very tight udders or sometimes following a difficult calving when the udder may have been bruised by the cow's own leg movements. Sometimes the blood has formed clots and then the diagnosis is easy. At other times it is mixed with colostrum, and it may be very difficult to decide if there is an acute mastitis present. Looking for a raised temperature, heat and pain from the quarter and general signs of health should distinguish between the two conditions, but if you are in any doubt I would strongly recommend that you infuse a tube of antibiotic. I know of no drugs which are regularly effective against blood in milk, and the only action is not to milk the quarter or only lightly relieve it so that the back pressure from the milk stops the blood flow.

Pea in Teat

Sometimes milk flow from the teat is obstructed by a small lump which floats around in the teat cistern but acts like a valve as soon as milk is drawn from the sphincter. This is called a *pea*, and consists of an accumulation of milk salts, fat and udder cells, in some respects like a kidney stone. I find the best way of removing these is to dilate the teat sphincter using a McClean's Knife and squeeze the pea out with a flush of milk, although if it is a large pea it may first be necessary to crush it into smaller pieces within the teat cistern. Sometimes the pea is attached to a membrane growing out from the wall of the teat cistern, or it is the membrane itself which is causing the blockage. In such cases, although milk flows easily through a cannula, as soon as the teat is drawn by hand the membrane obstructs the streak canal. I have never found any successful way of treating such cases.

Chapter 6

METABOLIC DISORDERS

A METABOLIC DISEASE, or metabolic disorder, is the name given to a group of illnesses in dairy cows which are caused by an over-exertion of their normal metabolism. These diseases are generally seen during early lactation, when milk yields are at a peak, and they are due to an imbalance between the *input* of the cow's food compared with her *output* in terms of maintenance, pregnancy and lactation. The four main metabolic disorders are:

Milk fever
Hypomagnesaemia
Acetonaemia
Fatty liver syndrome

For a better understanding of the mechanisms of a production disease, take the analogy of a cold-water header tank in the roof of a domestic house, as shown in figure 6.1. Water enters the tank via the input pipe and when it reaches a certain level its flow is shut off by a ball-valve. There will be various uses for the water; for example, one feed to the kitchen another to the bathroom and a third to the heating plant.

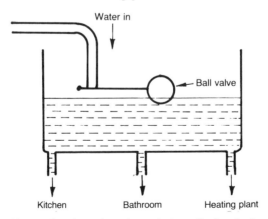

Figure 6.1   The cold-water header tank analogy—factors affecting the level of water in the tank.

When the ball-valve is open, water will enter the tank at a constant rate and the level of water in the tank will be determined by the rates of outflow; that is, to the kitchen, bathroom and heater. If the system was badly designed, it is possible that output will exceed input, in which case the tank runs dry and various problems occur (e.g. air-blocks, or the heating plant boils).

A dairy cow may be looked at in a similar way. Although she may have several feeds during the day, the rate of flow of nutrients from the rumen into her bloodstream (the *input*) is virtually constant. These nutrients, or *metabolites* as they are correctly called, are used for a variety of purposes (the *output*). Their main functions are for maintenance (for movement, warmth and tissue respiration), pregnancy (and the adult cow should spend about 75 per cent of her life pregnant) and, most important of all, milk production. For a dairy cow therefore the water tank principle can be rewritten as in figure 6.2.

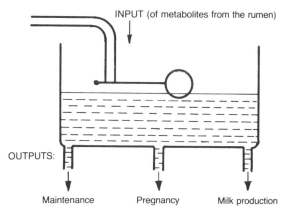

Figure 6.2   The water tank analogy used to explain the concept of production disease and metabolic profiles.

For a constant *input* of metabolites from the rumen, the level of 'water' in the tank (or in this analogy, the level of the metabolites circulating in the bloodstream) is governed by the overall rate of *output*. If output increases without any corresponding rise in input, the level of metabolites will fall until the tank is empty and this is when *metabolic disorders* occur.

Metabolic Profile Tests

We can take blood samples to measure the level of metabolites in the circulation and this is known as a *metabolic profile test*. The metabolic profile is an extremely useful technique for monitoring the nutritional and health status of dairy cows in that it tries to identify problems before they are seen as overt disease. The test measures the 'balance' between input, in terms of food, and output, based on the cow's requirements of nutrients for maintenance, pregnancy and lactation. Metabolic profiles are only an *aid* in the investigation of production diseases however and great care is needed both with the selection of cows to be blood-sampled and in the interpretation of results. Even so, they can give very useful information on herd problems, such as:

- unsatisfactory milk production or milk quality
- high incidence of metabolic diseases
- assessment of dietary energy and protein status
- investigation of suboptimal fertility
- mineral and trace element deficiencies.

One of the commonest mistakes made with metabolic profiles is that the wrong animals are sampled. For example take a herd where production is disappointing, the problem being that some cows fail to reach peak yield while others drop off rapidly from an early peak. Cows which have already fallen in yield have of course decreased their production to match the food intake being received, that is their output has dropped to balance input. Taking the analogy in figure 6.2, it is obvious that in this instance blood levels will return to normal. If you are trying to assess the nutritional status of your herd therefore, it is essential that at least moderate producing cows are chosen, otherwise the cause of the problem may be missed. Normally cows in the early lactation stage are sampled, for example at around four to eight weeks after calving. This is certainly the best group to examine when energy and protein balance are being checked, and there is also the advantage that cows at this stage of lactation are approaching the service period. However, there are occasions when you may wish to sample other groups of cows. When faced with a high incidence of milk fever or retained placenta, it would be best to look at the energy and mineral status of the dry cows and perhaps also a few animals immediately after calving, and analysis for magnesium and phosphorus might be particularly useful. Copper deficiency is best detected in pregnant heifers, since the requirements of copper for growth and pregnancy are greater than for milk production. Similarly, if you are investigating a possible fatty liver syndrome in your dairy herd, bloods are best taken from cows at seven to fourteen days after calving and analysed for glucose and GOT (an indicator of liver damage).

A fuller explanation of the metabolic profile test is outside the scope of this book and those interested should discuss it in detail with their veterinary surgeon. The metabolic diseases are described individually in the following section, when the concept of the 'nutritional imbalance' should become more apparent.

Milk Fever

The disease is best described by its technical name of *Parturient Hypocalcaemia*, which means a lowered blood calcium level around the time of calving. As figure 6.3 shows, the cow has a massive store of calcium in her skeleton (6,000 g) and plenty in the food in her intestine (100 g). She has only a small quantity (8 g) circulating in her blood however and this reservoir of

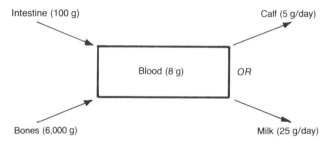

Figure 6.3   Calcium balance within the cow in pregnancy and lactation.

readily-available calcium is not sufficient to meet the tremendous change from the requirements of the calf in late pregnancy (5 g/day) to the requirements of milk production in early lactation (25 g/day).

Calcium flows from the blood into the milk and unless blood levels can be replenished from stores in the intestine and bones, blood calcium falls, leading to milk fever. The deficiency is only of a temporary nature, however, because the cow has ample reserves of calcium in her skeleton. She simply cannot get access to them quickly enough. In this respect milk fever is rather different from the other metabolic diseases. A few days after calving she soon learns to increase the rate of mobilisation of calcium from her reserves, aided by vitamin D and parathyroid hormone, and she is then able to cope with the demands of lactation. Older cows are much more susceptible to milk fever because the calcium reserves in their skeletons are less available. The condition is rarely seen in heifers, although it does sometimes occur six or eight weeks after calving when it may be associated with either a digestive upset or the cow coming on heat (i.e. into oestrus—see page 203). Channel Island breeds, particularly Jerseys, are more susceptible than any others.

Clinical signs

Calcium is used in the body to transmit electrical impulses from the nerves to the muscles, so the clinical signs of milk fever are essentially those of lack of muscle function. Classically, a cow which has recently calved will be found sitting and unable to rise, or possibly she is only able to half lift herself on her hind legs and then falls back to the ground again. Chapter Five (page 118) gave a list of the other possible causes of an inability to stand after calving and it should be read in conjunction with this section. The milk fever cow is quiet and sits with a characteristic 'S' shape in her neck (plate 6.1), rather than holding her head to one side in a slow bend, which is the position you would see in a normal cow (e.g. plate 5.20). Her coat feels cold, she is likely to be cudding either irregularly or not at all, and this makes her slightly blown. Her temperature will be below normal. The rectum will be full of faeces, making the anus bulge backwards. This occurs because there is insufficient muscle power to enable the cow to defecate, and is a feature clearly seen in plate 6.1. As blood calcium falls, intestinal movement also decreases and as a result,

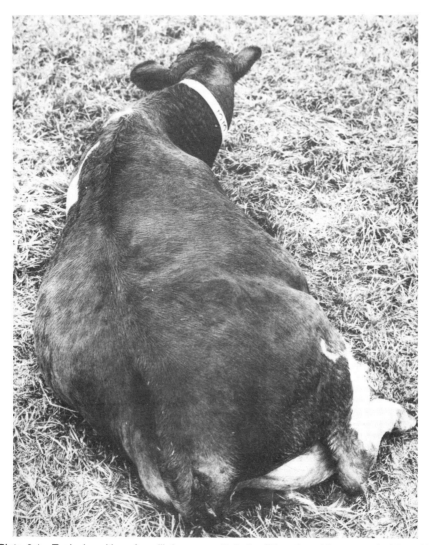

Plate 6.1 Typical position of a milk fever cow. Note the 'S' neck and the rectum bulging with faeces under her tail.

even less calcium is absorbed from the gut into the blood. Some cows develop a fine muscle tremor, seen as a 'shivering' especially over the neck and chest area. If left untreated, the muscle paralysis worsens and she eventually rolls over onto her side and lacks the power to sit up again. When she is on her side the normal rumen gases cannot escape, so she becomes bloated and death is caused by either excessive pressure on the heart or possibly by inhaling rumen contents which have been forced up into the mouth by the pressure of the gas.

Mechanisms controlling blood calcium levels

We have seen that the clinical signs of milk fever are caused by a sharp fall in blood calcium concentration. Milk fever only occurs in a relatively small proportion of cows however, so what are the mechanisms by which normal unaffected cows maintain their blood calcium levels at calving? Figure 6.3 shows that the cow can draw calcium from her skeleton and from the food in her intestine. Falling blood calcium levels trigger off a signal which leads to the release of parathyroid hormone. (The four parathyroid glands are found two on each side of the thyroid gland in the neck.) Parathyroid hormone has a small ability to stimulate calcium and phosphorus release from bone, but its main action is in the kidney where it converts a vitamin D precursor into the very active form of 1,25 dihydroxyvitamin D. It is this latter hormone which is mainly responsible for increasing the absorption of calcium from the gut and bone, and although all cows show increases in circulating levels of both parathyroid hormone and 1,25 dihydroxyvitamin D at calving, clearly some cows are unable to mount a response which is sufficient to prevent milk fever. The action of both hormones requires the presence of magnesium, and this is possibly why low magnesium intakes during the dry period lead to an increase in milk fever incidence.

Oestrogens inhibit calcium mobilisation mechanisms, and since oestrogen levels rise at calving, this would be yet another reason why milk fever occurs. It also explains why occasional cows develop milk fever six to eight weeks after calving when they come into oestrus.

Treatment

Calcium is given by injection, usually in the form of calcium borogluconate. Various regimes are used and the important feature is to make sure that the cow receives around 12 g of calcium in one dose. This may be given as 400 ml of a 40 per cent solution by *slow* intravenous injection—if given rapidly it can cause a fatal heart failure. The technique is described on page 351. Sometimes blood levels of phosphorus and/or magnesium are also low and if your vet thinks that this is a possibility, then proprietary preparations containing calcium mixed with phosphorus and magnesium should be used, for example, by giving two 400 ml injections of 20 per cent calcium borogluconate mixed with magnesium and phosphorus. There is less risk of heart failure using the 20 per cent calcium solutions intravenously and they can also be used subcutaneously. If 40 per cent solutions are given subcutaneously there is a risk of producing a sterile abscess under the skin, and this route of administration should therefore be reserved for 20% solutions only.

As soon as it is practically possible, the cow should be manoeuvred into a sitting position. If she was 'flat out' it would be better to try to get her upright while someone else goes to call for veterinary assistance and/or collect the calcium. Although it is very difficult when a cow is blown, *if* she can be sat upright, a cow with even severe milk fever will live for several hours. Bales of straw can be used as supports and it may be necessary to pull her head around with a halter. After the calcium has taken effect, the cow should sit upright reasonably well, although you must make sure that the hind legs are correctly positioned, as described on page 119. This is extremely important in order to prevent permanent nerve damage. The first signs that the calcium is working are often a belch, liberating ruminal gas, and defecation, as muscle power returns to the rumen and rectum respectively. It is said that if faeces flow from the blunt end of the cow soon after calcium has been administered to the pointed end, then the diagnosis of milk fever has been confirmed! Encourage the cow to start eating as soon as possible after treatment. This will supply additional dietary calcium and also promote gut activity to facilitate absorption of that calcium. It may even be worth giving a calcium/vitamin D drench (discussed under prevention) to prevent a relapse.

Usually the cow is standing again within a few hours of being given the calcium and the only preventive measure needed then is to make sure that the calf does not suckle too much and that the cow is not 'milked out' for one or two days, as this would stimulate increased milk flow and may precipitate another attack of milk fever. In a proportion of cases treatment may improve the general appearance of the cow, but she is still not standing six hours later. This is an instance where your veterinary surgeon should definitely be called. A thorough examination will be given to check that none of the other factors mentioned in Chapter Five are involved, and blood samples may be taken to see if magnesium or phosphorus levels are seriously low and possibly also to check for liver function and muscle damage. It may be that the cow simply needs a second dose of calcium, and this is often the case, with full recovery occurring one to two hours later. If she remains recumbent however, she should be moved on to a non-slip surface and nursed as described on page 119. Do not give excessive amounts of calcium at any one time. This can produce a temporary *hypercalcaemia* (high blood calcium), thus stimulating production of the hormone *calcitonin*, which in turn may produce a *hypocalcaemia* (relapse of milk fever) when the overdose of calcium is excreted.

Prevention and control
Spring- or autumn-calving herds, grazing lush wet pasture, may suffer an almost 100 per cent incidence of milk fever. There are three probable reasons for this. Firstly, grass contains a high level of calcium. If the dry cow has been having a high dietary calcium intake, because she only needs a very small amount (5 g per day) for the calf, her calcium mobilisation mechanisms (involving vitamin D and parathyroid hormone) become 'lazy'. When there is then a sudden increase in the calcium demand for lactation, she is unable to cope with it. If, on the other hand, instead of grass, she was fed on a low calcium diet during the dry period, her mobilisation mechanisms would be 'fit and active', because they have had to work hard to get enough calcium even for pregnancy. In this state she is more able to cope with the sudden demands of calcium for milk production.

Secondly, spring or autumn grass may contain low levels of magnesium and it has been shown that a marginal hypomagnesaemia (that is, low blood magnesium levels) can precipitate milk fever. The pasture may also be low in phosphorus, so that although calcium deficiency is the prime problem, low-grade magnesium and phosphorus imbalances are acting as exacerbating factors. Thirdly, during calving there is a period of gut stasis; that is, normal gut movements cease, and this reduces further the cow's ability to absorb calcium. One of the stimuli for the resumption of normal intestinal activity after calving is the presence of bulky food in the gut and, as all dairy farmers know, lush wet autumn grass passes through the gut fairly rapidly! The incidence of milk fever can be reduced by feeding a quantity of hay or straw to increase the 'bulk' in the intestine, thus improving calcium absorption, both by decreasing the rate of passage of food through the intestine and by providing a better stimulus for the resumption of gut activity after calving.

Some of the more important ways of controlling milk fever are therefore as follows.

- Low calcium intakes during the dry period. Rations as low as 20 g per cow per day have been suggested, but this is virtually impossible, especially if grass is part of the diet. However, it is not uncommon to put late-pregnant cows onto a sparse pasture and feed a special 'down-calver' concentrate (very low in calcium) as a means of control.
- Avoid excessive feeding or 'steaming up' precalving, so that the risk of fatty liver (see page 152) is reduced and the very high early flush of milk production does not occur. Conventional dairy cakes are especially bad in this respect because they contain high levels of calcium. Rolled barley would be a better alternative.
- Ensure adequate dietary magnesium and phosphorus intakes.
- Supplement with hay or straw.
- Provide a highly palatable diet to maintain appetite prior to and immediately after parturition, and at this stage supplement with high calcium products.

Other control measures which can be used are:

1. Inject very high doses (10 million units) of vitamin D eight or ten days before calving, to assist the calcium mobilisation from bones and intestine. The difficulty lies with predicting when calving will occur. The vitamin D takes 2–3 days before it is converted into an active form, and a second dose should not be given because of the risk of calcium being laid down in the arteries and elsewhere causing 'hardening', a process known as *metastatic calcification*. There is a much more potent and safer analogue—1,25, dihydroxy D3—but so far, supplies of this are not commercially available.
2. Give vitamin D mixed with 100–150 g calcium chloride, either in the feed or as a drench, for four or five days before calving. Calcium is absorbed better from acid gut conditions and this can be produced by adding ammonium and magnesium salts to the ration. These measures are not routinely practised however, because of the difficulty of treating cows very close to calving as a separate group.
3. If faced with an outbreak, or if certain cows are calving which are known to have had milk fever in previous lactations, it is worthwhile giving 400 ml of a 20 per cent calcium solution (possibly with a low level of magnesium and phosphorus) subcutaneously, immediately after calving. This will help the cow over her first critical four or six hours.

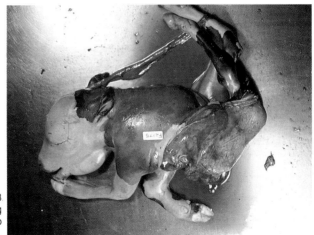

Colour plate 3
A schistome calf showing
additional limb
abnormalities.

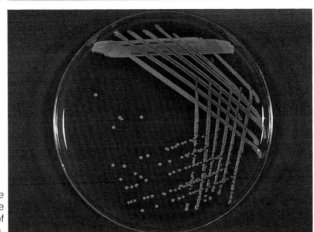

Colour plate 4   The white
lines and clumps on the
plate are colonies of
bacteria.

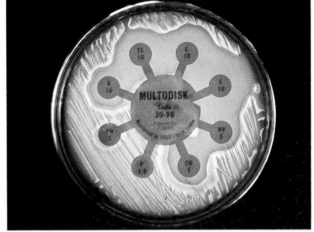

Colour plate 5   Antibiotic
sensitivity testing. If the
bacteria can grow up to
the disc, they are resistant
to the antibiotic contained
in the disc (penicillin and
ampicillin, P 1.5 and PN 2, in
this case).

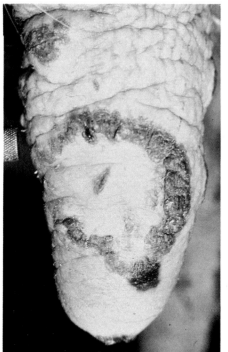

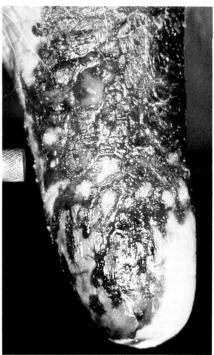

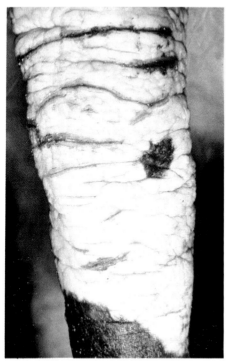

Colour plate 6 (*Above left*)   Pseudocowpox lesion. Note the typical circular pattern.

Colour plate 7 (*Above right*)   Bovine herpes mammillitis, a red raw teat after the initial blister has burst.

Colour plate 8   Teat chaps, deep infected cracks in the skin.

Grass Staggers (Hypomagnesaemia)

As its name implies, hypomagnesaemia is caused by a deficiency of magnesium in the blood. The disease occurs in beef cows on very bare pastures and in single-suckled calves, but here we will be confining our attention to the condition as seen in milking cows. The cow's daily requirements of magnesium are:

for maintenance	10 g
for lactation (e.g. 30 litres @ 0.6 g/litre)	18 g
Total requirement:	28 g/day

Grass may contain as little as 0.1 per cent magnesium in the dry matter however, so a cow grazing 16 kg DM per day would be receiving only 16 g magnesium, giving her an overall deficit of 12 g per day. There are virtually no stores of magnesium in the body and the cow must therefore receive a regular daily intake to avoid blood levels falling and hypomagnesaemia developing. Low magnesium is a feature of heavily fertilised lush modern swards. Pasture levels are further reduced by a high soil potash and a low pH since both factors decrease magnesium uptake by the plant. Uptake by the animal, that is absorption of magnesium from the intestine, is also influenced by pH, and it is reduced by the rapid passage of food (as occurs with lush grazing) and the formation of certain insoluble mineral complexes.

Clinical signs
One of the functions of magnesium in the body is to act as an electrical suppressant of nerve and muscle activity. The symptoms of deficiency are therefore the reverse of this, that is *excitability*. In the early stages the cow will have an erratic, slightly stiff-legged walk, with her head held high and her

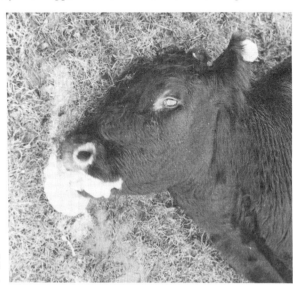

Plate 6.2 Hypomagnesaemia. Note the wild look in the eye and frothing at the mouth.

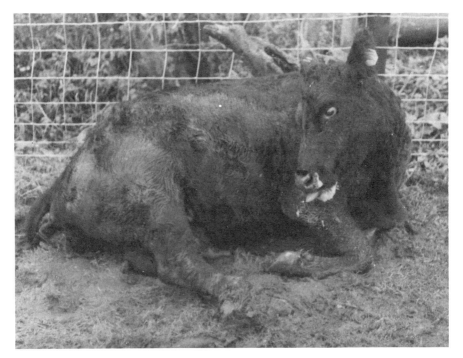

Plate 6.3 Following the administration of magnesium and sedatives, the cow shown in plate 6.2 was able to sit up, but she was still panting.

eyes wide and staring. If she is suddenly excited, or even if she is driven for any distance, she may fall over and go into *hypomagnesaemic tetany*: her legs will either be stiff and in spasm, or they will be paddling violently. Her head will be straight, her eyelids 'fluttering' if you approach them with your hand and she is likely to be frothing at the lips and 'chomping' with her mouth. The 'wild' eye and frothing are two features clearly recognisable in plate 6.2. A proportion of cows are simply found dead, the excitement having produced heart failure, but even then the presence of extensive struggling and paddling marks on the ground where she has been found lying may give a clue as to the cause of death.

Treatment
If hypomagnesaemia is suspected, try to avoid exciting the cow and precipitating a session of tetanic spasms. Magnesium therapy, usually as 400 ml of a 25 per cent solution of magnesium sulphate, should be given immediately. If you have some to hand, administer a bottle *subcutaneously*— if given intravenously it will precipitate a fatal heart attack. At the same time, and especially if the cow is showing spasms, veterinary assistance should be sought. Your vet will be able to administer sedatives to calm the cow, thus reducing the risk of a heart attack, and he will probably give a mixture of magnesium and calcium by slow intravenous injection, monitoring the heart

as he does so. He will also want to discuss the relevant control measures for the remainder of the herd.

Following the administration of magnesium and sedatives, the excitability of the cow is soon reduced. She should then be propped upright, putting her legs in the correct sitting position to avoid muscle damage (see page 119), and drenched with 60–90 grams of calcined magnesite, or some other similar preparation, to restore intestinal magnesium levels. Plate 6.3 shows the cow in plate 6.2 after magnesium therapy and sedatives. She was more relaxed and able to sit unsupported, although she was still panting from the spasms. Unfortunately she died from a heart attack less than two hours later.

Prevention and control
Magnesium is not stored in the body and control is based on providing a regular daily intake during the period of risk, that is whenever the cows are grazing lush young pasture. This occurs especially during May and early June, and can also be a problem in September. Outbreaks of disease are seen particularly following 'stress', for example on a very cold, wet day, when the cow's energy intake is also reduced. Hypomagnesaemia is also more likely to occur in cows which are mobilising large amounts of body fat and hence there may be an association with fatty liver syndrome. There are numerous methods of magnesium supplementation and you will need to choose the system best suited to your own farm routine:

1. Increase the calcined magnesite level in the concentrate to 60 g in 5.5 kg (2 oz in 12 lb). Unfortunately this reduces its palatability and may lead to refusal by some cows. Others, particularly those on a higher level of feeding, may scour. However, the main problem is that when there is ample grazing available, it is uneconomic to feed high levels of concentrate.
2. Magnesium bullets: these are large, cylindrical, metallic objects (plate 6.4) which, given by mouth, lodge in the bottom of the reticulum where they slowly dissolve, releasing magnesium at a controlled rate each day. Their weight keeps them in place, although in a small proportion of cows they are regurgitated with the cud and these animals are then at risk. Generally two bullets are given to reduce this risk and they supply magnesium to cover a two-month period.

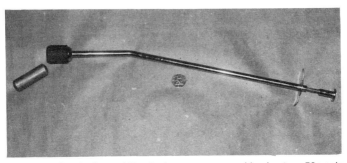

Plate 6.4 A magnesium bullet and the dosing gun compared in size to a 50p coin.

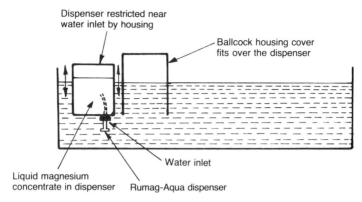

Note: Water flow rate into the trough must be adequate. If the dispenser falls onto its side it ceases to dispense.

Figure 6.4   The Rumag-Aqua dispenser, a method of adding magnesium to the drinking water.

3. Magnesium supplementation of the drinking water. This is probably the best method of control since the higher-yielding cows who need more magnesium will be drinking more water and will hence receive a higher intake of supplement. Usually a concentrated solution of magnesium acetate is used and this can be added to the water trough by hand, or by means of proportioners. The latter may be fitted to the mains supply, thus medicating the drinking water for the whole farm, or there are simple and relatively inexpensive devices which can be attached to individual water troughs. One such device is shown in figure 6.4. A much cheaper, but somewhat less accurate method is to use commercial magnesium chloride, which is approximately 50 per cent pure. A reasonable dose would be 60 g per cow per day, but this of course depends on what other sources of magnesium are available. Put the daily amount required by the herd into a fertiliser sack, add some water and then tie the top. Punch eight to ten holes in the sack, then place it in the water trough. The magnesium now diffuses into the water. It should be stressed that this is not an accurate method, but by supplementing the drinking water it does mean that all cows receive an additional intake.

4. Free-access high-magnesium minerals will undoubtedly help, but some cows will take far more than they need (probably because they like the taste of the salt added to it), while others will take nothing and be at risk. This is a good example of the fallacy of the statement that 'cows take whichever mineral they need' (for a fuller discussion of this method of mineral supplementation, see pages 299 and 307.

5. Pasture dusting: spreading calcined magnesite over the pasture every second or third day, using an artificial fertiliser distributor works quite well, although it is fairly laborious and entails driving over the grazing. It

should be applied at a rate which will provide an intake of 60 g per cow per day.

6. Improve the magnesium content of the sward. This can be done in four main ways, namely:

- Use a clover mixture, since clover has a much higher magnesium content than grass.
- add calcined magnesite to the soil at the rate of 5.0 cwt per acre. This only has any effect on sandy or low pH soils.
- avoid using high potassium fertilisers on pastures which the cows are going to graze in the spring and also avoid grazing pastures which have had heavy applications of slurry during the winter (slurry has a high potassium level). A high potassium content in the soil significantly reduces magnesium uptake by the plants and hence increases the risk of hypomagnesaemia.
- regular liming maintains the correct soil pH and improves magnesium uptake. A discussion on methods of increasing soil and pasture mineral levels, and on supplementation in general, is given on page 294.

Because of the risk of rapid death from hypomagnesaemia, some form of additional magnesium supplementation should always be given when the cows are grazing lush spring pasture. However, one of the problems is defining the period of risk and this can only be done by sampling those cows which are most susceptible, that is, the highest-yielding cows receiving no concentrate. Your veterinary surgeon can take blood samples to check magnesium levels, although analysis of urine is even better. Not only does urine analysis give advance warning of impending hypomagnesaemia, but it also indicates when magnesium supplementation is excessive, in other words, when it can be reduced or discontinued. In this way expense may be saved without putting the cows at risk. Mineral analysis on silage will identify the herds where winter hypomagnesaemia could be a problem.

Acetonaemia

Acetonaemia, which is also called *Ketosis* or *Slow Fever*, occurs in higher-yielding cows in early lactation. To appreciate why the disease occurs and also what causes the Fatty Liver Syndrome, we need to understand a little of the biochemistry of the metabolism of the cow. This is given in outline in figure 6.5.

High-carbohydrate 'starch' type foods, e.g. barley or sugarbeet, are broken down by the ruminal micro-organisms into a simple acid, *propionate*, and this is carried to the liver, where it is used to produce *glucose*. The main function of glucose is in the synthesis of milk and in fact the rate of milk production is largely determined by the rate of supply of glucose to the udder. This is why glucose is one of the metabolites measured as an indicator of energy status in the metabolic profile test (see page 138). Propionate has a second function, however, and that is its involvement in fat metabolism, or more precisely in the release of useful energy (E in figure 6.5) from fat. The cow in early

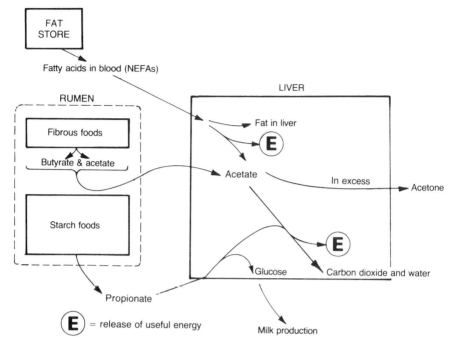

Figure 6.5   Energy metabolism in the cow.

lactation is unlikely to be able to consume sufficient energy in her diet to meet the needs of milk production and so she sends out an alarm signal to call on the help of her fat stores. Fat is broken into small blocks, the *fatty acids*. They can also be measured in the metabolic profile test when they are known as NEFAs, i.e. non-esterified fatty acids, and these are carried via the blood to the liver. Once in the liver they are broken down to *acetate* (or acetic acid) and this releases considerable quantities of useful energy E. However, the complete degradation of acetate to carbon dioxide and water with the release of further energy requires the interaction of propionate. The diagram also shows that fibrous foods (hay, etc.) are decomposed by the ruminal microorganisms into acetate and butyrate. These two metabolites pass directly to the liver; the butyrate is converted into acetate, and the overall effect is to further increase the cow's requirements for propionate.

If the cow is not being adequately fed, her total propionate production will be converted into glucose and used for milk production. There is still a signal going out for the mobilisation of fat to produce energy however, but because there is no further propionate available, fat metabolism cannot proceed beyond the acetate stage, and the excess acetate accumulates in the liver. After a while the liver is unable to store any further acetate, and to dispose of it two molecules of acetate are combined to produce *acetone*. The acetone passes from the liver into the blood, where it acts as an intoxicant to the cow, producing the symptoms of *acetonaemia*. The word literally means 'acetone in the blood', and it is effectively caused by an inadequate intake of 'starchy' food in a cow which is already mobilising body fat. Other ketone compounds formed from the excess acetate include *acetoacetate* and *beta-hydroxybutyrate*. The latter compound is also used as an indicator of energy status in the metabolic profile test. High blood levels of beta-hydroxybutyrate indicate a dietary energy deficit.

Clinical signs

Acetonaemia is seen primarily in higher-yielding cows and the first clinical sign is likely to be a partial or total refusal to eat concentrate, although she will probably continue to eat some hay or silage. She then becomes very dull and lethargic, and hence the name *slow fever*. After a short while, rumination virtually ceases, the dung becomes dry and hard, and milk production falls. In a small proportion of cows the acetone can affect the brain and these animals become excitable, froth at the mouth, lick objects excessively or stand with their heads raised and pushed into a corner. A common clinical sign is constipation, which is the result of excessive fluid loss from the body producing very dry dung.

The best diagnostic sign is the smell of acetone on the breath, which has a 'sharp' scent, like pear-drops. If you are in doubt, try sniffing the breath of a normal cow, then the breath of an affected cow and finally a bottle of nail-varnish remover, which is neat acetone!

Treatment

Because there are other conditions, for example, displacement of the abomasum (see page 324) which can lead to secondary acetonaemia, you would be well advised to seek veterinary advice for the diagnosis and treatment. The treatment prescribed will most probably consist of three components. Firstly drugs given by injection, to stimulate an increase in blood glucose levels and a boost to the rate of liver metabolism generally. These drugs would be of the anabolic steroid or glucocorticoid groups. Secondly, substances can be given by mouth to boost blood sugar levels and to improve metabolism. Probably the most common are sodium propionate and glycerol, which are chemically closely related. Reference to figure 6.5 shows how propionate can combine with the excess acetate in the liver, allowing its full metabolism to carbon dioxide, water and energy. This will not only reduce blood levels of acetone, but it will also allow the release of considerable quantities of energy from the acetate, and in so doing it overcomes the primary defect of acetonaemia. Glucose will only be beneficial if given by intravenous injection. If given by mouth it is decomposed by the ruminal micro-organisms.

Finally, altering the ration of sick animals and feeding them individually will help. Sometimes affected cows will eat barley, sugarbeet pulp or fodder beet, but not proprietary dairy cake, with its higher protein content. Molasses may also be palatable.

Prevention

As acetonaemia is caused by an energy intake which is inadequate to meet the demands of milk production, then clearly prevention and control of the disease are based on maintaining a correct diet. The ration must contain sufficient readily available energy to meet the needs of metabolism as described in figure 6.5; that is, a reasonable intake of cereal products or proprietary concentrate. If the forage is of poor quality (poor hay or silage), then additional concentrate needs to be fed to balance this and, as a rough guide, the M/D of the overall ration for a high-yielding early lactation cow should not fall below 10.5 MJ/kg Dry Matter. Especially dangerous are rations containing excessive fibre levels (see page 156), silage with poor palatability, e.g. with a butyric fermentation, or diets with a gross excess of protein. These factors could lead to outbreaks of acetonaemia, with quite large numbers of cows affected. If apparently normal cows from such herds were blood-sampled, for example as part of a metabolic profile, they would undoubtedly have low glucose levels, high acetones and high levels of non-esterified fatty acids (NEFAs) and beta-hydroxybutyrate in their blood.

Acetonaemia can also occur in individual animals and here it may be management which is at fault. Possible causes include inadequate feeding-space, so that the smaller cows or heifers get pushed away and do not receive their fair share. Secondly uneven distribution of the daily feeds can lead to some cows being unable to cope, while those with larger appetites can compensate. A third cause is cows which are overfat at calving because excessive fatness leads to reduced appetites in early lactation thus making them more susceptible to acetonaemia. This may occur as an individual or a herd problem.

Sometimes there is a primary failure of the liver, so that the cow is unable to carry out her metabolic functions correctly. Chronic liver fluke would be a good example, or the fatty liver syndrome which is covered in the next section. The conversion of propionate to glucose and the complete oxidation of acetate to carbon dioxide and water both occur in the liver cells, and hence liver damage can predispose to acetonaemia.

The Fatty Liver Syndrome

This has only recently been recognised as a clinical disorder and its cause has many similarities to acetonaemia. Research has shown that even normal cows can have quite a high proportion of fat stored in their liver cells immediately prior to calving. Then, with the stimulus of milk production, a signal is sent out calling for mobilisation of fat from the fat stores of the body to meet the energy deficit. This was explained with figure 6.5. When the fat arrives at the liver, there may already be a backlog of acetate and so surplus fat is stored in the liver cells until it can be used. Eventually the amount of fat stored reaches such a high level (up to 60 per cent of the space inside the liver cell) that its normal functions, including acetate metabolism and the conversion of propionate to glucose, are seriously retarded. This means that the rate of acetate utilisation is even further reduced and even more fat accumulates. All aspects of liver function are now affected and in the extreme case the cow simply degenerates into a condition of acute liver failure. A lesser degree of fatty liver seems to be common in many dairy herds. One survey showed that 40 per cent of the cows sampled at 1–2 weeks post-calving had more than one-fifth of the space within their liver cells occupied by fat.

Clinical signs
The severe disease of total liver failure is often precipitated by some other condition, quite commonly an unresponsive case of milk fever. While the cow is on the ground her appetite will be reduced and so she has to mobilise fat from her reserves to her liver to meet her energy requirements. Some animals continue to eat and drink and generally look bright. Others become dull and depressed and, after a day or two, stop eating—these may be the liver failure cases. Their eyes become dull and they cease to notice your approach or any other movements around them. They tend to sit with their head twisted around to one side, almost touching their hind feet, and they may then start to make small moaning and groaning sounds with each laboured breath. Any movements are inco-ordinated and severely affected animals roll over onto their sides and are unable to sit up, even with assistance. At this stage the prognosis is hopeless and no treatment will be of any value. Blood samples taken in the early stages would give very high GOT values, indicating liver damage.

Such severe manifestations of fatty liver are only the tip of the iceberg. Many cows are now known to be mildly affected, so that various important liver functions are depressed, simply because of the bulk of fat present in the liver cell. Probably the most significant of these is the effect on subsequent

Table 6.1   The effects of fatty liver on fertility and disease incidence

	'Normal' cows (less than 20% fat)	*Fatty liver cows* (greater than 20% fat)
1. Calving to:		
first ovarian activity	20 days	30 days
first observed oestrus	50 days	70 days
Services per conception	1.6	2.4
2. Incidence of disease in seventeen experimental cows:		
Ketosis	2	5
Mastitis	1	6
Retained placenta	1	1
Cystic ovaries	0	2
Milk fever	1	2
Total disease incidence	5 (in 9 normal cows)	16 (in 8 fatty liver cows)

(Taken from Reid I. & Roberts J. (1982), *In Practice*, 4, 164)

fertility. The protein *albumin* is manufactured in the liver. Its rate of production is depressed in cows with fatty liver syndrome and blood albumin levels fall. Research has shown that cows with low blood albumin levels after calving will have a reduced conception rate when they are served later in their lactation. Table 6.1 shows a survey which has grouped cows into those with 'normal' levels (<20%) of fat in their liver cells at one to two weeks post-calving and those with moderate to severe fatty liver (>20% fat). The difference in the subsequent fertility of the two groups is quite startling and a possible cause of this is given on page 232. Cows with fatty livers are also more susceptible to infectious disease and to metabolic disorders. This is clearly demonstrated in the second part of table 6.1 which shows the incidence of disease in an experiment in which eight cows developed fatty liver and nine cows remained normal.

Prevention
Cows should be fit but not fat in late pregnancy and must be fed well in early lactation to avoid excessive weight loss. Diet is therefore extremely important in control and these points have already been mentioned in relation to acetonaemia. Not only do overfat cows (body score 4.0 and above) have excessive fat in their liver cells, but they will also have reduced appetites in early lactation, thus exacerbating their energy deficit.

Acidosis

Acidosis could be considered as a metabolic disorder, although others would say that it is simply a digestive upset. Cattle fed all-forage rations have a pH in their rumen of around 6.0–6.5, and the products of micro-organism fermentation are acetate (70%), propionate (20%) and butyrate (8%) in approximately the proportions shown. Following a feed of concentrate, that is, highly fermentable carbohydrate, certain types of bacteria proliferate to produce lactic acid and this results in a fall in rumen pH. If the acidity reaches pH 5.0 there is likely to be a reduction in rumen motility, in other words the rumen stops contracting. This results in a loss of appetite for the cow, and she may not eat anything for one to two hours after a large feed of concentrate. More severe reductions in ruminal pH, for example to 4.5–4.0 or below, will result in quite severe signs of ill-health, and these are described in the 'over-eating syndrome' on page 320. At this stage the lactic acid concentration in the rumen will be so high that fluid is drawn in from the circulation by osmosis, blood pressure then falls and a state of shock begins to develop. Some of the lactic acid is absorbed from the rumen, and this has the metabolic effect on the cow known as *acidosis*. Apart from the reduction in her appetite the main clinical signs are panting (by breathing rapidly she is able to reduce the level of acidity in her blood) and laminitis. If the condition is allowed to persist in a chronic form, then the butterfat content of the milk will fall quite rapidly and can easily drop to 2.5 per cent or below. This is because butterfat is produced by joining acetate molecules end to end to form a chain and with a high carbohydrate fermentation, not only does the rumen become more acid but the amounts of acetate produced falls and propionate rises.

The cow normally overcomes excess acidity in her rumen by the buffering effects of bicarbonate and phosphate in her saliva, and it is only when her diet is poorly balanced that problems occur. Acidosis can be minimised in three ways. First, maintain a minimum of 40 per cent forage in the overall ration dry matter. To achieve this it may be necessary to provide highly palatable silage to encourage a high intake, as well as ensuring that excessive quantities of concentrate are not available. Second, space the concentrate feeds as evenly throughout the day as possible. This 'little and often' principle reaches its ideal in complete feeding systems. Third, using products such as sodium bicarbonate added to the concentrate at the rate of 12.5–20.0 kg per ton will help to counteract the lactic acid. This would probably only be worthwhile where large amounts of concentrate were being fed twice daily in the parlour to early lactation cows. However, if your buildings are designed so that this is your only feeding system, the use of sodium bicarbonate could have a significant effect on reducing the incidence of laminitis and on improving milk fats as well as producing benefits of an increase in overall dry matter intake and milk yield.

Factors Affecting Milk Quality

Milk quality is not strictly a metabolic disorder, but I have included it in this section because it is strongly influenced by diet and feeding practices. The average composition of typical Friesian milk can be given as:

Water	87.5%	
Butterfat (BF)	3.8%	
Solids not Fat (SNF)	8.7% = 3.3% protein	= 2.6% casein
		0.6% albumin + globulin
	4.7% sugar (lactose)	
	0.7% ash (minerals, including calcium)	

To a certain extent the levels of BF and SNF for a lactation are established during the first six to ten weeks after calving. If milk quality is poor at this stage, then it is quite difficult to achieve an improvement later in the lactation and it may not be until the following year that full correction occurs. Total yield is similarly affected.

Diet is probably the major factor affecting milk quality. Fibrous foods (e.g. hay and silage) are degraded by the ruminal micro-organisms to produce acetate, and butterfat consists of long chains of acetate molecules joined end to end. On the other hand, the rate of production of the protein component of SNF, which is also synthesised in the udder, is dependent on the availability of glucose, and therefore on the level of propionate production from 'starchy' foods in the rumen (see figure 6.5 and page 149).

Inadequate long fibre or excess concentrate in the ration leads to low butterfat levels. If silage is young and of a very high digestibility, the provision of 1–2 kg of hay or straw is beneficial. This applies especially when turning out to lush grazing in the spring or autumn. A minimum of 2 kg of long fibre is required for the average cow.

Conversely, diets with inadequate energy or excess fibre lead to low SNF. This is common in hay-fed herds unless the ration is supplemented with sugarbeet, potatoes, barley or some other energy source, although roots seem particularly beneficial. Surprisingly it is the protein fraction of the SNF which is reduced with low energy rations. Inadequate dietary protein, especially insufficient undegradable protein, can also reduce SNF, but has less effect than the energy content of the ration. Ruminal acidosis can also affect milk quality as described on page 154.

Protected fats, that is fats which have been treated to prevent them being broken down by the ruminal bacteria, can be added to the ration up to about 1.0 kg per cow per day, or about 7% in the concentrate. They pass directly into the small intestine, where they are absorbed and then used by the udder to produce butterfat. They will produce a rise in butterfat, but if too much protected fat is included, SNF levels will fall. Unsaturated fats (viz. oils) depress butterfat and SNF levels.

Part of the effect of nutrition on milk quality is determined during the dry period. Cows which calve down in poor condition may suffer a depression of around 0.1 per cent SNF and 0.2 per cent butterfat and this can persist throughout the lactation. You should aim to calve the cows fit but not fat, that is at a body score of 3–3½. Higher than this could lead to fatty livers.

Before leaving the effects of diet on milk quality, it ought to be pointed out that some of the factors which lead to high yields will automatically lead to a reduction in quality. Part of this is simply due to the dilution of milk. While you must consider the percentages of butterfat and SNF therefore, it is the overall milk yield that is likely to have the greatest effect on productivity, although payment systems over the past few years have placed increasing importance on quality, partly because a greater proportion of milk is being used for manufacture rather than liquid sales.

The main diseases affecting milk quality are parasitism and mastitis. Fluke, worms and even a very heavy louse infestation will all reduce butterfat and SNF, although the most common is the effect of liver fluke which reduces SNF levels.

A herd with a cell count of over 750,000 cells/ml is probably losing 750–900 litres per cow per year, 0.5% lactose and a smaller amount (0.3%) of butterfat. The control of cell count is covered in the section on mastitis. Both butterfat and the protein component of SNF are inherited and so breeding can have a significant long-term effect. Bulls should be chosen with a high milk-quality performance and poor cows should not be used for breeding. The genetic variation in butterfat is much greater than for protein however, and breeding for improved protein status is therefore likely to produce a slower response than breeding for butterfat. Milk quality is generally highest in heifers, falling with increasing age to about the fifth lactation, when it remains approximately constant. It is also lowest at peak yield (probably a dilution effect), although the improvement in quality in later lactation is greater in pregnant than in non-pregnant animals. A large number of cows reaching peak yield in November, combined with the final batch of late-calvers being dried off, is a common cause of a reduction in milk quality in autumn-calving herds. Aiming for a well-fed, young herd, paying attention to mastitis and parasite prevention and keeping a tight control on breeding and fertility should all help to maintain a satisfactory milk quality status.

Chapter 7

MASTITIS AND CONDITIONS OF THE UDDER

MASTITIS CONTINUES to be a major cause of economic loss to the national dairy herd and I suspect that, combined with teat injuries, it is one of the greatest aggravations to the herdsman. Although the incidence of infections caused by *Staphylococcus aureus*, *Streptococcus agalactiae* and *Streptococcus dysgalactiae* has decreased and the national mastitis cell count has fallen, this has been matched by a rise in the number of cases caused by *Escherichia coli* and *Streptococcus uberis*, known as environmental mastitis. A Mastitis Surveillance Scheme carried out on four hundred herds in England and Wales from 1979 to 1982 showed that an average herd of a hundred cows would have thirty-five cases of mastitis each year, defining a 'case' of mastitis as one quarter affected on one occasion. There is, of course, tremendous variation in the severity of mastitis, ranging from a few clots needing only one course of treatment, to an acute case in which the cow dies. However, the average cost of a case of mastitis based on the antibiotics used, milk discarded, reduction in quality and the reduced milking potential of the cow for the remainder of the lactation, was estimated at approximately £60 for each case at 1985 values. With approximately 2.8 million cows in Great Britain, this was a cost to the national herd of £59 million per year or £21 for every cow in your herd! Other surveys have shown an incidence of over fifty cases per hundred cows per year, which means that the overall cost would rise to £30 per year for every cow in your herd, viz. an average of £3,000 every year lost in mastitis alone for a hundred-cow herd.

MECHANISMS OF MILK SYNTHESIS

The structure of the normal teat and udder is shown in figure 7.1. Milk is produced by the gland cells lining the alveoli deep in the udder and it is stored in the alveoli, their ducts and in the udder cistern between milkings. The average composition of milk is given on page 17 (table 2.1) and again on page 155. Its components are derived from metabolites carried in the blood and it is said that 500 litres of blood must flow through the udder to produce each litre of milk. The gland cell synthesises a globule of milk fat in its cytoplasm and then extrudes it out into the alveolar space. As the globule passes through

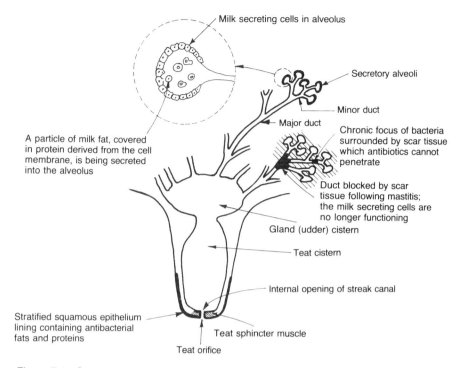

Figure 7.1   Structure of the udder and teat, showing some of the changes which occur in mastitis.

the cell membrane, it becomes coated with a thin layer of protein, and in this way the fat and some of the protein components of the milk are formed (see figure 7.1). Mastitis can damage the cell membrane, and fat globules may then be passed with an incomplete protein covering. In this form the fat can decompose, a process known as *lipolysis*, and this is why cows with mastitis often produce milk which has a bitter taste. The majority of milk protein (casein) is similarly synthesised in the alveolar cell cytoplasm and extruded into the alveolar space. Lactose (milk sugar) is produced by combining one molecule of glucose with one molecule of galactose and is extruded from the cell in a similar manner.

THE HORMONAL CONTROL OF MILK PRODUCTION AND LET-DOWN

Nutrition is clearly the greatest single factor affecting the level of milk production, and as is explained later in the chapter, mastitis can also influence yields. This short section deals primarily with the hormonal and managemental factors involved.

Hormonal Factors

The induction, or start, of lactation is controlled by a hormone called *prolactin* which is produced by the pituitary gland, situated at the base of the brain. Chapter 8 will discuss the factors which maintain high levels of progesterone during pregnancy. Immediately prior to parturition, blood progesterone levels fall. This allows prolactin levels to rise, and prolactin then produces the changes in the udder tissue needed to start milk production. In many species milk yield is maintained by high levels of circulating prolactin, and the higher the level of prolactin, the greater will be the level of milk production.

This is not so in the cow, however, where the continuation of milk yield appears to be controlled by a combination growth hormone produced by the pituitary gland, thyroxine produced by the thyroid gland in the neck and steroids from the adrenal glands situated beside the kidneys. When milk has been synthesised, oxytocin, yet another hormone produced by the pituitary gland, is needed to eject the milk from the udder. Oxytocin causes the contraction of small muscle-like elements (myoepithelial cells) surrounding the alveoli. This forces the milk down into the ducts and hence into the udder cistern and then to the teat cistern, where it is ready for withdrawal by the calf or the milking machine.

The overall process is known as milk let-down, and oxytocin is released from the pituitary gland by what is known as a reflex action, that is in response to a *consistent* stimulus which the cow associates with milking. This stimulus may be udder-washing or fore-milking, but neither are necessary. The cow can be trained to produce milk let-down (in response to oxytocin) simply by entering the parlour.

One point is important however. The stimulus for oxytocin release *must* be the same at every milking. If the proper stimulus is not provided, or if it is inhibited, then milk stays in the alveoli and only 50 per cent of normal production is obtained. Oxytocin has a very short duration of action. If the milking machine is not applied soon after the teat fills, the myoepithelial cells will relax, the alveoli enlarge once again and milk will be drawn back into the udder. It is absolutely vital that a constant routine is established in the milking parlour therefore, so that the cow knows precisely when the unit will be applied and she can train herself to 'let-down' accordingly.

In addition this whole process can be inhibited by the action of the hormone *adrenalin*, which is produced by the adrenal gland. Adrenalin is sometimes known as the 'flight or fight' hormone: in man it causes a thumping heart, cold hands and sweating, all of which are associated with fear. Anything which disturbs the cows—unusual noise, strangers, rough handling etc.—will lead to adrenalin release and may interfere with milk let-down and therefore overall production. It is adrenalin which produces the defecation associated with excitement—a phenomenon I expect every stockman will have witnessed! Treatment of milk let-down failure is also discussed on page 134 and 167.

Managemental Factors

Frequency of milking can have a marked effect on total production. If cows are milked only once daily, yields will fall by some 40 per cent, whereas milking three times daily can cause an increase of 10–15 per cent, depending on the herd. Because of the flatter lactation curve it produces, three times daily milking has to be continued until the end of lactation to obtain its full beneficial effect, however. The majority of farms milk at intervals of 14 hours and 10 hours, and trials have shown that this does not produce significantly lower production than precise 12-hourly intervals in anything but the very highest yielding herds. In the latter case it is possibly pressure of milk stored within the alveoli which becomes a factor limiting production. Machine stripping, that is additional manual pressure applied to the cluster at or towards the end of milk flow, may lead to a secondary release of oxytocin and may even train cows to 'hold back' some milk for this period. For the average yielding cow leaving *small* quantities of milk (e.g. 1–2 litres) in the udder is not too important in terms of overall yield, and if on one occasion a cow leaves the parlour only half-milked you will certainly not lose any more than a small part of the next milking's production, and possibly nothing if she is not a particularly high yielder. If a cow is consistently undermilked however, for example if only 60 per cent of the milk is withdrawn for 5–6 days, then this will result in a lowering of production. This effect can even be seen in an individual quarter, for example a quarter badly affected by teat-end damage, and this suggests that there must be factors in addition to oxytocin and the other central hormones, which are involved with milk production and release.

At the end of lactation the old milk-producing alveolar cells die off and are replaced by new tissue during, and especially towards the end of, the dry period. A dry period of 6–8 weeks is ideal, and if the cow is not dried off at all, the next lactation may be as much as 30 per cent lower. Situations such as this can occur when a bull is run with the herd continually and no pregnancy testing is carried out. In addition to having a very short or non-existent dry periods, some cows may conceive so soon after calving that both their 305-day lactation and annual production will be depressed.

What is Mastitis?

The word means simply 'inflammation of the mammary gland', but in common usage it is understood that the inflammation is caused by some infectious agent, usually by bacteria. Before discussing the disease in detail, the natural defences of the teat and udder will be examined, and this will give the reader an opportunity to understand the udder's reaction to infection.

Teat and Udder Defences

The teat has a number of ingenious defence mechanisms aimed at preventing the entry of bacteria and reducing the chances of mastitis (figure 7.1). The outer layer of teat skin, called stratified squamous epithelium, has a lining of dead cells, all impregnated with a hard, inert material called keratin, and this does not easily support bacterial growth. Only when the teat is cracked or chapped do large numbers of bacteria accumulate. Secondly the physical tightness of the teat sphincter muscle keeps the streak canal firmly closed and this helps to prevent bacterial entry. Third, the streak canal is also lined by stratified squamous epithelium, the superficial dead cells of which slough away and trap bacteria which may be invading. When milk flows out, both bacteria and dead cells are carried away from the udder. Perhaps most interesting of all, the epithelial lining around the teat end and through the streak canal contains lipids and proteins which have specific antibacterial activity. These protein molecules are even positively charged so that they can attract negatively charged bacteria towards them before damaging their membrane and destroying them.

The inside of the teat cistern is lined with a similar type of epithelium (but it is not keratinised) and this provides a further defence against certain types of bacteria, although others may be able to establish colonies in this area. If E. coli (an environmental organism, see page 182) reach this point, their toxins can damage the cells forming the epithelium, and this allows

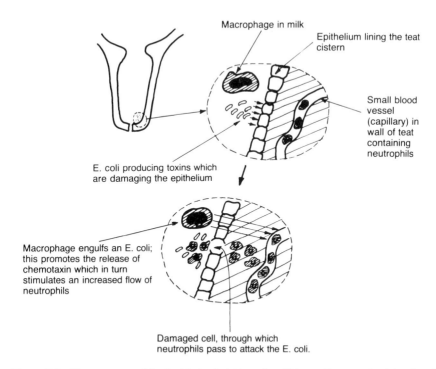

Figure 7.2 The response of the teat to bacterial invasion. This reaction can also take place in the udder cistern and ducts.

neutrophils (bacterial-killing white blood cells) to pour out through the damaged membrane to attack the bacteria. Macrophages are another type of bacterial-killing cell and they are already present in the milk. They can also destroy E. coli and, as they do, they release a chemical, *chemotaxin* which stimulates the release of further neutrophils from the circulation. These changes are shown diagrammatically in figure 7.2.

Although the whole process can be in operation in as little as four hours from the entry of E. coli, cows vary enormously in the rate at which their neutrophils can mount a counter-attack, and also in the ability of their neutrophils to kill bacteria. In one experiment, some cows were able to destroy 98 per cent of the E. coli infused into a quarter in as little as six hours, whereas other cows destroyed only 80 per cent. The clinical disease of E. coli mastitis is due to the production of toxins, so the faster a cow is able to mount a neutrophil response, the less likely she is to be severely ill. Research is even being carried out on bulls by taking a sample of their blood and monitoring the response of their neutrophils to chemotaxin and E. coli attack. In this way it may be possible one day to predict those bulls which will produce daughters with a rapid neutrophil response to E. coli; that is, those which are able to easily counteract E. coli mastitis. Neutrophils kill bacteria first by engulfing them into a vacuole, a cavity within the substance of the neutrophil, and then secreting toxic lysozymes onto them. In some cows the neutrophils are simply not so effective, whatever bacteria are involved. This variation in activity, which is probably genetic, is seen at any age and all stages of lactation, so heifer calves could be blood-sampled to assess their ability to withstand mastitis infection.

Staphylococci and streptococci invade the deeper parts of the gland and evoke a similar response of enlarged blood vessels and neutrophil attack. It is engorgement of the blood vessels which produces the hard, hot painful swollen quarter with mastitis, signs which every herdsman knows only too well. The smaller udder ducts may become blocked with clumps of bacteria, neutrophils and general debris, and by this stage the associated alveoli will no longer be producing any milk (see figure 7.1). The blockage may become almost permanent, and it will then be difficult for antibiotics to penetrate the foci of bacteria trapped inside. Some bacteria will periodically leak out during the course of the lactation, however, to evoke an inflammatory response in adjacent alveoli. This is seen clinically as a recurrent case of mastitis, but even if no clots are evident the cow will be intermittently shedding bacteria in her milk and will therefore be a danger to others.

The extent and the nature of the clots is often more of a reflection of the severity of the infection, rather than the type of bacteria present. Plate 7.1 shows milk being examined by stripping onto a black boot (possibly not the most hygienic practice!). Normal milk flows off fairly easily; if staphylococcal/ streptococcal clots are present they tend to stick to the surface, while 'milk' from a quarter infected with E. coli may be nothing more than a slightly brown-tinged clear fluid, which runs off without leaving a trace. A word of warning, however. These changes represent typical cases and it is *not possible* to be sure which bacteria are causing the mastitis simply by the appearance of

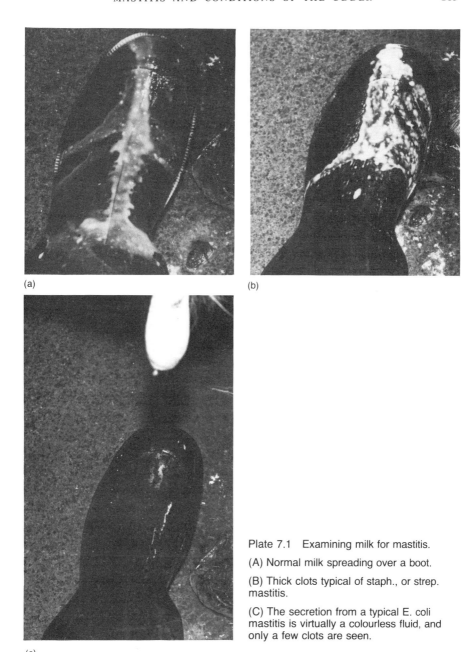

(a)

(b)

(c)

Plate 7.1   Examining milk for mastitis.

(A) Normal milk spreading over a boot.

(B) Thick clots typical of staph., or strep. mastitis.

(C) The secretion from a typical E. coli mastitis is virtually a colourless fluid, and only a few clots are seen.

the milk and the degree of illness of the cow. This is why your vet may want to sample a range of mastitis cases to see which are the most common organisms causing problems in your herd.

THE CONTROL OF MASTITIS

When penicillin was introduced in the 1940s it was assumed that with such an effective treatment, mastitis would soon be eliminated. This proved not to be the case. In fact mastitis is an interesting condition because many of the control methods which we can apply to other diseases are simply not relevant. For example:

- *Eradication*—will never be possible because there are so many different sources of infection.
- *Vaccination*—does not work because there are a wide range of bacterial serotypes involved and because immune systems in the udder are relatively poor.
- *Antibiotic treatment*—cannot be relied upon to eliminate infection because chronic foci exist which antibiotics are unable to penetrate.
- *Breeding resistant cows*—some success, but very slow.

The basis of mastitis control is therefore *herd management*, specifically aimed at reducing the level of bacterial challenge at the teat end and thereby reducing the rate of new infections. Mastitis can never be eradicated. However, if milking routines and hygiene techniques are improved so that the spread of infection is reduced, the number of new cases will decrease. This must be done within economic constraints: it is undoubtedly more cost-effective to accept a low level of infection within a herd than to spend large sums of money trying to eliminate the last few cases.

For mastitis therefore, all control measures are aimed at *prevention*. Broadly speaking there are three types of mastitis infection. These are:

1. Infections contracted from other cows (cow-to-cow transmission or contagious mastitis).
2. Infections contracted from the environment (environmental mastitis).
3. Infections in dry cows (e.g. summer mastitis).

As all three types require rather different control measures, they will be dealt with separately, starting with cow-to-cow transmission. Mastitis in the dry cow is included in a later section.

COW-TO-COW TRANSMITTED MASTITIS

The main bacteria involved in this group are:

Staphylococcus aureus—present in the udders of chronically infected cows and also in cuts and chaps on the teat skin.
Streptococcus agalactiae—found only in the udder (it can survive for 2–3 weeks away from the cow but *multiplication* occurs only in the udder).
Streptococcus dysgalactiae—in the udder and on teat skin lesions.

The main control measures for this group of infections are described in a five-point plan outlined by the National Institute for Research in Dairying and the Central Veterinary Laboratory at the end of their extensive field trials in 1969. Because the control measures are of such basic importance and are procedures that every herdsman should be carrying out as a routine, I will list them first and then explain why they are so important.

1. Keep the milking plant in good working order by regular maintenance and by correcting all faults detected at the twice-yearly machine tests.
2. Observe basic hygiene principles during milking and disinfect the teats immediately afterwards.
3. Check for clinical mastitis at every milking and treat all cases promptly and thoroughly
4. Give long-acting antibiotic to all cows at drying-off.
5. Keep records of clinical cases treated and cull those cows which have had recurrent attacks of mastitis in the same quarter.

By examining the various steps in the milking routine we can see how infection may be spread, and how the above measures help to control cow-to-cow transmitted (= contagious) mastitis.

The Milking Routine and How it Affects the Transmission of Mastitis

This will be dealt with under a series of headings, namely: the preparation of the udder; examination of foremilk; cleaning the clusters between cows; teat disinfection; the milking machine; teat-end impacts and other faults; the treatment of clinical mastitis; and the importance of records.

Preparation of the Udder

It is essential to adopt and maintain a constant routine for the cow in order to stimulate milk let-down (see also pages 134 and 161). If cows are nervous entering the parlour, or if there is some other change in their routine, let-down may be inhibited and teat damage similar to overmilking can occur for the first half to one minute after the unit has been applied, and until the teat fills with milk. Normally teats and udders are washed and this should be done with running water containing hypochlorite (250 ppm available chlorine) or iodophor (60 ppm available iodine) as a disinfectant. Buckets and cloths are especially liable to transmit infection and if they *must* be used they should be changed after every five cows. Mastitis organisms may be present on the skin of the teat or within the udder and these may contaminate the milker's hands when he is washing the udder or stripping the foremilk for evidence of mastitis. Cracks and chaps in his own hands may already be harbouring bacteria, however, and these may be a further source of *Staphylococcus aureus* mastitis infection. Whatever the origin of the bacteria on the milker's hands, they represent a potential source of danger to the next cow to be handled. The danger can be reduced by wearing rubber gloves (which are less liable to harbour bacteria) and by using a disinfectant in the water.

It is the *teats* which should be washed, rather than the udder and after washing the teats *must* be dried, using individual paper towels. If the teats are not dried, there will be a small drop of dirty water at the teat end and when the unit is applied this could be forced up into the teat, especially if there are vacuum fluctuations. Washing and drying the teats is also important in reducing the total bacterial count (TBC) of milk (see page 198).

Provided that the teats are clean and the TBC is low, an increasing number of herds have now discontinued washing. The action of entering the parlour and being given concentrates is sufficient to stimulate milk let-down, and omitting the washing certainly reduces milking time. There may be a small decrease in yield for the first few days after washing has been discontinued, but this is only temporary. The mastitis risk is also reduced, but there is an increased possibility of sediment and other contamination which might contravene the Milk and Dairies Regulations. An intermediate between the two extremes, and probably the best procedure, is to use a 'dry wipe'. This removes the dust and debris from the teat premilking, it provides some stimulation for let-down and it also enables a physical check to be made for the presence of mastitis. Of course, if the teats are obviously dirty, then they will have to be washed, but because washing removes the normal layer of protective fatty acids and also the 'natural' bacteria from teat skin, unnecessary washing is undoubtedly detrimental. When the teats dry off they lose some of their natural elasticity and pliability, and this can exaggerate teat chapping. The answer is clearly to house and manage cows so that they keep clean and teat washing is not required.

Checking the Foremilk

The early detection of clinical cases of mastitis is extremely important for three reasons. First, affected cows can then be milked after the rest of the herd, or perhaps with a separate cluster, thus avoiding the risk of transfer infection. Second, prompt treatment can be given, thus reducing the risk to

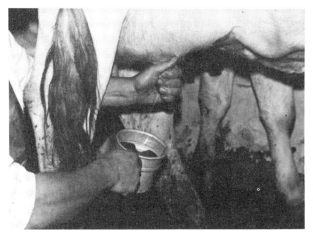

Plate 7.2 Stripping foremilk is the most effective way of detecting clinical mastitis (Photo: MMB).

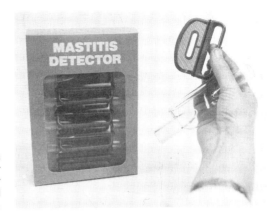

Plate 7.3   An 'in-line' mastitis detector. When clots appear on the screen, the detector can be pulled out, washed and re-inserted into the line.

other cows as well as increasing the prospects of full recovery. Third, infected milk can be discarded: if it passes into the bulk tank, not only does this contravene the contract with the Milk Marketing Board, but it can also cause a massive increase in the cell count and the total bacterial count of the milk.

The best way of detecting clinical mastitis is by stripping foremilk into a strip-cup (plate 7.2), but this is clearly a very onerous task. In an average herd where there are only thirty-five cases of clinical mastitis per hundred cows per year, the herdsman would have to strip almost seven thousand teats to find one case of mastitis! At this rate the risk of transmitting mastitis bacteria from teat chaps and subclinical carriers by repeated and unnecessary handling must be close to the risk of mastitis spreading by failure to detect a clinical case quickly enough. Simple stripping onto the floor of the parlour during the washing/wiping process is a useful alternative to the strip cup, although mastitis is not so easily detected by this method, and there is also the risk of spreading mastitis organisms into the environment. To avoid handling the teats there is an Ambic detector device (plate 7.3) which can be fitted into the long milk tube. Clots are easily seen on a filter screen (although you must look for them) and milk can by-pass the filter when it is blocked, so that flow rates are not impeded. With the Ambic detector, milk from a new case of mastitis will still enter the bulk tank at the first milking, but even this is far better than no foremilk examination at all. The importance of *early detection* and *adequate treatment* of clinical mastitis cannot be overstressed, since both factors greatly reduce the risk of spreading disease to other cows.

Cleaning of Clusters between Cows

When the cluster is removed from a cow the liners may be contaminated by mastitis organisms which have arisen from either the teat skin or the infected milk of a subclinically infected animal. One way of reducing the spread of mastitis would be to clean the clusters between each cow, either by flushing with water; by dipping them into hypochlorite and then flushing; or by pasteurisation (that is circulation with water at 85°C). There is no doubt that a combined disinfection and heat treatment of clusters would reduce significantly the spread of mastitis organisms, but at the moment it is not included as a routine in a 'package' of mastitis control measures, partly because of the cost (hot water) and partly because of the time involved (allowing the disinfectant to act). This is a good example of how the practical costs and problems of a mastitis control procedure may outweigh its advantages. However, if you are faced with a herd outbreak of staphylococcal/streptococcal mastitis it would be an excellent control measure to put into operation in the short term, even if you only did it after removing the clusters from clinical cases or from cows which had had mastitis earlier in their lactation.

Teat Disinfection

The most common method of disinfecting the teats between milkings is by teat dipping and to understand the benefits it must first be appreciated how new infections enter the udder. Some bacteria are undoubtedly forced directly up into the teat sinus by the machine and the factors responsible for this will be dealt with later. More commonly however, the milking machine or the hands of the milker physically transfer bacteria from an infected cow and deposit them onto the teat of a 'clean' cow. These bacteria then start to grow or 'colonise' cracks in the teat skin (colour plate 8), areas around the teat sphincter being particularly dangerous. Eventually if they can overcome all the teat defence mechanisms (see page 162), they may grow up into the udder itself and a new case of mastitis is established. This process may take several days, it is by far the commonest method of cow-to-cow transmission and it is *virtually eliminated* by disinfecting the teats between milkings. Conventional teat dips completely cover the teat in a film of disinfectant and kill the bacteria which were transferred to the teat during milking.

Most dips are formulated to persist for only two to three hours, but this is quite sufficient to exert their bacterial-killing action. Chlorhexidine probably persists for slightly longer (four to six hours). There are three basic types of material used:

hypochlorite—there should be not less than 10,000 ppm (1.0%) and prefably be 40,000 ppm (4%) available chlorine;
iodophor—not less than 5,000 ppm (0.5%) available iodine;
chlorhexidine—containing not less than 5,000 ppm (0.5%) chlorhexidine gluconate.

Hypochlorite is the cheapest and may be quite adequate for use in the summer. However, it quickly loses its potency if it gets dirty from the cows splashing mud or slurry onto their teats, or from contamination in the teat dip cup. This is why any remaining dip should be discarded at the end of each milking and the cups should be washed. Iodophors and chlorhexidine are less affected by contamination and in addition they can be mixed with *emollients*, that is substances like glycerine or lanolin which improve the condition of the teat skin. Concentrations of 10% glycerine or 2.5% lanolin are used, although these can be increased if 'chapping' is a severe problem. Very high concentrations of emollients, that is above 20%, will reduce the bacterial killing action of the dip, however, and as bacteria growing deep in the crevices of the skin tend to make the chaps worse, a balance is needed between the emollient and bacterial-killing effects. If hypochlorite is to be used with an emollient, it should be added immediately before milking to avoid excessive inactivation of the disinfectant.

Teat disinfectants are most commonly applied by dipping the teat into a cupful of liquid. To make the process easier, several different types of cup have been devised, the best probably being an anti-spill cup, an example of which is shown in plate 7.4. Teat dipping should be carried out with care.

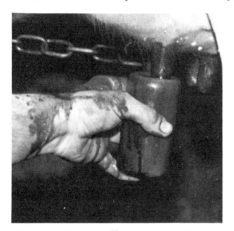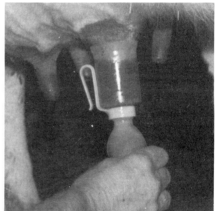

Plate 7.4   Teat dipping. The conventional cup shown in the left-hand photograph is overfull, and although the teats are well covered, dip has been splashed onto the operator's hand and indicates wastage (photo: MMB). The right-hand photograph shows an antispill cup.

Make sure the cup is deep enough to accommodate the whole length of even the largest teat (approximately 12 cm). If the cup is too full, immersion of the teat results in wastage of dip, whereas insufficient dip means that the teat does not get adequately coated. The whole teat needs to be covered with dip, because cracks could occur at any level. Spraying methods are also used and provided they are carried out conscientiously, they give a reasonable coverage to the teat and the dip is always clean. However, it is easy to coat only half the teat, and disinfectants with a high emollient content cannot be used. Sprays also use more ingredients and are therefore more expensive. Automated sprays, situated at the exit to the parlour and activated by a photo-electric cell as the cow passes, are also available. Teat disinfection is most effective if it is carried out as soon as the teat-cups are removed, ideally within thirty seconds, so that a film of dip covers the inside of the streak canal as the sphincter is closing. This cannot be achieved by the automated methods. On average teat dipping uses approximately seven litres of dip per cow per year, so although there are considerable advantages, the procedure has a significant cost attached to it.

In summary then, teat disinfection has three important functions:

1. It kills bacteria transferred from an infected cow via the milker's hands or the machine, and in so doing it prevents the establishment of a bacterial colony at the teat end.
2. If mixed with an emollient it keeps the teats supple and prevents 'chapping' and other lesions which could harbour *Staphylococcus aureus* and *Streptococcus dysgalactiae*.
3. Teat chaps with bacteria growing in them are slower to heal and so the antiseptic properties of teat disinfectants also promote the healing of teat lesions.

The overall effect of teat disinfection is to halve the rate at which new infections become established, and as such it is of considerable long-term benefit.

Teat-end Impacts

The milking machine can transfer bacteria from the infected skin or milk of one quarter, either to another quarter in the same cow or to the udder of a second cow. In fact the first of these options is by far the most likely and this is due to a reverse flow of milk hitting the teat end, producing a phenomenon known as an *impact* of milk. Look at figure 7.3. The diagram on the left shows the squeeze phase of the pulsation cycle, when the teat is being rested and no milk is flowing. When vacuum is reapplied to the pulsation tube, the liner starts to open to recommence the extraction of milk from the teat. The vacuum at the end of the teat now reaches a peak and milk flows back from the claw to hit the teat end fractionally before milk starts to flow out from the teat itself. This momentary reverse flow of milk from the claw produces an *impact* and of course it can easily carry with it infection from one of the other quarters. Admittedly many of the bacteria would be washed away again by the flow of milk from the teat itself, but some are not, and research has shown that milking plants producing a high number of impacts cause far more

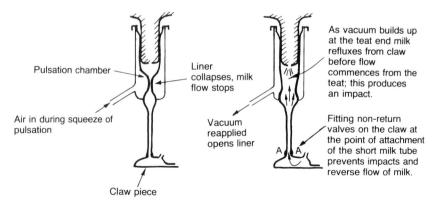

Figure 7.3   Teat-end impacts.

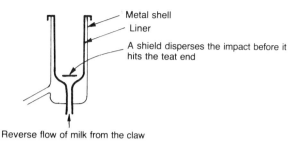

Figure 7.4   Teat shield in liner.

mastitis. One of the ways of preventing this is by means of teat *shields* or *deflectors*, fitted into the base of the liner. An example is given in figure 7.4. The reverse squirt of milk is now deflected towards the sides of the liner so that teat-end impacts under force cannot occur.

Reverse flow can still occur, however, and the end of the teat may still get bathed in infected milk. An alternative and much more effective system is to fit non-return valves into the claw at the point of entry of each short milk tube (point A, figure 7.3). If impacts now occur they are only with milk from the one quarter, and there is no risk of infected milk passing back from other quarters via the claw. Trials at the NIRD have shown a 15 per cent reduction in new infection rates using teat shields and a 20 per cent reduction in clinical mastitis with the ball-valve claw.

Teat-end impacts can be increased as a result of faulty milking techniques. If air is allowed to enter the liner beside the teat, then again milk rushes up from the clawpiece. This could occur if the cows are nervous and restless, perhaps because they have sore teats or possibly because the unit has already been left on too long. It could be the result of badly fitting liners which 'slip' during milking, or it could occur when the cow is being machine stripped. Machine stripping is rarely carried out now. There is ample evidence to show that leaving the last one or two litres of milk in the udder has no effect on total lactation production, whereas the accidental inlet of air while machine stripping will produce teat-end impacts and predispose to mastitis. For a similar reason, that is to avoid impacts, the vacuum should always be switched off before removing the cluster. Many modern parlours have automatic cluster removal and provided they are correctly adjusted, they will be beneficial in leading to a reduction in mastitis.

Probably the worst feature of the plant for producing teat-end impacts is excessive vacuum fluctuation, especially if the fluctuation is at the teat end. Vacuum fluctuations in the whole plant are usually the result of a faulty regulator valve, and as a result of their inspections of milking plants on farms the Milk Marketing Board mastitis technicians reported that poorly maintained vacuum regulators, leading to excessive vacuum fluctuation, were by far their commonest finding. The regulator should be cleaned at least once a week. Any dirt or corrosion means that it may 'stick' and this can lead to fluctuating vacuum. Another common cause of fluctuation was inadequate vacuum reserve of the pump and this occurred particularly when an existing parlour was enlarged or if vacuum-operated feeders or gates were added, but the same vacuum pump was used.

An important feature of the clawpiece is the presence of a small air-bleed, a hole approximately 0.8 mm in diameter, which allows the entry of air. The reason for this is that a mixture of air and milk will flow more evenly along the milk tube and away from the claw. If the air-bleed is blocked, milk leaves the claw in 'plugs' and this leads to excessive vacuum fluctuation at the teat end. Even with an air-bleed, claws can get clogged when milk flow rates are high, so there has been a trend in recent years to increase the internal volume of the claw. A full discussion of all the causes of vacuum fluctuation would be outside the scope of this book; however, high-level recorder jars and even the nature of the pipe runs can have quite an effect. I think it is sufficient for the reader to understand the significance of teat-end impacts, their relation to mastitis and the way in which vacuum fluctuations can produce them. It is then up to him to call in the specialist on milking machine function for the twice-yearly test or as a check when problems occur.

Other Milking Machine Faults

The teat is a very sensitive structure and if it is to function correctly and act as a reasonable barrier to the entry of mastitis organisms, it must be maintained

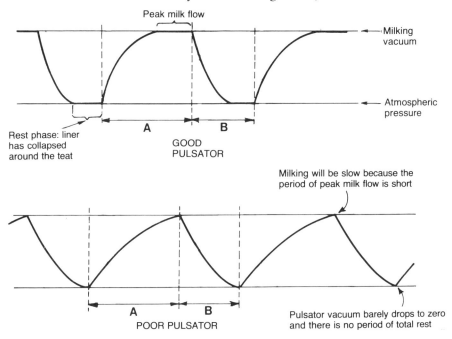

Figure 7.5 The pulsation curves of good and bad pulsators. The pulsation ratio is the ratio of A:B, viz. milk flow: rest periods.

in a healthy state. Pulsation during milking allows proper blood flow around the teat and if the pulsators do not allow sufficient rest, teat-end damage will occur. The top drawing in figure 7.5 shows the curve produced by a good pulsator. The vacuum outside the liner (in the pulsator chamber—see figure 7.3) rises quite rapidly to induce milk flow and then falls to zero to rest the teat. The liner has now collapsed and blood flow is being restored. The second curve shows a pulsator which barely reaches atmospheric pressure and certainly gives no rest period. This is bound to cause teat damage. Pulsators can also be adjusted to give varying periods of milking time to resting time (A:B in figure 7.5). A ratio of 2:1 is generally satisfactory. Higher than this (e.g. 3:1) produces a faster milk flow rate but may allow insufficient rest and can cause teat end damage.

Similar lesions can be caused by too high a vacuum, excessive vacuum fluctuations or simply because the machine is left on too long, that is by overmilking. Immediately after milking you may be able to see the tell-tale white rings at the top of the teats to show that the liners were too tight. If this situation is allowed to continue, the normal smooth end of the teat becomes roughened because the sphincter is being drawn out (plate 7.5 and colour

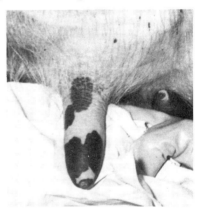

Plate 7.5   An everted teat sphincter, the result of
overmilking or a faulty machine.

plates 9 and 10) and this produces a hard, dry and cracked area around the base of the teat. Not only is this a good site for bacterial multiplication, but it also reduces the defence mechanisms of the teat against penetration by mastitis organisms. If the condition is allowed to develop it may become infected with bacteria such as *Fusiformis species* and it is then known as 'blackspot' (colour plates 11 and 12).

Poorly fitting liners can also be dangerous. If they are too large they may fall off, or they may allow air to suck in, producing teat-end impacts and slow milking. If they are too small, they constrict blood flow and increase teat-end damage. Liners should be soft-mouthed so that they hang on teats of varying sizes without causing problems, and they should be changed regularly. If they are allowed to become old and worn, when air enters the pulsation chamber during the rest or squeeze phase (to restore blood flow—see figure 7.3), the liner slaps against the side of the teat producing pain and teat damage. The pain may reduce let-down and in so doing lead to overmilking and further teat-end damage.

Liners which are cracked and worn are more difficult to clean and are therefore more likely to harbour bacteria and to transmit them from one cow to another. If there is an accumulation of 'milk stone' roughening their inner surface, this can cause teat chaffing and predispose to mastitis.

In summary then, even the normal milking machine is a major factor in transmitting mastitis organisms, but when it is not functioning correctly the risks are considerably greater. The most important features of the machine in relation to causing mastitis are:

1. Teat-end impacts.
2. Vacuum fluctuations.
3. Inadequate claw bleed; small-volume claws.
4. Overmilking; poor pulsation and other factors leading to teat-end damage.
5. Poorly fitting liners; worn and cracked rubbers.

The herdsman should regularly check that the oil level in the vacuum pump is adequate and that the belts are tight; that the vacuum regulator is functioning properly and is regularly cleaned; that all pulsators are operating correctly; and that leaking, cracked and worn rubbers are replaced. A regular, twice-yearly check on machine function, combined with routine maintenance, are essential parts of any mastitis control programme.

Treatment of Cow-to-Cow Transmitted Mastitis

The important points in the treatment of mastitis are: the early detection of clinical cases; the application of the correct antibiotic; continuing its use for the recommended period of time, and discarding contaminated milk. There are approximately sixty different brands of mastitis tubes on the market, many being the same drugs but produced by different manufacturers. The choice of product for your regular use should be a matter of discussion with your veterinary surgeon. He will know the type of problem on your farm and should be able to prescribe a suitable drug, although you will know the products which seem to give a better response. The technique of administering intra-mammary antibiotics is described on page 371. As a general rule, streptococci are always sensitive to penicillin, whereas a proportion of staphylococci will not be, and the synthetic penicillins (e.g. cloxacillin or ampicillin) or antibiotic combinations (e.g. penicillin and streptomycin) may have to be used. However, E. coli, pseudomonas and klebsiella (these organisms are dealt with in the environmental mastitis section) are totally resistant to penicillin, and other drugs such as the tetracyclines, streptomycin or neomycin must be employed. I think it is important to have only one, or at the most two, preparations in routine use on your farm. The initial choice of drug should depend on the results of a bacteriological examination of mastitis samples and the herdsman should routinely take his own milk samples for mastitis. Cleanliness is vital of course, to avoid getting false results. A good routine for milk sampling is as follows.

- Wash and dry the teat.
- Discard the first few squirts of milk: they may contain bacteria which have been growing in the teat sphincter, but which are not causing mastitis.
- Rub the end of the teat fifteen times with a swab soaked in methylated spirits (plate 7.6).
- Only then should you open the sample bottle, keeping the lid facing downwards and the opened bottle almost horizontal. This prevents particles of dust and bacteria dropping into the bottle.
- Finally, with the bottle between the horizontal and 45 degree angle, squirt in one jet of milk and replace the cover immediately (plate 7.7).
- Label the bottle with your name, the identity of the cow, the date and the quarter affected.

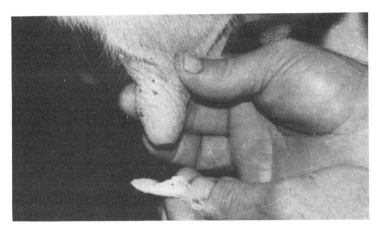

Plate 7.6   Swabbing teat end before taking a milk sample.

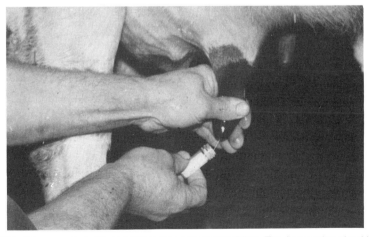

Plate 7.7   The sample bottle is held at an angle during filling. The first squirts should be discarded as they may contain bacteria from within the streak canal.

The sample needs to be taken to the laboratory as soon as is reasonably possible, although a delay of up to twenty-four hours is acceptable, provided that it is stored in a refrigerator. At the laboratory the milk is smeared across a blood agar plate and left to grow in an incubator at 37°C for twenty-four hours. Bacteria can be seen growing as small white clumps and sometimes their appearance alone is sufficient to identify them. Colour plate 4 shows typical colonies of *Staphylococcus aureus*. To confirm their identity, however, they should be stained and examined under a microscope. Antibiotic sensitivity tests are performed by covering a second blood agar plate with a suspension of bacteria and then placing on small paper discs, each impregnated with a different antibiotic. After a further twenty-four hours incubation this second plate is examined. If the bacteria have grown up to the edge of the paper disc, then the antibiotic contained in it is not killing them. If there is a 'zone of growth inhibition' around the disc, however, then that antibiotic *may* be effective for treating the cow. Colour plate 5 shows a typical example. This strain of *Staphylococcus aureus* is sensitive to all drugs tested except penicillin (P 1.5) and ampicillin (PN 2). I said 'may' be effective as a treatment because there are many other factors which can affect its action, such as the ease with which the product can penetrate the udder. Often the small ducts leading to the alveoli (figure 7.1) are blocked with pus and debris and the antibiotic is simply unable to penetrate to the site of the infection. Although the clots disappear, the cow is left with a focus of infection in the udder. She is then a *chronic carrier*, or we may say that she has a *subclinical infection*. This situation is especially common following *Staphylococcus aureus* infection, although it can also occur with *Streptococcus agalactiae* and *dysgalactiae*. Certain strains of staphylococci may even continue to live after they have been engulfed by the neutrophils or macrophages of the udder (see page 164). Whilst inside these cells they are protected from the action of antibiotics. When the macrophage dies, however, the bacteria are released and can start multiplying again. This is another cause of the chronic carrier cow and of mastitis which seems unresponsive to treatment. As we have already seen, subclinically affected cows are a risk to themselves in that the mastitis may recur or spread to another quarter and they are also a danger to the other cows in the herd.

Mastitis Records

I am a firm believer in recording the incidence of all types of disease on a farm but it is particularly important for mastitis. General disease monitoring is discussed on page 237. The type of mastitis recording system is not too important, but you *must* carry out the following procedures.

• Record every case of mastitis, giving the cow, date, quarter affected and tubes used.
• Record repeat treatments, so that chronic carriers are easily identified. Table 7.1 shows two types of recording systems. In the top method it is obvious that cow 42 has had several attacks in the left hind quarter. The

Table 7.1   Two types of mastitis records. The first system most easily identifies the problem cows

Cow	date	quarter	date	quarter	date	quarter	date	quarter
79	22.2.84	LH						
42	25.2.84	LH + RH	3.4.84	LH	15.5.84	LH + RF	23.7.84	LH
83	2.3.84	LF						
14	15.3.84	LF	17.6.84	RF				
27	12.5.84	RH + LH						
176	25.6.84	RH						
9	3.7.84	LF						
17	14.8.84	LH						
101	21.8.84	RH						

cow	date	quarter
79	22.2.84	LH
42	25.2.84	LH + RH
83	2.3.84	LF
42	3.4.84	LH
14	15.3.84	LF
27	12.5.84	LH + RH
42	15.5.84	LH + RF
14	17.6.84	RF
176	25.6.84	RH
9	3.7.84	LF
42	23.7.84	LH
17	14.8.84	LH
101	21.8.84	RH

same information is present on the second chart, but it is by no means so obvious. Even better is to keep records on individual cow cards. The whole lifetime history of the cow is then available, and the information can be used for culling and even selection decisions.

• Periodically analyse the records to calculate your own mastitis performance.

If we define a case of mastitis as one quarter affected once, then I would suggest that you aim to be below the following target figures:

• 25 per cent of the cows affected once or more each year
• thirty-five cases per hundred cows per year
• 4.5 tubes used per case treated.

These figures represent only average performance. Many people can achieve better results than this, although some will be far worse and must put more effort into mastitis control. The data relates to all types of mastitis, of course. It does not only apply to cow-to-cow transmission.

Look through your mastitis records just before drying-off. Cows which have had four cases or more in one quarter in a lactation ought to be culled.

They are likely to have such a deep-seated chronic infection that a cure is impossible and they will remain a risk to others, even after dry-cow therapy. Cows which have had two or more cases could be given a second dry-cow tube into the quarter two to three weeks after the first.

Dry Cow Therapy

Dry cow therapy plays an extremely important role in the control of cow-to-cow transmitted mastitis. Although clots and clinical signs may disappear, probably half the cows treated for mastitis during their lactation remain carriers. This is especially true for staphylococcal infections. In addition there will be a second group of animals which pick up infection but never show any clinical signs—they went straight into the subclinical phase. Both groups provide an important reservoir of infection for the other cows in the herd, and both are best treated during the dry period, when the udder tissue regresses. This is known as *dry cow therapy*. Special long-acting antibiotic preparations can be used because there are no problems with milk-withholding periods. In addition it is a far more effective time for treatment than when the cow is milking. It is an especially important opportunity to eliminate chronic *Staphylococcus aureus* infections and the dry-cow antibiotic used should therefore be chosen with this organism in mind. In addition, many new infections are picked up soon after drying-off and these could cause mastitis either in the dry period or in the next lactation. For example, on one trial at the NIRD, 25 per cent of quarters were infected in cows at drying off. Although 5 per cent of these quarters naturally overcame their infection, another 10 per cent became infected during the dry period, so that at calving 30 per cent of quarters were infected. Dry-cow therapy increases the number of quarters which lose their infection during the dry period and it also reduces the rate at which new infections become established.

There has been a suggestion by some that continued use of dry-cow therapy reduces udder infections to such a low level that it lowers the cow's resistance to E. coli mastitis. This theory has not been conclusively proved either way. It certainly does not seem to be the case as far as results from our own practice is concerned and my advice to the reader would be to continue with dry-cow treatment for all cows. I suspect that the advantages far outweigh the disadvantages. Dry cow therapy is doubly important during July to September, when there is a risk of summer mastitis (see page 189).

Cell Count

Before leaving the subject of contagious mastitis we ought to mention cell counts. When bacteria attack the glands in the alveoli (figures 7.1 and 7.2), cells from the blood (neutrophils) make a counter-attack. Some of the normal udder cells are also shed as a result of the infection. It is these blood cells and udder cells which together lead to an increase in the overall cell count of the milk. Mastitis leads to udder damage and therefore reduced milk production. The figures in table 7.2 produced by the MMB show almost 900 litres per cow difference in production between herds with the lowest and highest cell counts. In addition there will be a significant deterioration in milk solids (see page 156).

Table 7.2. Milk production related to cell count

Annual mean cell count ('000/ml)	Annual average production (litres/cow)	Difference from lowest cell count herds
< 250	4,973	—
250–499	4,782	−191
500–749	4,637	−336
750–999	4,205	−768
> 1,000	4,078	−895

(Source: J. Booth, MMB.)

The cell count is a good guide to the incidence of subclinical mastitis caused by *Staph. aureus*, *Strep. agalactiae* and *Strep. dysgalactiae*, although it is totally unrelated to the incidence of E. coli and other environmental infections. In addition there will be a rise in cell count in late lactation due to cells being shed by normal udder tissue and this is also unrelated to mastitis. Even a single cow with clinical mastitis whose milk unknowingly enters the bulk tank, can produce a significant rise in the overall herd cell count. Results should be interpreted with caution therefore and a rise in the cell count for one month should elicit no action apart from carefully checking for clinical cases while waiting for next month's result to see if the trend continues.

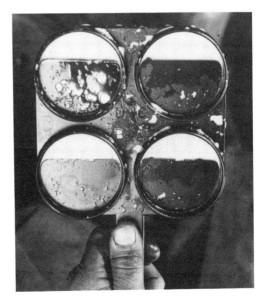

Plate 7.8 The California Mastitis Test, CMT. One squirt of milk from each quarter is delivered into trays A B C + D; an equal volume of reagent is added and the plate is gently rocked. In tray D the mixture has turned gelatinous indicating a high cell count.

If yours is a herd with a high cell count, it may be worthwhile taking individual cow samples in an attempt to identify the chronic carriers—that is, those cows which are acting as the reservoir of infection. An alternative is the *California Mastitis Test* (CMT) or *Whiteside Test* which uses a special chemical to detect milk which has a high cell count (concentrated Dettol is quite effective!). Plate 7.8 shows the CMT being carried out. Milk from each quarter is squirted onto a tray with four separate dishes. An equal volume of reagent is added and the tray is rocked from side to side for mixing. If the milk forms a thick, gelatinous clot, then it has a high cell count. The test is only a guide to the level of subclinical infections, but one survey showed that 85 per cent of positive CMT tests yielded bacteria, whereas only 15 per cent of CMT negative milks were infected. The great advantage of the CMT test is that it is very cheap and easy to perform. Ideally it needs to be done three times at monthly intervals. Cows which show a strong positive each time are chronic carriers.

Environmental Mastitis

So far we have been discussing control measures effective against mastitis transmitted from cow to cow. The other major source of mastitis infection is from the *environment* and the two main bacteria involved are:

- *Streptococcus uberis*: this organism is found in the mouth, vulva, teats and faeces of the cows, as well as the environment. Once away from the animal, it usually dies off fairly rapidly. It is probably the most common cause of environmental mastitis, and the clinical signs are generally less severe than with E. coli.
- *Escherichia coli*: enormous numbers are present in the faeces and pass out to contaminate the environment. Given ideal surroundings (and these are discussed later) they can multiply to even greater concentrations away from the cow. Disease may be severe and even fatal.

Clinical Signs of E. coli Mastitis

Although it is a common belief that E. coli mastitis is a particularly severe condition, in reality it can give rise to a whole range of symptoms. For some cows there may be simply an enlarged and slightly painful quarter with white stringy milk clots. Apart from this, the cow will be eating well and have a normal temperature. At the other extreme, a cow may be normal at one milking but dead from mastitis before the next. The variation in clinical signs is related to the dose of infection received and to the stage of lactation of the cow, and it also depends very much on the response of the udder to the E. coli challenge, as described on page 164. Some cows mount a tremendous cellular (neutrophil) attack on the bacteria, so that within four to six hours of the initial E. coli arriving at the udder, all of them have been killed off. By the time the herdsman sees the affected quarter, even though it may be hard, hot and painful, he is simply dealing with inflammation and healing, and in such cases a milk sample for bacteriology would probably be sterile. At the other extreme, some cows seem unable to produce such a prompt cellular response, and in consequence the E. coli population in the udder reaches very high numbers. In these cows the affected quarter may remain soft and the milk may be only slightly altered (it may simply appear thinner) but the cow herself is very ill. She may be shivering, shaking and scouring before there are any visible changes in the milk, and these more generalised symptoms are the result of toxins released by E. coli. What is considered 'typical' E. coli mastitis is somewhere between these two extremes. The cow has a swollen, hard, hot and painful quarter, she has a raised temperature and is off her food. Within twenty-four hours, and sometimes sooner, the milk changes to a straw-coloured liquid. Antibiotics and other drugs will be needed for the first few days, but there is little point in overtreating. I would certainly recommend discontinuing treatment after five to six days, even if the milk has not returned to normal. A proportion of quarters will be lost for the remainder of the lactation. The cow should not necessarily be culled, however, because the majority of quarters lost from E. coli return to milk at the next lactation. This is in marked contrast to summer mastitis, where lost quarters never recover.

Clinical Signs of Strep. uberis Mastitis

As stated on page 164 it is impossible to identify precisely the type of mastitis on clinical signs alone, although each organism may have a few characteristic features. Strep. uberis often produces a hard, hot swollen quarter and the cow may be dull and off her food for twenty-four hours with a very high temperature, but the more generalised signs of illness seen with E. coli do not occur. Treatment with penicillin is generally very effective, especially in terms of reducing the cow's temperature and restoring her appetite. It may still take several days or even a week before normal milk returns to the affected quarter, however.

Control of Environmental Mastitis

Because the environment is the source of infection, transmission of bacteria by the milker and the milking machine is less important and dry-cow therapy is ineffective as a control measure. Infection enters the teat between milkings and hence control of infection must be based on:

- reducing the challenge of infection from the environment;
- maintaining the natural defence mechanisms of the teat.

These two measures will be considered separately.

Reducing the Challenge from the Environment

The problem starts with the cow's own faeces. Each gram, a quantity no bigger than your little fingernail, contains between one and ten million E. coli bacteria and this figure can be even higher for an early-lactation cow fed on a high-concentrate/low-fibre ration. Systems must therefore be designed and managed so that they result in the minimum contact between the cow's teats and her faeces. This is why environmental mastitis normally declines dramatically in the summer months—the cows are no longer crowded and so there is a reduced risk of faecal contamination.

Some of the factors which can reduce the incidence of environmental contamination and hence E. coli mastitis are as follows. Cubicle passages should be scraped at least twice daily, preferably during milking and before the cows are dispersed. If permitted, cows tend to lie down immediately after milking and if they can walk back along clean passages they are less likely to carry contamination onto the cubicle beds. Ideally they should be excluded from the cubicles until thirty minutes after milking to allow the teat sphincter to close fully. Cubicle beds should also be cleaned. Wet and soiled material should be removed at least twice a day before scraping the passages, then if necessary fresh bedding should be applied before the cows return from milking. Make sure that the cubicle dimensions are correct for the size of your cows, so that they are comfortable and dung in the passage and not on the bed. Although limestone or earth floors are cheaper, I prefer to see a well-laid concrete base with a four-inch even fall from front to back and without a lip at the curb. The choice of bedding material must be a compromise between comfort, cost and hygiene. Sawdust may be a dangerous material to use for bedding, as table 7.3 shows. The coliform levels in the bedding and on the teats were much higher with sawdust than when shavings or straw were used. Other workers have shown that sand as cubicle bedding supports an even lower coliform population, although it may be less comfortable, more abrasive on the teats and can cause problems when handling the slurry. Chopped straw, applied fresh daily with a hand-propelled machine into a lip-less cubicle seems the best alternative. A small quantity of slaked lime sprinkled onto the beds twice weekly acts as a drying agent and a disinfectant. A word of warning, however: the level of E. coli in bedding material is not necessarily related to the degree of visual soiling. Unused sawdust may already contain high E. coli numbers if it has been allowed to get wet. It is the *dampness* of the bed as much as the degree of faecal soiling which affects the overall E. coli numbers, and this is why slaked lime is beneficial. It acts as both a drying agent and a disinfectant. Care is needed, however, because excess lime could damage the teats. Cubicles which have wet and soiled depressions at the rear of the bed are particularly dangerous.

When fresh bedding is added, E. coli numbers rapidly build up to a specific level and then remain constant (unless the bed gets wetter or dirtier) irrespective of how long the cows are housed. The practice of thoroughly clearing out the cubicles and re-bedding them during the winter period has little to recommend it therefore, unless additional efforts are made with regard to cleanliness after the re-bedding. Especially dangerous is the mixture of milk, faeces and bedding which is sometimes seen where the cow has been lying. Milk provides nutrients for E. coli, and the cow's udder warmth, so that bacterial numbers can multiply to very high levels, for example one thousand million E. coli per gram ($1,000 \times 10^6$) in the very area where the cow's teats

Table 7.3   The coliform populations supported by different types of bedding, and their effect on the coliform numbers obtained as a teat swab

	Total coliform count in cubicle bedding	Mean No. of coliforms obtained from a teat swab
sawdust	52.0×10^6	127
shavings	6.6×10^6	12
straw	3.1×10^6	8

(Rendos, Eberhart & Kesler J Dairy Sci 58 1492)

are lying. This is at least one hundred times higher than the level found in faeces, and twenty times higher than the levels shown for sawdust in table 7.3. As early-lactation cows are not only the most susceptible to E. coli mastitis but they also have the highest faecal E. coli levels and are the animals most likely to be leaking milk, it is a good idea to keep them in a separate group. They can then have their cubicles cleaned and re-bedded at least once a day and the passages scraped twice daily.

Overcrowding should be avoided. Cows which are packed together, rushed through passageways or simply have inadequate space are more likely to get faecal contamination of the teat ends. Overcrowding can also lead to inadequate ventilation and increased humidity, both of which may predispose towards a build-up of E. coli. Calving boxes should be kept as clean as possible. The dry cow is almost completely resistant to E. coli infection, but this changes abruptly at calving when she reaches her most susceptible stage. Cleanliness in calving boxes is therefore essential and, if faced with a severe outbreak of down-calving mastitis, consider calving outdoors. Many farms have inadequate calving facilities, and the practice of a single calving yard, used by the whole herd during the calving season, should be discouraged. Ideally each cow should have its own box, where the straw bedding should be kept meticulously clean and dry (see also page 98). The shorter the period of winter housing the less will be the risk of E. coli mastitis. There are more outbreaks of environmental mastitis, and often of greater severity, if October and November are warm and humid and this is particularly so in cows which have already been housed since August.

Teat Defences against Environmental Mastitis

The mechanisms were described on page 162. Research has shown that the cow is most susceptible to infection in the first hour after milking: figure 7.6 shows the effects of wiping a culture of E. coli across the teat sphincter. Immediately after the end of milking, 35 per cent of quarters developed mastitis, whereas this fell to only 5 per cent if the culture was applied to the teat end within an hour of the next milking. The practical implication of this is to try to keep cows clean *and* on their feet for at least thirty minutes after milking. This can be done by shutting them away from the cubicles, or by providing them with a fresh feed as they leave the parlour. Some cows will

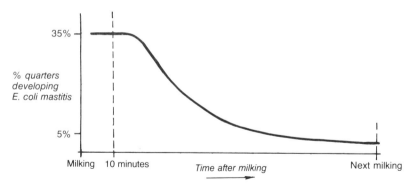

Figure 7.6   The importance of teat sphincter closure and E. coli mastitis. Thirty-five per cent of the teats which were exposed to a culture of E. coli in the first ten minutes after milking developed mastitis, whereas this fell to only 5 per cent immediately before the next milking.

have just taken a large concentrate intake, however, and will not want to eat anything further.

Current teat dips persist for two to three hours and as such they will give some protection during this critical phase of post-milking challenge. Newer products are being tested which may give full bacteriological cover for the whole of the period between milkings, however, and if they prove successful they could be a significant advance in the control of environmental mastitis.

The milking machine can reduce the effectiveness of the teat-end barrier and hence predispose to environmental mastitis. Overmilking, excessive vacuum fluctuations and the other factors described on page 175 cause eversion and damage to the teat sphincter (see plate 7.5), and this reduces its resistance to E. coli challenge. Cows in early lactation have a higher incidence of sphincter damage, and this suggests that it is at least partly dependent on the level of production. Combined with the high coliform count of their faeces, it puts this group particularly at risk. One survey showed that cows with pointed teats were almost twice as likely to develop teat orifice damage as cows in the same herd with round or flat teat ends, although there was no difference recorded in the incidence of mastitis between the two groups. General hygiene is important: if the liners are so dirty that they are con-taminated with environmental organisms, then impacts (described on page 172) can force E. coli up into the teat ends. Similarly if cows have to be washed, running water containing a disinfectant should be used and it is *essential* that the teats are wiped dry before applying the machine; that droplet of dirty water at the teat end could be teeming with bacteria. Provided that the teats are not grossly soiled, the risk of mastitis is reduced if teats are dry wiped and not washed. Any unhygienic milking practice leading to faecal contamination of the teats will increase the risk of environmental mastitis.

The final teat factor to be considered is the natural design of the sphincter itself. When called to treat severely ill cases of down-calving mastitis I have always felt that there is a certain type of cow—a very easy milker with an open teat end—that is most often affected and research has shown that there is a relationship between peak milk flow rate and susceptibility to mastitis. Other cases of genetic susceptibility were described on page 164. Unfortunately speed of milking has many advantages, probably sufficient to outweigh the disadvantages of an increased risk of environmental mastitis.

I have dealt with the causes of mastitis and their control at some length. You will note that all control measures are aimed at reducing the exposure of the udder to infection—even to the extreme of removing potential carriers from the herd. Mastitis should be considered as a herd problem and not a condition of individual cows. This is why the keeping of records and their analysis to produce objective data for the incidence of disease is so important.

The following series of headings is a summary of the chapter so far:

Clinical Mastitis

(1) *Contagious = cow-to-cow transmitted*: Staph.; Streps. agalactiae and dysgalactiae
(2) *Environmental*: E. coli; Strep. uberis

Control of contagious mastitis
1. Good udder preparation and maintain healthy teats.
2. Proper machine function
   —large volume claws with air-bleeds.
   —correct pulsation.
   —soft and uncracked liners.
   —avoid vacuum fluctuations.
   —teat shields or ball-valve claws.
3. Early detection and thorough treatment of clinical cases.
4. Teat disinfection.
5. Dry-cow therapy.
6. Cull persistent offenders.

Control of environmental mastitis
1. Dry teats which have been washed.
2. Strict hygiene with bedding.
3. Keep faecal contamination of the teats and environment low.
4. Maintain healthy teat end defences by correct machine function and use.
5. Teat disinfection.

Antibiotic Residues in Milk

One of the more expensive aspects of mastitis is the milk which has to be discarded from cows under treatment. There are several reasons why milk contaminated with antibiotic should not be sold. These are:

1. *Public Health.* Some people are allergic to antibiotics, especially the penicillins, and even fatalities have been known to occur. If, in this health-

conscious age, milk gains a public reputation for containing antibiotics, liquid sales could decline quite rapidly.
2. *Interference with manufacturing.* Antibiotics can destroy the bacterial cultures used in yoghurt and cheese manufacture.
3. *Legality.* It is a contravention of both the MMB contract and the Milk and Dairies Regulations to sell contaminated milk.

From October 1982 all farms have had their milk tested at least once each week, and the test, which is based on adding milk to a culture of antibiotic-sensitive bacteria, can detect levels down to 0.02 units of penicillin per 1.0 ml of milk. Other types of antibiotics (e.g. neomycin) and certain sulphonamides are less easily detected. Most test failures are simply due to not discarding the milk for the recommended length of time following intramammary antibiotic treatment. This may be deliberate or accidental, for example cows under treatment were not easily or accurately identified, or inadequate records meant that the herdsman or the relief milker was not sure when he could start to re-use milk from a treated cow. Ideally mastitis cows should be milked after the rest of the herd. Not only does this mean that they will not be spreading infection to others, but it also reduces the risk of accidental transfer of contaminated milk into the bulk tank. An alternative is to have a separate cluster fitted onto a bucket or a churn which is kept in the pit. The cluster can be left soaking in disinfectant between mastitic cows, and this prevents the spread of mastitis as well as ensuring that all antibiotic milk is discarded. If cows under treatment do have to be milked into the jars during the middle of milking, the jars should be drained and then rinsed with clean water before continuing onto the next cow. Even then, leaking fittings could allow enough antibiotic milk into the bulk tank to lead to a test failure.

The other common reason suspected for test failures stems from dry-cow therapy. The contract with the MMB states that milk should be withheld for the first four days after calving, and if this is not done there is a risk of

Table 7.4 Reasons suggested for antibiotic test failures

Reason	Percentage
Poor records or none	32
Not withholding milk for the full period	32
Calving early/short dry period	15
Accidental transfer of milk	14
Prolonged excretion	12
Contamination of recorder jars	9
Withholding milk from treated quarters only	8
Lack of advice on withholding period	6
Mechanical failure	6
Recently purchased cows	3
Milking through jars	1
Use of dry-cow preparation during lactation	1

(Survey of farmers in 1981. Source: J. Booth, *In Practice*, July 1982.)

antibiotic contamination. Cows which calve early pose a particular problem especially if dry-cow therapy has been administered in the preceding four weeks. Table 7.4 shows a list of reasons suggested by farmers as to why their milk had failed the test. The figures add up to more than 100 per cent because several farmers gave more than one reason for a test failure. Poor records and inadequate withholding periods seem to be the main causes. Although withholding milk from treated quarters only was given as a reason for eight failures, it seems unlikely that sufficient antibiotic could diffuse from one quarter to another to lead to significant contamination of the bulk milk, and some other cause is more probable. There is slightly more antibiotic diffusing to the quarter on the same side than to the quarters on the other side, but either way the amounts are minimal. The terms of the MMB contract state that all milk should be discarded from a cow under any form of antibiotic or oestrogen therapy, however.

Summer Mastitis

This is a condition seen especially in pregnant cows and heifers, although it can also occur in non-pregnant animals, young calves and occasionally even in steers. The first sign that something is wrong may be that the animal is standing apart from the others and perhaps she is walking rather stiffly. Careful examination of the udder shows that one or more of the quarters is hard, hot, swollen and, especially in a heifer, it will be very painful, so take care when handling her. If milked, a yellow, custardy material is produced which normally has a foul smell, although the absence of the smell does not completely rule out summer mastitis. Another characteristic, and one which is often not mentioned, is that the teat sinus becomes thickened. Squeeze and roll one of the other teats between your thumb and forefinger: you will find it feels soft and empty. In the quarter affected by summer mastitis the teat seems thicker, as if it has a fibrous cord through the teat cistern. Only heifers are affected in this way. Sometimes heifers calving down with a blind quarter have a similar thickening of the teat and I suspect that these have had a low-grade summer mastitis which was not detected (see page 134 for a further discussion of blind quarters). In the early stages the affected animal will be running a high temperature, due to septicaemia and toxaemia. Untreated cases may abort or even die, while others may develop a permanent arthritis from infection localising in the joints. Recently it has been shown that even if calves are born alive they will probably be stunted and have a reduced viability.

The cause of summer mastitis
There are four bacteria involved:

- *Corynebacterium pyogenes* (78%)
- *Streptococcus dysgalactiae* (17%)
- *Peptococcus indolicus* (85%)
- A micrococcus (74%).

The percentages express the number of times each organism has been found associated with summer mastitis (J. Bramley, personal communication). Pure cultures of any one of these bacteria applied to the teat end will not produce disease, but mixed cultures will, especially using Peptococcus and C. pyogenes. Infection is transferred to the teat end by females of the sucking fly *Hydrotaea irritans*, also known as the sheep head-fly. H. irritans lives near woods, small copses and around wet, boggy ground. Immature flies overwinter in the soil, and the adults roost in trees and bushes from where they fly out to feed. There is only one generation of adults each year and they are found during July, August and September. These are therefore the three worst months for summer mastitis and disease occurs most commonly when the weather is warm and humid, with humidity being the most important factor. This is because high winds (above 20 km per hour) and heavy rain inhibit the activity of the flies. Although it carries infection, H. irritans probably cannot cause disease on its own. There must first be damage to the end of the teat, either by biting flies, or by the cow walking over sharp grass, thistles or thorns, or even by licking her own teats excessively. H. irritans then comes to feed on the small drops of blood or serum which are oozing from the tip of the teat and in so doing transmits summer mastitis infection.

Treatment
Unfortunately, by the time summer mastitis has been noticed, the quarter has usually already been lost and treatment is mainly aimed at reducing the illness in the animal, thereby preventing abortion. Occasional quarters do recover, however, especially if the cow or heifer calves soon after. Your vet will probably use penicillin, given both by injection and as tubes in to the quarter, although some say that it is pointless applying any intramammary treatment. Summer mastitis is effectively an abscess in the udder and, as such, *drainage* is vital. It is best achieved by regular stripping until the quarter dries up, although this can take several weeks and may be painful to the animal so some farmers prefer to have the end of the teat amputated to allow natural drainage.

Prevention of summer mastitis
Prevention consists of two parts, firstly dry-cow therapy and secondly fly control. Dry-cow antibiotic gives good protection, but it persists for only three weeks, so a second or even third infusion may be necessary for cows with a long dry period. However, with such cows additional care needs to be taken to avoid antibiotic contamination of the milk after calving. Dry-cow tubes can also be given to heifers, especially if they are 'bagging up' although they again need to be at least four weeks before calving to avoid antibiotic problems. The only difference in technique is that the tip of the dry cow tube is placed against the outside of the heifer's teat sphincter, rather than through the streak canal as you would normally do for a cow. For both cows and heifers it is essential to clean the end of the teat first, so as to avoid introducing other infections.

Fly control
In dairy herds fly control has several advantages in addition to summer

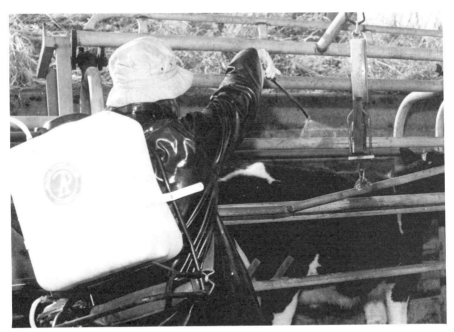

Plate 7.9 Fly spray applied with a knapsack-spray.

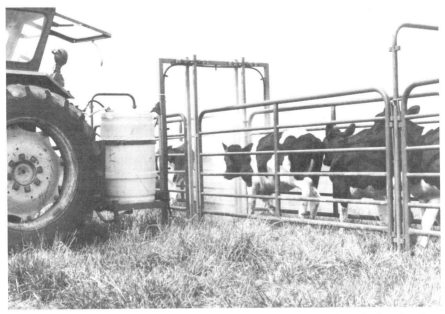

Plate 7.10 A spray race. Because cattle rush through, there is a tendency for less than the recommended amount to be applied.

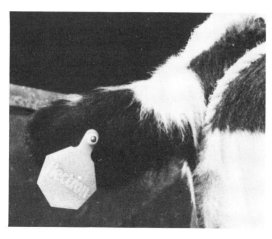

Plate 7.11   Flectron ear tag. It is impregnated with the insecticide cypermethrin which slowly dissolves in the sebum on the animal's skin and then flows over its body.

mastitis prevention. If the cows are irritated by flies they tend to bunch together in the shade rather than graze and this will reduce their milk production. They may be restless when being milked and perhaps kick off the clusters, or, even worse, they can tear their teats when kicking at flies. This is particularly common in older cows with pendulous udders close to calving, because there is often a drip of colostrum on the end of the teat which attracts the flies. In heifers fly control is an important preventive measure against New Forest Eye.

There are now several chemicals on the market which claim to give protection against flies for two, three or even four weeks. They can be applied by knapsack sprayer (plate 7.9) or using a spray race (plate 7.10) although it can be difficult to get the manufacturer's recommended dose to stay on the animal. Alternatively you can use a large plastic ear tag (plate 7.11) which has been impregnated with an insecticide (cypermethrin in 'Flectron' tags and fenvalerate in 'Tirade' tags). As the animals groom themselves they wipe the tag across their coat and the natural oils in the skin (the sebum) dissolve the cypermethrin, to give a complete body covering. There is a flow of body oil passing over the skin of the animal, especially from the shoulder backwards, and a complete coating of insecticide is achieved within twelve hours of applying the tag. Unfortunately this flow of sebum does not continue onto the teats, and this is probably one reason why experience with the tags has shown that they reduce fly numbers but do not control them totally and some cases of summer mastitis will still occur, even when a tag is used in each ear. One of the best methods of fly control for summer mastitis and certainly the cheapest is to use a persistent insecticide contained in a thick jelly (Rycopel Ltd). It has to be smeared onto the udder every two weeks, but it is easily applied once the heifers or cows have been rounded up.

The favourite landing place for H. irritans is along the animal's abdomen and on its udder, so this is the important area to cover with fly repellant. It is simply not sufficient to spray insecticide over their backs and then feel pleased that fewer flies are seen on their heads and shoulders. The fly is attracted by any discharge and very large numbers will be seen on the end of an affected teat. It is important that animals with summer mastitis are removed from the remainder of the group, therefore, because they will be acting as a reservoir of infection for the others.

Finally, try to avoid grazing heifers and dry cows near woody or wet areas during the summer months. If you have had a bad outbreak of summer mastitis in a particular field in one year, you know it must be a good breeding place for H. irritans and should therefore be avoided in future years.

Uncommon Causes of Mastitis

We have dealt with the common causes of mastitis and their control, but there are a few odd infections which may not fit into the standard pattern. A word of warning however: by definition these infections are not particularly common and if you have a difficult mastitis problem in your herd it is more likely that environmental organisms or cow-to-cow transmission is involved. I will list the names of the unusual infections and give a few notes on their significance.

Corynebacterium bovis, Staphylococcus epidermidis and micrococci
These three can be dealt with in one group. They rarely cause clots or any other clinical signs, but they can lead to a high cell count. They are controlled by teat-dipping and dry-cow therapy.

Mycoplasma
This mastitis usually leads to a hard, hot quarter and flocculent changes in the milk, although some cows may show virtually no symptoms at all and act as carriers. Because it is not a true bacterial infection, normal antibiotics are ineffective in treatment and the mastitis may remain for a week or more. (Mycoplasmas are closely related to bacteria however, and certain drugs, e.g. erythromycin, tylosin or spectinomycin, may help in treatment.) Some cows recover on their own, while others have to be culled. Mycoplasmas can also cause inflammation and swelling of the joints leading to acute lameness. The fetlocks are commonly affected. Lameness and mastitis are not necessarily seen in any one herd at the same time.

Yeasts
Yeasts are another group of non-bacterial infections which can cause mastitis. They produce changes similar to Mycoplasma, although the cow invariably has a significantly raised temperature. Yeasts are common in the environment, and this is the source of infection. They are totally unresponsive to antibiotics, and iodine therapy may be needed for treatment. They may even be introduced when infusing intramammary antibiotic against a normal bacterial mastitis if careful aseptic precautions are not used.

Leptospira hardjo (the cause of leptospirosis)
Leptospirosis causes a rise in temperature, the cow may be off her food and the small amount of milk present is rather thick, almost like colostrum. One of

the most prominent clinical signs is the sudden and massive drop in yield and hence the names 'milk drop syndrome' or 'flabby bag' are sometimes used. Treatment with streptomycin is generally effective, although the cow may take several days to recover. There is now a good vaccine available against *Leptospira hardjo* and you should ask your vet if it is worthwhile or cost-effective for your herd. The disease is dealt with in more detail in Chapter Twelve (page 341).

Pseudomonas

Pseudomonas normally leads to a slightly thickened quarter and white 'lumpy' clots in the milk which would be indistinguishable from staphylococcal/ streptococcal infections. The bacteria grow *inside* the udder cells however and this largely protects them from the action of antibiotics which tend to be mainly in the extra-cellular fluid surrounding the tissues and only reach low concentrations inside the cells. Response to treatment is therefore very poor. Many cases continue for days or weeks, or they may appear to recover but then recur a few days later. Pseudomonas can grow in the header tank which feeds the udder-washing equipment and also in improperly cleaned milking machines. These are the most probable sources of infection where no antiseptic is being used, or if the plant-cleaning routine is inadequate. In freshly calved cows Pseudomonas can cause a very severe or even fatal mastitis and the symptoms of this are identical to an acute E. coli infection (described on page 182).

Klebsiella

This organism also causes a very severe mastitis, with udder changes similar to those caused by E. coli in the fresh calver. Treatment is often unsuccessful. The infection is associated with sawdust as a cubicle bedding, especially if the sawdust was damp and heated up before it was used.

Bacillus cereus

Another organism which can produce a whole range of clinical signs. The commonest is a mild hardening of the quarter, with thin milk and very small clots. However, it can sometimes cause an acute *gangrenous mastitis*: the skin over the affected quarter turns blue and feels cold, the milk changes to a thin, port-coloured liquid, sometimes mixed with gas, and the cow is desperately ill. Even if she recovers from this onslaught, the whole of the quarter may slowly fall off over the next one or two months, leaving a festering sore. In my opinion such cases are best culled as soon as they are diagnosed. A specific strain of *Staphylococcus aureus* can also cause gangrenous mastitis. *Bacillus cereus* is found in dust and outbreaks have also been associated with feeding brewer's grains.

DISEASES OF THE TEAT

We defined mastitis as an infection of the udder. In addition there are a few conditions of the teat which are worthy of note, some being infections and others simply physical damage.

Pseudocowpox

This is a paravaccinia virus infection and probably the commonest teat lesion seen in cows. It is usually seen as a circle of small haemorrhagic spots or scabs, often with normal skin in the centre (colour plate 6), although some- times the blister which precedes this may be noticed. Being a virus infection, there is no specific treatment, although teat dip will help to prevent secondary bacterial infection and if mixed with an emollient it will promote healing. Hypochlorite also has a non-specific viral-killing action if in direct contact with the virus, although of course it is difficult to use with emollients (see page 170). If you have a severe outbreak you would be wise to milk the affected cows last to reduce the rate of spread of infection. Usually there are only a few cases in each herd however, often in recently introduced heifers, because these have little or no immunity. Immunity to pseudocowpox is relatively short-lived anyway, and because of this some herds may experience waves of infection and disease every six to twelve months. Gloves should be worn to prevent the development of *milkers' nodules*, small warts on your hands and fingers which are caused by the virus. The virus is also closely related, if not identical to, the Orf virus which causes scabs on the lips and nose of sheep and which can also affect man.

Bovine Herpes Mammillitis

This is another virus infection, but fortunately much less common because the disease is very severe. Large and very painful blisters develop on the teat and they may be so sore that milking is virtually impossible. When the blisters burst, a raw scabby area is exposed (colour plate 7) and this may take two or three weeks to heal. Cannulas may have to be used for milking. Heifers are most susceptible, and even the skin of the udder may be affected. At this stage it looks similar to a severe photosensitisation, but affecting only the teats and sometimes the skin of the udder. I have known freshly calved heifers to be so badly affected that they have had to be culled because they were impossible to milk. Luckily immunity is good, lasting four or five years and herd outbreaks are relatively rare. Teat dipping and separation of affected animals are the only useful control measures.

Teat Warts

This is the third virus infection and again it is heifers which are by far the worst affected, this time yearlings and in-calvers. Warts may appear as fleshy lumps or they may be of the feathery type. Both are shown in plate 7.12. Feathery warts are the easiest to deal with because most of them can be quite easily pulled off and the teat dressed with an antiseptic cream or teat dip. With either type of wart you could ask your vet to send a specimen to a laboratory to have an *autogenous vaccine* prepared. The vaccine, which can be injected either into or under the skin (i.e. intradermally or subcutaneously), is probably only 30 per cent effective, but sometimes heifers are so severely

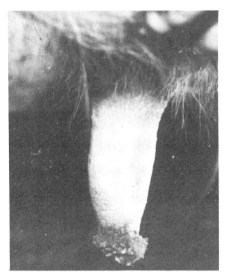

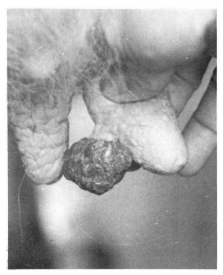

Plate 7.12(a)   The 'feathery' type of teat
wart which can easily be pulled off if the root
is small enough.

Plate 7.12(b)   The 'fleshy' type of teat wart.

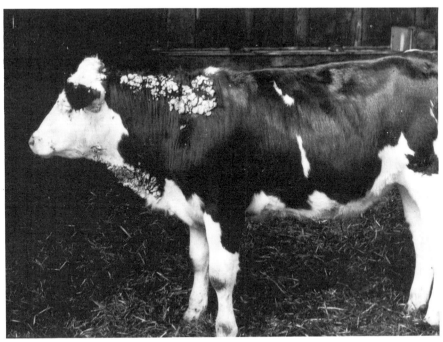

Plate 7.13   Warts on the head and neck. These normally disappear spontaneously, but
vaccines can be used.

affected that any help is welcome. The virus is thought to be transmitted by flies, so attention to fly control (described on page 190) is important. Warts may spread all over the body, with the head, neck and belly being particularly badly affected (plate 7.13). They occur mainly in 1–2 year old cattle and most cases spontaneously recover during the next summer at grazing. If they become so large that they ulcerate and develop a secondary bacterial infection, a vaccine can be prepared and this is much more effective than vaccines against teat warts.

Teat Chaps

This is the name given to cracks and splits in the teat skin. Typical examples are seen in colour plate 8. They become infected with bacteria which makes them sore, and of course they act as reservoirs of infection of the mastitis organisms *Staphylococcus aureus* and *Streptococcus dysgalactiae* (see page 166). The best treatment is teat dip or an ointment which has both antiseptic and emollient properties. Chaps occur particularly in the spring and autumn, when cows have to walk through muddy gateways and when there are cold winds. Teat skin does not have the sebaceous glands found elsewhere in the body. This means that when dry, the normal pliable and elastic properties of the skin are soon lost, its keratin layer cracks, and chaps soon form.

Milking Machine Damage

A faulty machine can interfere with the blood supply to the teat during milking and this leads to cracks and chaps. Excessive vacuum fluctuations and overmilking may also produce prolapse of the teat sphincter, as shown in plate 7.5 and colour plates 9 and 10.

Blackspot

This is the name given to a lump of proud flesh which develops on the end of the teat and interferes with milking (colour plate 11). There is no single specific cause, but it is most probably the result of a combination of machine damage (see also page 175), possibly chilling of the teats from bad weather and a secondary infection with the bacterium *Fusiformis necrophorus* (which also causes foul of the foot). Teat dipping and antiseptic ointments are the best treatment and sometimes the teat has to be rested, by letting the milk flow through a cannula. Colour plate 12 shows a teat at the healing stage.

Cut Teats

Sometimes herds experience 'outbreaks' of deep gashes into their teats. The cut tends to run half-way round the teat or more; it is at the lower end towards the sphincter and it may penetrate into the canal. A typical example is shown in plate 7.14 and I know that the sight of this fills any herdsman with gloom. You will obviously need your vet to attend to the damage, but it may be worth

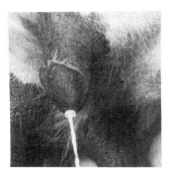

Plate 7.14 Typical cut teat. A cannula allows the milk to run, but it increases the risk of mastitis. This wound would probably be best dealt with by anaesthetising the teat, amputating the loose flap of skin with scissors and then milking the cow normally without a cannula.

looking at a few of the possible causes. The cut is most probably caused by the teat being stepped on, either by the cow itself, or by another cow. To try to prevent further cases you should look at possible overcrowding, cows being rushed about, poor cubicle design, insufficient cubicle numbers, inadequate dunging passage width and slippery floors. It is also possible that you have a high proportion of older cows with pendulous udders, where the teats are more at risk.

TOTAL BACTERIAL COUNT OF MILK (TBC)

Whereas *cell count* measures the number of cells in the milk and is used as an indicator of the degree of subclinical mastitis, the Total Bacterial Count (TBC) is a measure of the number of bacteria present. Bacteria in the milk come from either the cow or the milking equipment. If they originate from the cow, they will either be associated with mastitis (and hence there is some relationship between TBC and cell count), or will have come from the outside of the teat. Teat chaps and the other lesions described on page 197 will all increase the TBC, as will washing the teat without wiping it afterwards. The use of an antiseptic in the udder wash is important in reducing the TBC as well as being a mastitis control measure, although avoiding washing is probably the best answer for both conditions. The clay-type of mud from gateways and kale fields contains relatively few bacteria, and if possible should be removed by dry wiping rather than washing.

Bacteria occur in the plant because the cleaning system is inadequate and this may happen particularly if there are any blind ends, cracked rubbers or other areas which can harbour infection, or it may be simply that you have increased the size of your parlour but kept the original cleaning system, and there is now an inadequate supply of hot water to sterilise the whole plant. Your local Dairy Husbandry Adviser will be able to check these points with you. General hygiene in the parlour is important. If the equipment gets dusty between milkings or, even worse, if faeces are splashed into the teat cups, then this is bound to raise the TBC. Bacteria multiply very quickly at warm temperatures and so the sooner the milk is brought down to 4°C the better. Plate coolers may be an advantage in reducing the TBC for this reason, although of course it is far more logical to identify the source of the bacteria and deal with the problem that way.

Milk from a cow with streptococcal mastitis can be teeming with bacteria and if this is allowed into the bulk tank it will significantly raise the herd TBC. For example, if the milk from one cow with an active case of streptococcal mastitis is allowed into the bulk milk of one hundred others, this alone is sufficient to raise the TBC from 10,000 to 70,000 per ml. This is by far the most common cause of a sudden increase in the TBC which returns to normal by the next test. It is also a disadvantage of the in-line mastitis detectors (plate 7.3) since infected milk may have already reached the bulk tank before the mastitis is recognised.

In 1982 a system of milk payments based on the TBC was introduced. This resulted in a sharp fall in the average TBC for the national herd, and as many of the measures to maintain a low TBC will also help in mastitis control, perhaps payment for TBC will provide an incentive to indirectly reduce mastitis incidence in the future.

Chapter 8

FERTILITY AND ITS CONTROL

AFTER FEEDING, fertility is the factor which has the greatest effect on the economics of dairy farming. Maintenance of good fertility is to a large extent governed by management, and this means that the individual farmer or herdsman has a very important part to play in its control. First let us look at the economics. The *calving interval*, the overall measure of herd fertility, is the period between one calving and the next and should be 365 days, that is exactly one year. At 1985 values, agricultural economists quoted a loss of more than £2.00 per cow for each **day** that the calving interval is extended beyond 365 days. Figures such as these, quoted in abstract, often have relatively little meaning, however, and the following gives an idea of how the amount is calculated.

The example is based on 1985 figures, so I would urge the reader to insert current-day values to calculate a more accurate cost. Take a rather mediocre cow giving a 305-day lactation of 5,470 litres, with a calving interval of 365 days. Averaged out to include a 60-day dry period, this gives her a potential milk production of 5,470 ÷ 365 = 15 litres per day. Other assumptions are:

1. a milk price of 14p/litre;
2. a concentrate price of £150 per ton (15p per kg);
3. high-level concentrate use, e.g. 0.4 kg/litre over the whole year;
4. a calf value of £73.00 (20p per day [£73.00 ÷ 365]).

At this level of concentrate use (0.4 kg/litre) and concentrate price (15p/kg), it can be seen that the concentrate cost to produce one litre of milk is $0.4 \times 15 = 6.0$p. The margin of milk over concentrate is therefore $14.0 - 6.0 = 8.0$p per litre (milk price minus concentrate cost equals margin). Our simplified example assumes that the maintenance costs and overheads of the cow—grazing, forage, labour, etc.—will remain constant whether or not she is pregnant and that the profit comes from milk production. Every day over 365 days that she does not become pregnant is therefore a day of lost production—in our example a loss of:

15 litres/day at a margin of 8p/litre
$= 15 \times 8$
$= 120$p per day *lost*.

Even the calf is worth 20p per day (£73 ÷ 365) over the year, so the overall cost is 120 + 20 = 140p per cow per day lost. In practical terms, an individual cow loses time in three-week cycles from a missed heat or a failure of conception, hence—

Cost of 21-day cycle = 21 × 140p
= £29.40.

This figure is much lower than the true value of £2.00 per cow (£42.00 per cycle) per day quoted earlier, because it does not include the additional costs of disturbance of the calving pattern, higher replacement rates and other factors. As well as inserting present-day figures for milk price, concentrate costs and calf value, I would also urge the reader to try different levels of yield. A cow giving 8,205 litres in her 305-day lactation, for example, could be losing a potential margin of 210p per day, or £44.10 per 21-day cycle, at 1985 values. There is a tendency by some to allow high-yielding cows a longer calving interval because, it is said, they are milking so well that you will never get them in calf and anyway they will keep producing at a high level later in lactation. This is a fallacy. As figure 8.1 shows, most milk is given at peak lactation and a cow which has two 'peaks' over an 18-month period will perform much better than a cow which was left unserved because she was a high yielder. This is an extreme example, but it illustrates the point very well.

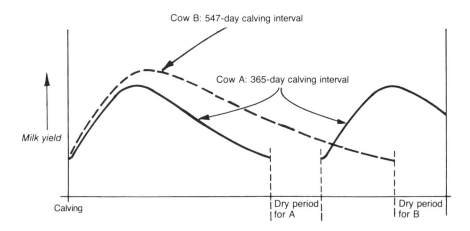

Figure 8.1   The effects of calving interval on milk yield. Cow A had a 365-day calving interval and therefore achieved two peak yields in an 18-month period. Although cow B peaked at a higher level and milked extremely well, her overall milk production was lower.

THE COMPONENTS OF THE CALVING INTERVAL

The calving interval is defined as the period between one calving and the next and it is the overall measure of fertility status. There are several distinct stages however and these need to be identified before we can discuss the factors affecting fertility.

Take calving as the starting point. After calving the cow must overcome any uterine infections. She must then begin her ovarian cycles, to come on heat and ovulate every 21 days, and she must cycle regularly without any abnormalities. In a herd using artificial insemination she has to be *seen* to be bulling so that she may be presented for AI, and this is known as *heat detection*. After service the egg must be fertilised and then the developing embryo must attach itself or *implant*, onto the wall of the uterus. These two processes of fertilisation and implantation, are together known as conception. Good conception rates, that is avoiding large numbers of repeat services, are very important in fertility control. Once the foetus has become established in the uterus, there is still the possibility of early foetal death or, at a later stage, abortion, which is defined as the premature expulsion of the calf. If all these hurdles can be overcome, then birth occurs and the calving interval has been established. In summary then, the determinants of the calving interval are:

1. Elimination of uterine infection.
2. Commencement of regular oestrous cycles after calving.
3. Visual observation of oestrus, that is heat detection.
4. The combined effects of fertilisation and implantation to give conception.
5. Avoiding early foetal death.
6. The production of a full-term calf, that is without abortion.

Each of these factors will be dealt with in detail later in the chapter, but to enable a better understanding of the processes involved, I would first like to explain some of the physical and hormonal changes associated with the oestrous cycle.

THE OESTROUS CYCLE

This is the name given to the sequence of physical and hormonal events which culminate in the behavioural signs of the cow being 'on heat' or 'on bulling', or 'in oestrus', approximately every three weeks. *Puberty* is the age at which an animal becomes sexually mature; that is, when oestrous cycles begin. In heifers the onset of puberty can vary from as little as six to as much as eighteen months old, with nutrition being the biggest single determining factor.

Figure 8.2 gives the basic anatomy of the cow's reproductive tract and this was described in detail on page 94. At birth, the ovary contains all the eggs the cow will need for her reproductive life (some 75,000 eggs are present in each ovary!) and from puberty onwards one egg is passed down into the uterus every 21 days, interrupted only by pregnancy and a short period of

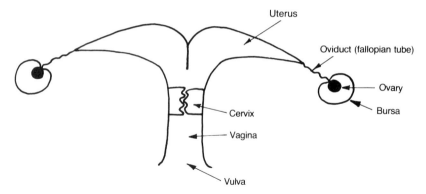

Figure 8.2   The reproductive tract of the cow.

ovarian inactivity in early lactation. When it is ready to be shed, the egg is contained in a small fluid-filled sac on the surface of the ovary called a *follicle*.

At the end of oestrus the follicle bursts and releases the egg into the oviduct. This is known as ovulation (see figure 8.3). The egg then passes down to the junction of the oviduct and uterus, and this is the point where fertilisation may take place.

Immediately after ovulation, glandular tissue begins to form in the base of the ruptured follicle and it grows until there is a mass protruding from the surface of the ovary called the corpus luteum. It is sometimes known as the 'yellow body' because of its colour, or simply abbreviated as 'the corp' and is clearly seen in plate 5.1. This structure can be felt from day four or five onwards, and it is what your veterinary surgeon is feeling for when he is assessing whether or not a cow is cycling. From its shape and size he will also

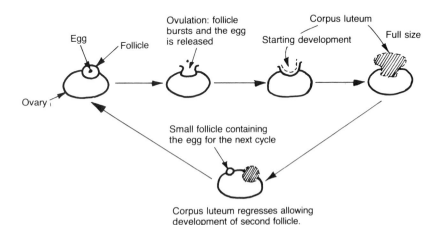

Figure 8.3   Changes in the ovary during the oestrous cycle.

be able to give you some idea of how many days past the previous bulling the cow is at the time of examination and this will help you to know when to watch for her next heat. If the cow conceives, the corpus luteum remains in the ovary for the whole of pregnancy. However, if she does not conceive it decreases in size from day 16 onwards and this allows the development of a second follicle.

As the follicle expands and matures in preparation for ovulation, it produces increased quantities of the hormone *oestrogen*. It is the action of oestrogen in the body which causes the physical changes associated with oestrus including, for example, enlargement of the vulva, passage of the 'bulling slime' and, of course, mounting behaviour.

A few days after ovulation, the corpus luteum begins to produce the hormone *progesterone* and this has almost the opposite effect. It suppresses the signs of heat and it prepares the uterus to accept a fertilised egg, now known as the developing ovum. If fertilisation has occurred, the ovum will begin to attach itself to the wall of the uterus twelve to fifteen days after ovulation. This process is known as implantation and although it is not completed for another twenty days, the placenta is already forming and pregnancy is established. The corpus luteum remains in the ovary throughout pregnancy and continues to produce progesterone, some of which passes via

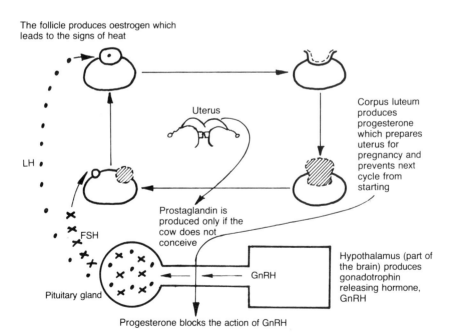

Figure 8.4 Hormonal changes during the oestrous cycle.

the blood to the brain and prevents the start of a new ovarian cycle. The hormonal changes are shown diagrammatically in figure 8.4. Two of the hormones responsible for the initiation of ovarian cycles are:

> *Follicle stimulating hormone*   *FSH*
> *Luteinising hormone*   *LH*

They are shown as crosses and dots respectively in figure 8.4. Both are manufactured in the *pituitary gland*, which is situated at the base of the brain, and they pass to the ovary via the bloodstream. Both are needed to stimulate follicle development, but luteinising hormone also specifically leads to rupture of the follicle and this causes ovulation. Although LH and FSH are manufactured in the pituitary gland, their release is controlled by an additional hormone, gonadotrophin releasing hormone (GnRH) which is produced in the hypothalamus of the brain. Progesterone prevents the action of GnRH and it therefore indirectly blocks the release of LH and FSH. Although these two hormones are being produced in the pituitary gland throughout the cycle it is only when progesterone levels fall and GnRH becomes activated that surges of FSH and LH are released in the bloodstream to stimulate the development of the next cycle.

If the cow does not become pregnant the uterus produces a hormone, *prostaglandin*, at about day 16. Prostaglandin leads to the dissolution and regression of the corpus luteum. Progesterone levels then fall and GnRH becomes activated in the brain. LH and FSH are released from the pituitary gland, a new follicle develops, ovulation occurs and a second oestrous cycle is started.

Action of Fertility Cycle Drugs

Many of the hormones which we have described are also available as injectable preparations and you may find it interesting to know which types of drugs your vet uses for fertility treatments. Oestrogen can be used to stimulate ovarian function in cows which have not started cycling after calving. It has two disadvantages, however. Firstly there is a danger of cystic ovaries developing after treatment and secondly the cow may only show the *behavioural* signs of oestrus, without going through any of the ovarian changes which lead to pregnancy. More commonly FSH or LH are used, or GnRH can be given to stimulate the release of FSH and LH which is naturally produced. LH (or GnRH) can also be used on the day of service to ensure that ovulation occurs and it is sometimes called a 'holding injection' for repeat breeders. This is described in more detail on page 235. To superovulate donor cows prior to embryo transfer, large doses of FSH are injected (usually in the form of PMSG) so that multiple ovulations occur. Several doses of semen are then given by AI and the resulting developing embryos (there may be between five and fifteen present) are flushed out of the donor cow six days after insemination, by means of catheters fed into her uterus. One embryo is then placed into the uterus of each of the recipient cows, these having been previously synchronised so that they are also six days past their last oestrus. The donor cow can either be superovulated and 'flushed' again, for several occasions if required, or she may be served at the next heat and left to carry a natural pregnancy.

Prostaglandin, either the natural hormone or a synthetic product, is an extremely commonly used drug. When given by intramuscular injection it causes the dissolution of the corpus luteum, progesterone levels fall, GnRH becomes activated, FSH and LH are released and the cow comes into oestrus three to four days after injection. These changes can be followed in figure 8.4. Prostaglandin can only act if there is a corpus luteum in the ovary however, and the corpus luteum is only sensitive to prostaglandin during days five to fifteen of the cycle. One word of caution: prostaglandin will lead to the regression of the corpus luteum whether or not the cow is pregnant, and if given to a cow at less than 150 days or greater than 250 days of pregnancy it is highly likely that she will abort. Your veterinary surgeon will therefore want to carry out a rectal examination of the cow prior to the administration of the drug and you should also check your records to ensure that there is no possibility of the cow having been served in the preceding six weeks, since pregnancies of this age or less may not be detectable by rectal examination.

Another commonly used drug is the Progesterone Releasing Intravaginal Device (PRID). This is a flexible plastic coil (plate 8.1) impregnated with the hormone progesterone and it is inserted into the cow's vagina using a special applicator (plate 8.2). The progesterone is absorbed by the cow and blocks her GnRH activity, so that although the corpus luteum regresses naturally, a

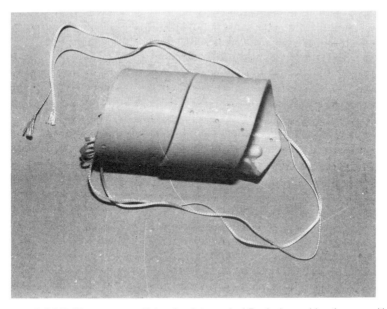

Plate 8.1   A PRID (Progesterone Releasing Intravaginal Device), provides the cow with a significant level of progesterone for twelve days. The small capsule in its right-hand end contains oestradiol benzoate.

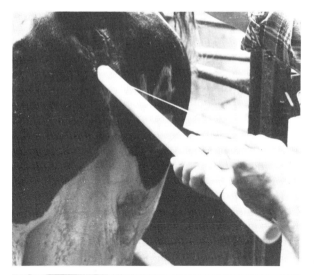

Plate 8.2   The PRID being inserted into a cow's vagina.

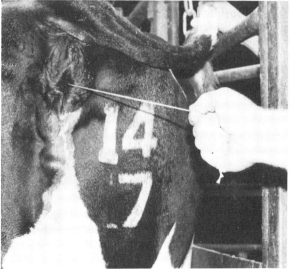

Plate 8.3   The PRID is removed twelve days after insertion by pulling on the string left hanging from the vagina.

new cycle cannot start because no FSH or LH can be released. The PRID remains in the vagina for twelve days, after which it is removed (plate 8.3) by pulling the string which was left hanging from the vulva. Removing the PRID leads to a sudden reduction in progesterone levels, GnRH becomes activated, the FSH and LH which has been manufactured by the pituitary during the previous twelve days is released and passes to the ovary, and the cow comes into oestrus two or three days later. These hormonal changes can again be followed in figure 8.4. The small capsule of oestradiol benzoate at the tip of the PRID (plate 8.1) helps to remove any remaining corpus luteum tissue which would otherwise have reduced the effect of the progesterone drop.

Both prostaglandin and the PRID can be used to synchronise the onset of oestrus in groups of cows or heifers, thus allowing fixed-time AI and eliminating the need for heat detection. This will be covered in more detail later in the chapter.

Cystic Ovaries

In figure 8.3 we saw that the normal follicle ruptured to release the egg (the process of ovulation) and this was followed by the growth of the corpus luteum. Sometimes however, instead of rupturing, the follicle continues to enlarge and this forms an ovarian cyst (figure 8.5). If oestrogen is produced,

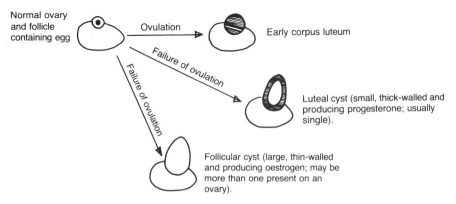

Figure 8.5   The development of cystic ovaries.

the cow is said to have a follicular cyst and she shows signs of excessive oestrus behaviour. The cow is sometimes said to be nymphing, or we say that she has become a nymphomaniac. These cows will come into oestrus at irregular intervals, perhaps every eight to twelve days or even more frequently and they may stay on heat for three to four days instead of the normal twelve to eighteen hours. They may also become active whenever any other cows in the herd are bulling. If left untreated, they develop a very high tail head and their pelvis may creak as they walk, due to oestrogen relaxing the supporting ligaments. Eventually masculinisation develops and the cow starts roaring and pawing the ground like a bull.

Sometimes instead of a follicular cyst developing, a layer of progesterone-producing tissue may grow on the inside of the cyst wall and this is known as a luteal cyst (figure 8.5). The progesterone produced by the luteal cyst blocks GnRH activity, ovarian cycles cease and the cow is never seen on heat. She is now in the true state of *anoestrus*, which simply means *without ovarian activity*. The differentiation between follicular and luteal cysts is not always an easy matter. Only the extreme forms have been described and some intermediate stages occur, with possibly a change from follicular to luteal activity. Differentiation is important, however, since it affects treatment. Luteal cysts can be treated with prostaglandin. On the other hand, for follicular cysts your vet may use LH or GnRH, a PRID or a combination of LH and progesterone. Even then treatment may not be successful. Diagnosis of the type of cyst is best made using milk progesterone samples (see page 211).

Normally about 4 per cent of cows develop cystic ovaries each year, although in some herds they can become quite a problem. The condition is partly inherited—I can remember treating a cow and two of her daughters for cysts on one farm and on the same day! In Sweden, cystic ovaries once occurred in 10 per cent of all cows, so they introduced a careful selection policy to ensure that bulls used for breeding were not derived from cows which had had cystic ovaries. This has reduced their national incidence to 5 per cent, much the same as the current level in Great Britain. Stress is thought to be another factor involved. Stress causes a variety of hormonal upsets and is associated with duodenal ulcers in man. It has been suggested that a cow under stress does not produce enough GnRH in the brain (figure 8.4) and this leads to an inadequate release of FSH and LH. A follicle is produced and the cow comes on heat, but there is insufficient LH to cause ovulation. In dairy cows stress arises from a variety of factors; for example, overcrowding, insufficient numbers of cubicles, being continually rushed rather than being handled slowly and quietly, too many movements (scraping, feeding, bedding) during the day, inadequate feeding-space and so on. Nutrition has also been suggested as a cause of cystic ovaries, particularly in high-yielding cows underfed at peak, but to my knowledge there is no direct proof of this. Others have suggested that manganese deficiency may be involved (see page 303), and factors such as B-carotene deficiency, fatty liver syndrome and the presence of certain oestrogenic toxins in the food have all been suggested as possible predisposing causes. Cows with fatty livers (see page 152) have been shown to have much higher levels of circulating prostaglandin than normal cows, and this could interfere with their oestrous cycles and subsequent fertility.

Failure to Cycle

Most cows have started some oestrous cycle changes in their ovaries by about three weeks after calving, although the first *visible* heat may not be seen until four or five weeks. However, a few cows remain with inactive ovaries until sixty days or more after calving and you will need to get your vet to attend to these. They are true anoestrous cows (see page 209). He will carry out a rectal examination to make sure that there are no abnormalities on the ovary and then he will give a suitable treatment, for example a PRID. The action of the PRID is described on page 207.

Failure to cycle is most commonly seen in first calved heifers which have lost excessive bodyweight during the first few weeks of lactation—in other words, it occurs as a result of underfeeding. It is also seen in suckler cows and in this case the continued presence of the calf seems to inhibit ovarian activity. In some high-yielding cows (about 3 per cent) ovarian cycles start but then stop again. The commonest cause of cows not seen bulling is poor heat detection, but the possibility that the cow has stopped cycling should not be overlooked and you should get your vet to check for this. The syndrome is referred to as the 'long low progesterone' or 'anovulatory' phase and its importance has been identified by means of serial milk progesterone sampling (see figure 8.11).

PREGNANCY DETECTION

Milk Progesterone Tests

In figures 8.3 and 8.4 we saw how the corpus luteum is present in the ovary between one heat and the next and that it produces the hormone progesterone. Progesterone circulates in the blood and passes into the milk and measurements of *milk* progesterone levels can be very useful in several areas of fertility control. Figure 8.6 shows the milk progesterone of a cow which had her first heat (oestrus) at thirty days after calving. When she is on heat there is

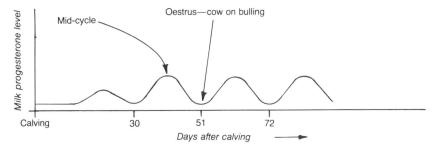

Figure 8.6   Milk progesterone in a normal cycling cow.

no corpus luteum present in the ovary and so milk progesterone levels fall to zero. Levels rise to a peak during the middle of the next cycle and then return to zero twenty-one days later (now fifty-one days after calving) at the following oestrus. Figure 8.7 shows the same cow, but this time she was successfully inseminated at day 51. Because pregnancy was established, the corpus luteum stayed in the ovary and she did not come on heat at day 72. The dotted line shows how the cycles would have continued if the insemination had not been successful. This is the basis of the *milk progesterone pregnancy test*. A milk sample is taken twenty-four days after insemination—at twenty-four days because the cow could well return to service at 21–24 days and there is no point in sending a milk sample to the laboratory at day 21, only to find that the cow comes bulling one or two days later. Even if she came on heat at day 19–21 but was not observed, milk progesterone levels would still be low at day 24.

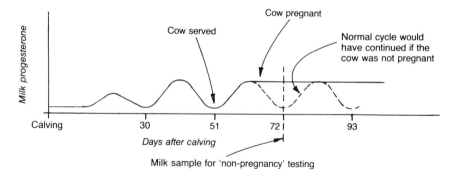

Figure 8.7   Milk progesterone levels in pregnancy.

A high milk progesterone level at twenty-four days after service indicates pregnancy and a low level indicates that the cow is not pregnant, and that she was on heat at 19–24 days but that oestrus was not observed. The accuracy of the test is very good for cows which are *not* pregnant (i.e. low progesterone levels), but only 80–85 per cent of the cows which had high progesterone values will be pregnant when examined manually at eight weeks after service. Because of this many prefer to call milk progesterone an indicator of *non-pregnancy*.

Some of the reasons for the false positive results are given in figures 8.8, 8.9 and 8.10. The first cause is early embryonic death (figure 8.8). The cow was pregnant when she was milk-sampled at twenty-four days after service, but she then lost her calf and came on heat fifty-four days later. Irregular return intervals such as these are a good indicator that early embryonic death has occurred.

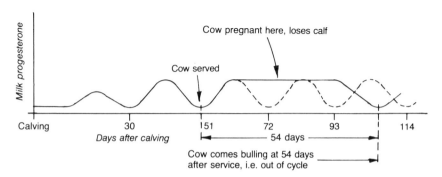

Figure 8.8   Milk progesterone and early foetal death.

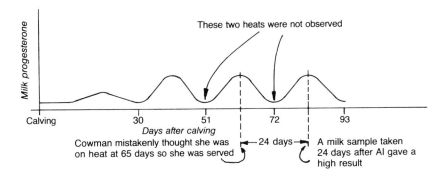

Figure 8.9   Milk progesterone and poor heat detection.

A second cause of false positive results is incorrect heat detection. In figure 8.9 the graph shows the cow's normal cycles. The cowman missed her heat at day 51, but mistakenly thought she was bulling at 65 days so had her served. Unfortunately he also missed her true heat at 72 days and so he took a milk sample twenty-four days after serving her. Of course by this stage the cow was in the middle of her next cycle, so the milk sample came back with a high progesterone level, a 'positive' result, but we know that the cow could not have been pregnant. Because his heat detection was poor, the cowman had missed both of the true heats at days 51 and 72.

This type of situation is more common than you may think. Surveys have been carried out in which all cows presented for AI have been milk sampled. If they are truly on heat the progesterone levels should be zero. In fact results have shown that around 10–15 per cent of cows presented for AI are *not on heat.* Clearly the conception rate of these cows will be zero and this shows how

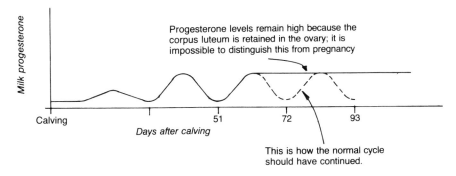

Figure 8.10   Milk progesterone and retained corpus luteum.

heat detection and conception rates are closely linked. Herds with a high proportion of *negative* milk progesterone results (viz. returns at 21 days were not observed and so the cow was milk sampled at 24 days) are likely to have a poorer conception rate, as well as a larger number of false positive milk progesterone results.

The third category of false positive results covers factors *other than pregnancy* which hold the cow in mid-cycle, that is maintain the corpus luteum in the ovary. Pregnancy is obviously the main reason for a 'persistent' corpus luteum, but a type of uterine infection known as a *pyometra* (see page 231) and a luteal cyst can have the same effect and sometimes the cow simply stays in mid-cycle for no apparent reason (figure 8.10). The later situation is sometimes called a persistent corpus luteum, or simply prolonged luteal activity.

On other occasions a cow may start cycling and then stop, but without any corpus luteum in the ovary. This would give the long low milk progesterone or anovulatory pattern shown in figure 8.11 It will not confuse the milk pregnancy test however, because the result of low progesterone, that is, 'not pregnant', will be correct anyway. These cows are often seen 'messing about', almost coming on heat but not quite and you will need your vet to check for cystic ovaries.

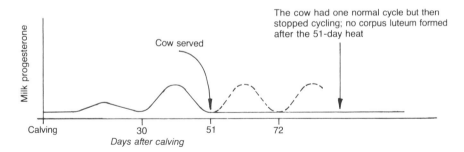

Figure 8.11   Long low progesterone or anovulatory phase.

Sampling for milk progesterone
Samples must be taken into bottles containing a special preservative (usually potassium dichromate) and these are best obtained from the laboratory which is going to carry out the analysis. It is most important that a sample of well-mixed whole milk is taken. Progesterone is concentrated in the fat portion of the milk, so if the bottle is filled with strippings (which are high in fat) at the end of milking, the progesterone content will be erroneously high. This could lead to a positive result when in fact the cow is not pregnant. If, on the other hand, milk is left to stand in the jar, fat rises to the top. A sample now taken from the bottom of the jar could give a falsely low progesterone result, which might say 'not pregnant' when the cow has in fact conceived.

Pregnancy Diagnosis—Other Methods

The milk progesterone test has already been described, although this is more of an indicator of non-pregnancy. The three other major methods of pregnancy detection are rectal examination, oestrone sulphate in milk and ultrasonic probes. Your vet will be able to detect pregnancy by rectal examination from approximately seven weeks onwards. In heifers with small compact uteri it may be possible to detect as early as five weeks, but older cows can present problems at this stage. Feeling through the wall of the rectum he will compare the size of the uterine horns. The pregnant side is larger and at six weeks the placental membranes may be felt enclosing a bag of fluid. It is most important to distinguish this uterine enlargement from a pyometra (page 231) or simply failure to return to a normal size following a previous pregnancy. At eight weeks the calf can be felt, approximately the size of your thumb nail, and by twelve weeks cotyledons (see page 96) are developing.

The advantages of a manual rectal examination are its accuracy, that pregnancy can be detected from seven weeks onwards or even less, that an assessment of the stage of pregnancy can be made, and that if the cow is not pregnant possible reasons why can be given by examining the ovaries. The risks to the cow are minimal, and abortion will only occur if the very young calf (eight to ten weeks pregnant) is grasped and squeezed between the finger and thumb. This is almost impossible to achieve accidentally.

Oestrone sulphate is a hormone produced only by the pregnant uterus.

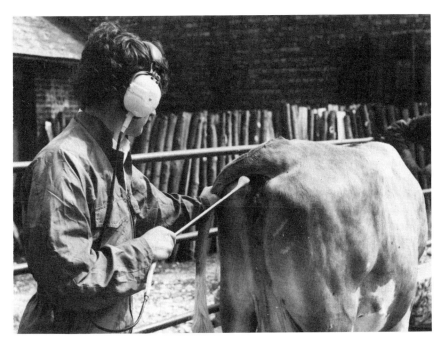

Plate 8.4   Using an Ultrasound rectal probe to detect pregnancy (Photo: Medata Ltd).

Significant quantities can be detected in the milk from 105 days of pregnancy until calving. The test, currently offered only by the MMB, is very accurate and has the advantage over milk progesterone that milk samples do not need to be taken on a specific day. It cannot be used for early pregnancy detection, however.

The mechanical detector probe is a device which is inserted into the rectum. It emits a beam of ultra-sound which is subjected to a small change in frequency when it is reflected from a moving surface such as the foetal heart or pulsating maternal or placental blood vessels. The reflected ultra-sound is collected by the same probe and converted into audible sounds which are monitored by means of headphones (plate 8.4). In experienced hands the manufacturers claim that pregnancy can be detected as early as six weeks, and even an external probe, placed against the cow's side, should detect the foetal heart from four to five months. There are often many extraneous sounds which can also be heard however, and considerable experience is needed before a high degree of accuracy is attained. The device is very popular in sows, possibly because the stockman gets more experience with using it.

HEAT DETECTION

'Heat' or 'on bulling' is the expression given to the behaviour shown by the cow when she is in oestrus, that is when she has a mature follicle in her ovary and is about to ovulate. In herds using artificial insemination it is vital that heat detection is accurate and for this we need to know the signs of heat. These can be roughly divided into early, mid and late.

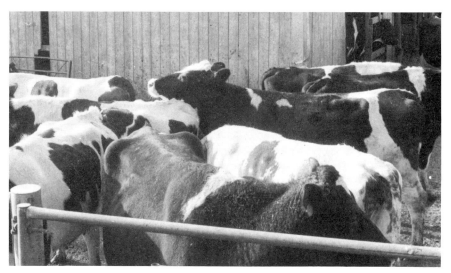

Plate 8.5   Signs of heat: chin resting. This cow may have only been going to push past the others. She was in fact on heat.

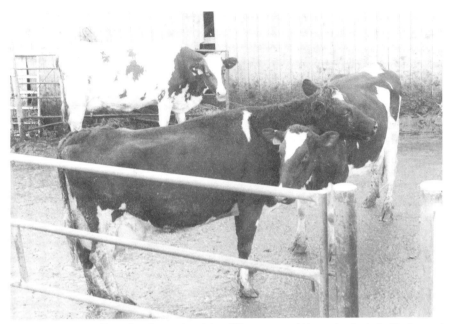

Plate 8.6   Signs of heat: bunting and nudging. Either cow could be on heat—in fact both were!

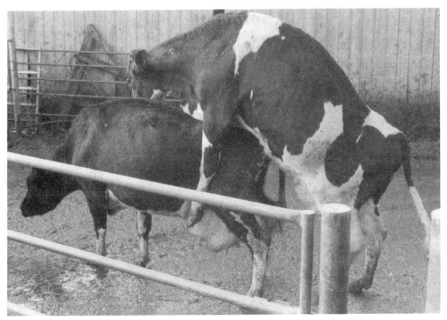

Plate 8.7   Signs of heat: standing to be mounted. It is the underneath cow which is definitely on heat.

Early signs of heat
The cow becomes restless, perhaps standing apart from the main group; she may be looking around in the parlour instead of eating her concentrate and her yield will be down. She may lick or sniff the urine and vulva of other cows or simply rest her chin on another cow's back as shown in plate 8.5. There is no way of telling whether this cow is on heat or whether she is only trying to push past. Sometimes there is some playful bunting and nudging behaviour (plate 8.6). In all the activities where two cows are involved, it could be either cow coming on heat. In the early stages, our cow may try to jump others, but she will not stand to be mounted.

Mid signs of heat
Standing to be mounted (plate 8.7) is the most sure and positive sign of heat and you should always look for this. It is the cow standing underneath which is on heat, unless they are mounting head to head, in which case it is the top cow (plate 8.8). All the early signs of sniffing, nudging and chin resting may still be present, possibly slightly more intensely, and they are often a preliminary to mounting. You may see some enlargement of the vulva and later slime will be passed, known as the 'bulling string'. This is often seen hanging from the vulva, particularly when the cow is sitting in the cubicles. The mucus is produced in the uterus, and released as the cervix opens when oestrus approaches. If you do not see the slime itself, look for signs of clear tacky mucus stuck around the tail at the level of the vulva.

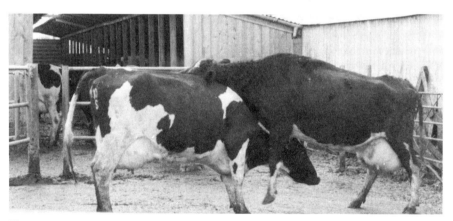

Plate 8.8   Signs of heat: mounting head to head. Now it is the top cow which is on heat.

Late signs of heat
The cow will now be less restless and will no longer stand to be mounted by others. You should be able to see the marks where she has been ridden however, for example, areas of raw skin on the tailhead or on each side of the tail, and there may be muddy marks down her flank. If you see fresh blood on the tail or mixed with the bulling string, you could well be too late: she may have been on heat yesterday or even the day before. Some say that blood on

the insemination catheter is a sure sign that the cow will return to service. This is not true, although it may indicate that she was inseminated fairly late in heat.

Heat Detection Rate

This is an assessment of how good you are at spotting heats. Assume that you have an autumn-calving herd, that you intend to start serving on 5 December and on that date there are fifty cows eligible for AI. By 26 December (twenty-one days later) you have served forty of these. Provided that they were all cycling normally, this means that your heat detection rate was forty out of fifty, or 80 per cent. Compared to many large farms this is very good: 60 per cent is an average figure and although 40 per cent is poor, it is by no means uncommon. So why is the rate so low?

The problem

People such as Dr Esslemont and his colleagues from Reading University have watched dairy cows continually, day and night, for twenty-five days or more. They found that most cows came bulling, but that for some the heat periods were very short and this was especially so in the dark and cold days of the winter. For example, 20 per cent of cows were on heat for less than six hours, with some showing heat for as little as two hours; 20 per cent were mounted less than six times, and there was an average of twenty minutes between mounts. So if a cow came on heat at 11 p.m. she may well have finished by 5 a.m. and detection would be almost impossible. They also found that more cows came on heat during the night hours of 10 p.m. to 5 a.m.

Improving Heat Detection

You can do more for your overall herd fertility by improving heat detection than by any other single action. Some of the important factors are as follows:

1. Observation. Everyone on the farm should be on the look-out for cows on heat and the herdsman should set aside specific times of the day for heat detection. As the average interval between mounts is twenty minutes this should be the minimum period he spends watching. More cows come on heat at night, so go and have a look around last thing in the evening, before you go to bed. This may not be a particularly welcoming thought on a wet winter's evening, but it will pay dividends in terms of heat detection. Watch the cows when they are resting—you are much less likely to spot bullers when they are being moved around for milking, feeding or scraping the passages.

On many farms there is a small corner of the yard, perhaps half-way between the cubicles and the outside feeding area, where a group of cows congregate when one of them is on heat. This is known as the 'buller group' or the 'buller area' and if you can identify a favourite haunt such as this it makes heat detection much easier. An example is shown in plate 8.9. The three cows on the right-hand side of the gate eat and sleep in the cubicle house behind

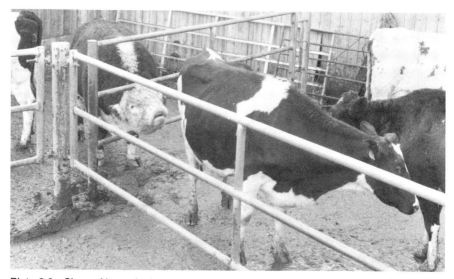

Plate 8.9 Signs of heat: the bull running with the dry cows on the opposite side of the gate makes this empty area very attractive for the buller group.

them. The bull is running with the dry cows, but of course oestrous cows are attracted towards him. This small area of empty yard is just outside the parlour and ideal for the buller group. Note the bull's facial expression—a similar attitude is often adopted by cows when they are sniffing the vulva of a cow in oestrus. Plates 8.5 to 8.9 were all from the same area.

The other aspects of observation include almost any change in the cow's normal behaviour. She may come into the parlour last rather than with an earlier group. Her milk yield is likely to be down—one survey in New Zealand showed that cows which had a 25 per cent reduction in yield at one milking followed by a 25 per cent compensatory increase at the next were highly likely to be in oestrus, and these changes were sufficient to make insemination worthwhile. Cows on heat may stand away from the feeding area and bellow over the gate, and when in the parlour they may be restless, shuffling their feet, looking around and not eating their food.

2. *Records* play a vital role in heat detection. If you have a visual display board like the one in plate 8.10 you can see which cows *should* be on heat over the next few days and they can be watched especially carefully. It also helps with the 'buller group'. There are three cows in plate 8.9. The cowman jotted their numbers down on a pad and in the office he found that only one of them was due on heat: one had just calved and the other one was already pregnant. He now needs to go back and watch the suspect cow much more carefully.

3. *Cow identification.* You may see a cow jump when she is too far away for you to be sure which cow it is. Clear markings, preferably at both the front

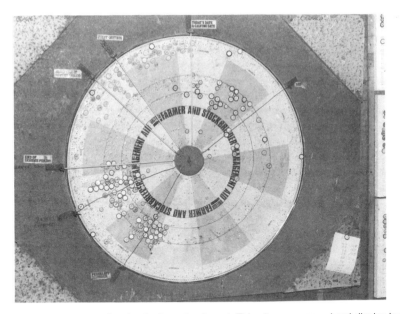

Plate 8.10 An example of a circular breeding board. This gives an easy visual display but some other written record is also necessary.

(ear tags or collars) and rear (freeze-branding) of the cow make it less likely that mistakes will be made. This is particularly important if you look at the cows last thing at night and have to leave a message for someone to keep the cow in for AI on the following day, or if you want other farm staff to assist with heat detection.

4. Healthy cows are more likely to show signs of heat than animals which are thin due to underfeeding or disease. I think that lameness is especially important here: cows with bad feet spend far more time lying down and are bound to be difficult to catch bulling. Some say that specific minerals and trace elements are also involved; for example, calcium, phosphorus, manganese, copper and iodine. While there may not be any conclusive proof of this, there are so many hormonal changes involved in the oestrous cycle that it must be logical to provide a properly balanced ration and thus avoid nutritional stress.

5. Housing can also play a part. Overcrowding has been mentioned as a factor increasing the incidence of both lameness and environmental mastitis and I am sure that cows which are packed into small, poorly ventilated and often purpose-built cubicle houses which give very little room for movement are much more difficult to spot when on heat. I like to see at least one open yard for a loafing area, somewhere where the 'buller group' can become active, without the risk of them treading on the teats of other cows. This is one advantage of having the feeding area reasonably separated from the cubicles or bedding area.

6. Regular veterinary visits. Although they are not specifically aimed at heat detection, routine fertility visits play an important part (see page 237 for a fuller description). Cows which have not yet been seen on heat are identified for special attention, whereas others can be confirmed as pregnant and need not be watched so closely.

7. Heat detection aids. There are a few devices which can be used to help you identify a cow on heat. The first, and I think the best of these is the *Kamar Heat Mount Detector*. This consists of a small clear plastic tube (plate 8.11) with a fine hole at one end. It is enclosed in an opaque plastic shield fixed to a piece of cloth and the device is glued to the tailhead of the cow (plate 8.12),

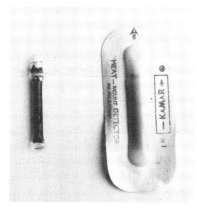

Plate 8.11   A Kamar Heat-Mount Detector. The plastic tube on the left is from inside the opaque capsule. The fine hole in its upper end allows the ink to be squeezed through.

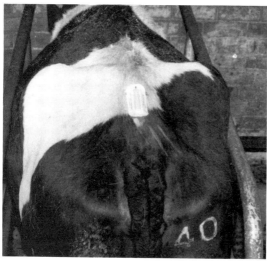

Plate 8.12   The Kamar is glued onto the tail-head, with the arrow pointing forwards.

making sure the arrow is pointing forwards. If the cow walks under a rail the ink in the inner tube is pushed to the back but cannot escape. If she is mounted by another cow however, the weight and thrusting action of the mounting cow forces the dye forwards, through the fine hole and into the outer casing. The white opaque plastic now turns a brilliant red colour, as shown in colour plate 13, indicating that the cow is on heat. False positives do occur, for example due to an oestrous cow mounting a Kamar cow when she is not in a position to escape. The plate probably shows a definite oestrus however, because the sides of the Kamar are dirty and the hair on the cow's tail arch has been rubbed forwards.

Tel Tail paint is used in a similar way. A thick layer of paint is applied as a band along the tailhead so that it flattens the hairs of the coat which are running backwards at this point. This dries and hardens, but when the cow is mounted by another, the paint cracks up, or is rubbed off altogether. With the paint therefore, you have to remember which cows were marked and then act as soon as the paint has gone, whereas the appearance of a bright red Kamar is much more obvious. With either device you must remember that they are only an *aid* to heat detection: you should then consult your records to see if the cow is supposed to be on heat and look to see if she is showing any other behavioural signs or rub marks.

The other two heat detection aids worthy of note are closed-circuit television cameras, so that the cows can be watched from the comfort of your kitchen or living-room and sniffer dogs. Apparently dogs can be trained to sniff out and identify cows on heat: perhaps they could also sort the cows and phone the AI! Pedometers, devices strapped to the cow's leg to register movement, have been used but they have not proved successful.

SYNCHRONISATION OF OESTRUS

As its title suggests, synchronisation of oestrus means that the oestrous cycle is being manipulated such that all the cows or heifers in a group come bulling at the same time, and they can then all be inseminated on the same day. Synchronisation therefore removes the need for heat detection. It can be a very useful technique for heifers. If they are running outside, insemination on one day makes handling much easier and batch calving can also be a big advantage. Using Friesian semen means that an additional group of Friesian heifer calves could be available and this is especially useful in an expanding herd (see also page 226). Synchronisation can be used in cows to overcome the problems of heat detection.

Prostaglandins

Two drugs are used, PRIDs or prostaglandins. The hormonal action of the PRID and its intravaginal application were described on page 207. Prostaglandins (PG) act only if the cow is between day 5 and day 15 of her cycle, that is when there is a mid-cycle corpus luteum present.

An injection of prostaglandin dissolves the corpus luteum, progesterone levels fall and the cow comes bulling in three to four days (see figure 8.4 and page 207). Two injections of prostaglandin are needed to synchronise oestrus in a group of cows or heifers the second being given eleven days after the first. The reasons for this are as follows: At any one time the cows will be at varying stages of their cycle, from 0 to 21 days, so following the first injection only those at 5–15 days of their cycle will respond, to come bulling three to four days later. This is shown in figure 8.12.

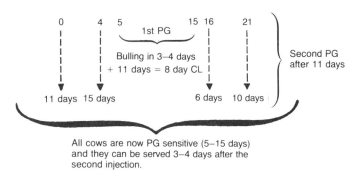

Figure 8.12   Prostaglandin synchronisation of heat.

The second injection for synchronisation is given eleven days after the first, and figure 8.12 shows the various stages of the cycle which the cows will be spanning at that stage. Cows which were originally at 0 and 4 days will now be at 11 and 15 days of their cycle respectively. Cows which responded to the first injection came bulling in three to four days, so after eleven days they will be seven to eight days into their next cycle (11 − 3 = 8 days). The cows which were originally at 16 days did not respond to the first injection, but came bulling naturally five days later, so after eleven days they are 11 − 5 = 6 days into their next cycle. Similarly, those cows originally at 21 days will be ten days into their next cycle. From this it can be seen (figure 8.12) that eleven days after the first injection, all of the cows in the group will be between 6 and 15 days of their cycle and are therefore sensitive to prostaglandin. Following the second injection they will all come bulling within three or four days and the group can be inseminated on both days.

An alternative is to give one insemination after seventy-eight to eighty hours. Although this may result in a very small reduction (e.g. 3–4 per cent) in conception rate it is probably much less than the cost of an additional insemination. This is the standard way of using prostaglandin for synchronisation, but there are several other systems. For example, you can inject the whole group on day one and then serve all cows seen on heat. There should be a surge of inseminations at the third and fourth day after injection, and hopefully a steady trickle thereafter. Those which have not been observed by day 11 are given a second injection and served blind three and four days later. You would be best to discuss with your vet the system most suited to your herd.

PRID

The cost of a PRID (see page 207) is approximately the same as two injections of prostaglandin, although the PRID is more difficult and therefore more expensive to administer. Only one veterinary visit is required, however, since the herdsman would normally remove the PRIDs, whereas two visits are required with prostaglandin. On a cost basis therefore the two treatments are approximately equal. Prostaglandins act only on cows which are already cycling, whereas a PRID will also stimulate ovarian activity and may cure any cysts present. PRIDs may cause a foul-smelling white discharge in a proportion of animals. This is of vaginal and not uterine origin, and it is due to irritation by the PRID. It does not seem to have any effect on conception rate even though it looks rather unpleasant, and in most cases the discharge disappears a few days after the PRID has been removed.

Effective Synchronisation

Whichever system is used, there will be a small proportion of animals which fail to synchronise. The problem is worse with cows, because their normal cycle lengths are much more variable. Only 90 per cent of normal cows have cycle lengths of eighteen to twenty-four days. In other words, 10 per cent of quite normal cows have cycles of less than eighteen days, or more than twenty-four days. The enthusiastic reader might like to substitute these cycle lengths for those in figure 8.12 and see for himself how a proportion will then fail to synchronise! If you are *sure* that a cow is standing to be mounted one or two days after she has already received a double AI, then she *must* be inseminated for the third time, because she clearly failed to respond to the synchronisation process.

Synchronisation of oestrus has provided a useful opportunity to study some of the factors affecting conception rate. Very good results are possible, but it is essential to ensure that the animals are on a rising plane of nutrition from four weeks before until three weeks after insemination, to ensure good fertilisation and implantation. Grazing heifers, or those on hay or silage, should be supplemented with 1½–2 kg of barley, and early lactation feeding of dairy cows needs to be such that weight loss over this period is minimised. Stress should definitely be avoided, so the idea of inseminating the heifers when they are being handled for worming or tuberculin testing is definitely not on, neither should they have their ration suddenly changed (for example, with housing) part way through the treatment.

When synchronisation was first introduced, a few people expected it to be a cure-all; insufficient attention was paid to husbandry, poor results were obtained and the technique fell out of favour. Because of the problems of heat detection however, it can be an excellent way of starting the service period to get good batch calving and trials have shown that it is cost-effective to do this. Table 8.1 shows the theoretical performance of one hundred cows with good heat detection (80 per cent) and conception (60 per cent) rates. Even then, only forty-eight cows ($100 \times 0.8 \times 0.6$) would be pregnant at the end of three weeks. If synchronisation was used, there may be a small proportion of cows which fail to respond (say 5 per cent) and conception rates may fall slightly (again, say 5 per cent) but the overall performance at the end of three weeks is significantly better. If heat detection was poor (say 50 per cent), then table 8.1 shows that the benefits of synchronisation are considerably greater. In fact if heat detection was poor, conception rates would also be poorer for the reasons given on page 230, and so even fewer than thirty cows would be pregnant after three weeks.

Table 8.1   Comparing the performance of normal observation and synchronisation in one hundred cows at the start of the service period

	Heat detection rate (%)	Conception rate (%)	Cows pregnant after 3 weeks
Observation and AI			
—Good heat detection	80	60	48
—Poor heat detection	50	60	30
Synchronisation	95	55	52

One of the most important aspects of maintaining a tight calving pattern is to introduce heifers into the herd at the start of the calving period. With almost unavoidable problems of early lactation weight loss, it is only too easy to let cows 'slip' around the year a few weeks, and it is therefore logical to introduce heifers into the herd in a tight batch as early as possible. Oestrus synchronisation helps to achieve this. In addition, if Friesian semen is used, the heifers will produce a valuable extra crop of Friesian heifer calves. These calves are being born at the very start of the calving season so that when they are introduced into the herd two years later they are well grown, better able to compete with the cows and will probably get back in calf faster in their first lactation. Although calves from heifers are smaller, there is good evidence to suggest that at least part of the size difference is made up during rearing.

Surveys have shown that, provided the bull is carefully selected, there are no more problems calving heifers at two years than when they are older. It is also said that the bigger heifer which can attain a higher forage intake is more likely to get overfat and produce an oversized calf, especially if she is fed concentrates precalving in addition to liberal intakes of grass. If proven bulls are used, there is also a good argument that obtaining an additional crop of Friesian heifer calves from heifers is increasing the rate of genetic selection by one generation. As the heritability of milk production is only 45 per cent it may be more profitable to introduce well-grown heifers into the herd at the start of the calving season rather than trying hard to get a Friesian calf from a late calver just because she is a high yielder.

CONCEPTION RATES

So far we have dealt with ovarian cycles and the importance of heat detection. Having served our cow, we hope that she will become pregnant. The proportion of cows which hold to service is known as the *conception rate*. This may be expressed as the conception rate to first service, the conception rate to all services, or inversely as the number of services per conception. A good figure would be 65 per cent conception to first service, although 55 per cent is probably average for the national herd and figures of 40 per cent or less are by no means uncommon.

These are *conception* rates however, and they will be significantly higher than final calving rates. Research has shown that if you took a hundred cows a few days after insemination almost 90 per cent of the eggs shed would have been fertilised and are developing as embryos, but many of these die in the early stages so that by 21 days the number of living embryos has fallen to 75 per cent; that is, 15 per cent have been lost already, and at least 25 per cent of the cows would return to service. When your vet carries out a manual pregnancy test at about 50 days, a further 10 per cent of embryos will have been lost partly due to failure of implantation at 30–35 days, and only 65 per cent of the cows are likely to be detectably pregnant to the first service. Allowing a 5 per cent loss from abortion plus occasional deaths and casualty slaughter of pregnant cows this gives an eventual calving rate of 60 per cent. The stages are shown in table 8.2. In poor fertility herds losses will be very much higher than this.

Table 8.2　The fate of one hundred bovine eggs in a herd with good fertility

	Losses
100 eggs shed	
	10 fertilisation failure
90 fertilised ova	
	15 early embryonic mortality
75 survive to 21 days	
	10 implantation failure/embryonic mortality
65 survive to 56 days	
	5 abortions/deaths/culls
60 cows calve	
Total calvings 60	**Total losses 40**

Early Embryonic Mortality

The cause of the high rate of early embryonic mortality, or early foetal death, has been the subject of considerable speculation and research. Recently, using refined genetic techniques and chromosome analysis, it has shown that part of the loss during the first twenty-one days is due to 'non-viable embryos'. In other words, if these embryos were allowed to develop into a full-term calf, the calf would be so badly deformed that it could not live a normal existence. Early embryonic mortality is therefore a method of eliminating such calves in the early stages and this must be an advantage to the survival of the species. Older cows have a higher rate of genetic abnormalities and embryonic mortality than heifers and it is worth comparing this with women, where there is an increased incidence of certain genetic birth defects with age, and where up to 30 per cent of miscarriages are thought to be due to chromosomal abnormalities.

Other causes of embryonic mortality include stress (over-crowding, poor handling, fighting for food, lameness etc.), sudden changes in diet during the first twenty-four days of pregnancy and certain nutritional deficiencies, of which energy is the most likely. Poor heat detection, leading to the insemination of cows which are already pregnant, may also cause foetal death. This problem is compounded by the fact that about 5 per cent of cows show standing heat when they *are pregnant* and it is impossible for the herdsman to know whether or not a bulling cow is pregnant. Unless he has already had her checked for pregnancy, he is almost certain to have her inseminated, thus running the risk of aborting an established foetus.

Serving too Soon after Calving

If cows are served too soon after calving, conception rates will be lower. This is thought to be due to the uterus not having settled down properly after the previous pregnancy and not being ready to accept the embryo for implantation. Figure 8.13 shows that you need to delay service until seventy days post-calving in order to achieve the best conception rates and if you serve at 35–40 days, conception rates may fall to 40 per cent. Under average farm conditions, however, I would recommend that cows are served after 55 days. The overall measure of fertility is the average period from calving to conception, however, since calving to conception plus gestation length (281 days) gives the calving interval and the gestation length is constant.

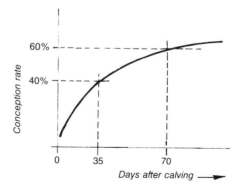

Figure 8.13   Conception rate varies with the interval from calving to service.

Table 8.3 **A theoretical comparison of the overall calving-to-conception (C–C) interval of 100 cows, where serving started at 50 days after calving and achieved a 60% conception rate (top group) with another 100 cows served from 34 days onwards and achieving an only 40% conception rate**

	No. cows served	No. cows conceiving	Mean C–C interval	No. cows not pregnant
1st service	100	60	60	40
2nd service	40	24	81	16
3rd service	16	10	102	6
4th service	6	4	123	2
5th service	2	1	144	1*
Mean C–C 72.7 days (= 353.7 days CI)				
1st service	100	40	44	60
2nd service	60	24	65	36
3rd service	36	14	86	22
4th service	22	9	107	13
5th service	13	5	128	8
6th service	8	3	149	5
7th service	5	2	170	3
8th service	3	1	191	2*
Mean C–C 72.3 days (= 353.3 days CI)				

* these cows would be culled as infertile

Although the mean calving intervals are almost identical, the first group is the preferred situation because its spread of calvings for next year will be much tighter and there are far fewer services per conception (1.7 compared with 2.5 for the second group).

Table 8.3 shows that if you begin with one hundred cows you get almost the same overall calving-to-conception (C–C) interval by starting the service period at 34 days and accepting only a 40 per cent conception rate, as you do by waiting until 50 days post-calving to get a 60 per cent conception rate. Assuming that it takes twenty-one days to serve all the cows in a group, if the serving of one hundred cows is started at 34 days post-calving then the average calving-to-first-service interval (and calving-to-conception interval for those which hold to service) will be forty-four days. Similarly, if serving is started at 50 days post-calving then the average calving-to-first-service interval will be sixty days (viz $50 + (21 \div 2) = 60$).

Table 8.3 assumes that the conception rate remains constant throughout the service period in both groups. However, if the 40 per cent rate is due entirely to serving too soon after calving, then by the second service conception rate may have risen towards 60 per cent and the figures will not be strictly accurate. The table also shows that one normal cow would need five services starting at 50 days post-calving, whereas three cows would need eight services starting at 34 days. Although the calving-to-conception intervals are very similar, the 50-day starting point is the preferred result, because it will give a tighter calving pattern the following year, there will be fewer culls and fewer insemination fees. For example 1.7 inseminations were required for each conception in the first group, but this rose to 2.5 services per conception by starting at 34 days. If your herd already has a poor conception rate, however, you may be forced to start serving at less than 50 days, although there is then a risk that this may depress conception rates even further.

Other Factors Affecting the Conception Rate

So far we have identified two of the most important factors affecting conception rate, namely early embryonic mortality and serving cows too soon after calving. The third factor is *poor heat detection*. The reasons why this affects conception rate were given in detail on page 213 and I suggest that this section is now referred to again. If heat detection is poor, many of the cows are not seen when they are bulling. In addition, other cows are inseminated when they are not on heat. Their conception rate is of course zero, but even worse, if they had been served previously, insemination when they are not on heat could terminate an already established pregnancy, thus reducing conception rates even further.

Some of the other factors which can affect conception rates are given in the following:

Timing of insemination

If you see a cow bulling this morning, should you inseminate her today or tomorrow? In Britain you cannot call for the AI service after 10.00 a.m. and so I would recommend that you serve a cow the *same day* as you see her on heat and not the following day. We have already seen that heat is a very variable period, lasting from three to thirty hours. Ovulation (that is the bursting of the follicle and shedding of the egg into the fallopian tube) always occurs twelve hours *after* the end of standing heat, irrespective of when heat started. Once shed, the egg remains viable for only six hours, whereas sperms can survive for up to thirty hours in the uterus. It is therefore much better to have the sperm waiting for the egg. In fact sperm has to spend a few hours in the uterus to undergo a process known as *capacitation* before it is capable of fertilising the egg. When you see a cow standing to be mounted you cannot have any idea of whether she is just starting heat, just finishing, or how long the heat period will last. The only sure way is to have her inseminated, so that the sperms are ready and waiting for ovulation to occur. However, if the cow is still in 'standing heat' the following morning, or even late the same evening, then it is best to have her inseminated for a second time. This is especially true if the inseminator came early in the morning rather than during the afternoon. Figure 8.14 shows how poor timing of insemination leads to reduced conception rates. Although cows served early or late in oestrus *may* conceive, their chances of doing so are much less, and the best conception rates are obtained by serving a cow when she is actually in standing heat.

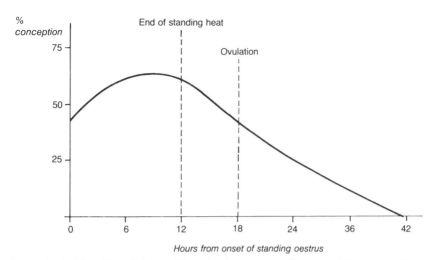

Figure 8.14   The effect of timing of insemination on conception rates. This cow was in standing oestrus for twelve hours and ovulated twelve hours later. If standing oestrus had lasted for twenty-four hours conception rates during the first six hours would have been much poorer.

Figure 8.14 also shows that there is a greater reduction in conception rate by serving them too late in heat rather than too early.

Poor handling facilities
If the inseminator has to chase your cow around the yard and then stand her in the front of a herringbone parlour where she can wriggle from side to side, you cannot expect him to do a perfect job. The cow should be well restrained, ready and waiting for him and preferably left with an adequate supply of food and water. It is not an easy task to pass the insemination catheter through the cervix and into the uterus. The cow needs to be on the same level as the inseminator and restrained so that she cannot move forwards or sideways. If the cow is excessively excited and stressed this may upset her hormonal mechanisms so that ovulation or fertilisation may fail to occur anyway.

Endometritis
Sometimes known as 'the whites' this is an infection of the inner wall of the uterus (endo- = inside; -metr- = uterus; -itis = inflammation of). When a cow is on heat the cervix opens and the uterus contracts expelling the bulling string, so if there is any discharge present, then this is the time when it is most likely to be seen. In more severe cases there may be a continual discharge, visible as white mucoid globules on the tail or at the vulva. Sometimes the uterus is full of pus but no discharge is produced. This is called a *pyometra*. Prostaglandin is the treatment normally given. It brings the cow into oestrus, thus emptying the uterus. At the same time the increased levels of circulating oestrogen associated with oestrus boosts the activity of the bacterial-fighting cells (neutrophils) which are lining the uterus.

Uterine infections may occur following a retained cleansing, an assisted calving (particularly if you are not careful with your hygiene), or simply dirty calving boxes. Sometimes herd outbreaks occur, when almost every cow may have a discharge. I have known this to be associated with underfeeding and excessive weight loss in early lactation, particularly in heifers. Presumably this is because nutritional stress decreases their resistance to infection, and in addition, ovarian cycles, which would clear up the endometritis, fail to start. Endometritis may also be associated with some of the factors leading to a high incidence of retained placenta (for example hypocalcaemia, excessive interference at calving, mineral and trace element imbalances), even though the number of retained cleansings is normal. Alternatively it may be a sequel to a more acute metritis (see page 129).

Sometimes when your vet examines a cow he can find no pus or any other evidence of uterine infection, but on careful palpation there may be a thickening of the fallopian tube (see figure 8.2) or 'adhesions' of the bursa to the ovary. This could be due to stretching and tearing at calving, although it may also be associated with the physical damage caused by an earlier metritis or endometritis, especially if the infection was not attended to promptly. If the bursa is fused or 'adhesed' to the surface of the ovary, then this will make it more difficult for an egg to pass down the fallopian tube at ovulation, thus reducing the chances of conception and possibly making the cow infertile.

Fatty liver syndrome
This is described in Chapter Six on 'Metabolic Disorders', on page 152. Cows with fatty liver have low albumin and glucose levels in their blood and their conception rates will be reduced. They are also more susceptible to retained placenta and uterine infections, and this may have a secondary effect on conception rate.

Specific infections
Poor conception rates caused by infections with such organisms as *Brucella abortus*, *Trichomonas foetus* and *Campylobacter* (previously known as *Vibrio*) are fortunately less common in Britain nowadays. However, as bulls are being used more often in dairy herds, particularly as 'sweepers' at the end of the service period, the possibility of campylobacteriosis (vibriosis) should not be overlooked. Your vet would need to take special samples of vaginal mucus or washings from the bull's prepuce to check for this organism.

Stress
Social stress cows is an interesting condition but rather difficult to define. It is quite easy for a cow introduced into a small herd of 40–50 others to come into contact with each one of them and soon establish her own position in the 'pecking order'. The chances of meeting 250–300 cows over a few days is much less however, and the situation becomes almost impossible if cows are being taken in and out of the herd all the time. In this situation our cow will be continually meeting new faces and possibly having to fight to establish her superiority (or otherwise) with them. This is a clear example of stress, and it is

becoming increasingly apparent that if group size goes above a hundred cows or if group composition is constantly changing, then the cows will be adversely affected. If they are given a midday feed there may be a 200 per cent variation in individual food intake, and this could be even greater if trough space is inadequate. Factors such as inadequate numbers of cubicles, blind-ending passageways from which submissive cows are unable to escape or simply inadequate loafing areas, are further examples of stress.

In addition to reducing fertility (by delaying the onset of oestrous cycles or by reducing conception rates), stress increases the animal's susceptibility to disease and decreases its milk production. Good animal management therefore has an important bearing on fertility.

Nutrition
Eating is probably the most important activity of the dairy cow, because without food she cannot milk or grow. Many aspects of feeding can have an effect on fertility and some have been mentioned already, for example, inadequate feeding-space can cause stress and lead to an increased incidence of early embryonic mortality, as well as causing difficulties with heat detection; general underfeeding and weight loss in early lactation may be associated with uterine infections; an energy deficit in overfat cows immediately after calving may lead to fatty liver syndrome; excess calcium or inadequate magnesium intakes during the dry period cause an increased incidence of milk fever and this in turn may lead to more endometritis and reduced conception rates.

Earlier in this chapter we saw that the physical and hormonal changes in the ovary associated with oestrus are extremely complex. The hormonal balance needed to maintain pregnancy has not been discussed but it is equally as intricate. It is likely that minerals and trace elements affect only minute aspects of these events and so it would therefore be illogical, if not naive, to expect nutrition to have a precise and consistent effect on overall fertility. The exact relationships have yet to be established and my own approach to a herd fertility problem is to examine the diet and to correct as many of the abnormalities as possible. This may seem rather unscientific, but fertility control is a dynamic process. At any one time it is influenced by a wide variety of factors and if we can help the cow to overcome some of her nutritional imbalances, then she may well cope with the remainder and the herd can once more return to reasonable fertility. These are general comments. There are certain aspects of nutrition which are more positively correlated with conception rate however and which need to be discussed in a little more detail.

Energy balance
It is well accepted that conception rates are improved if cows and heifers are served on a rising plane of nutrition. This is very difficult to achieve in early lactation. Figure 8.15 shows how milk yield reaches a peak well before the cow achieves her maximum appetite capacity and so some weight loss is bound to occur. The problem is more acute with first-calved heifers which not only have to compete with older cows for food, but they also need an additional allowance for growth. This occurs at a time when they are changing

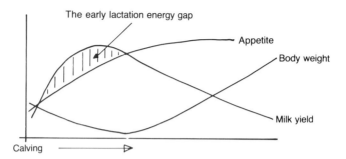

Figure 8.15   In early lactation milk yield peaks before a cow reaches her maximum dry matter intake. The energy gap leads to weight loss.

their front teeth, making eating even more difficult. If nutrition is adequate, weight loss may have stopped by the time the cow is ready to be served and there may even be some weight gain. This is especially true by the second or third service if the cow repeats.

Energy balance can be measured in a variety of ways. Conventionally the quantity and quality of the food being eaten is compared with the cow's requirements for milk production and a diet balance sheet is prepared. Secondary checks are always worthwhile, however, and measurements such as body weight loss, body condition score, the bulk milk protein content and blood glucose levels in the metabolic profile test (see page 138) will all help in the assessment of energy status. Several people have shown a specific correlation between blood glucose levels and conception rates. Energy balance may affect those cows in a herd which were being served when there was just a short-term problem.

Figure 8.16 is a Cu-sum graph of conception rate. The cows are arranged in order of service date along the horizontal axis, the bottom of the graph. Starting from zero in November, if a cow conceives the plot moves up one

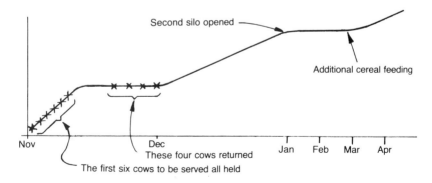

Figure 8.16   A Cu-sum graph of conception rate.

square. If the next cow does not conceive, the plot moves along one square, but remains horizontal. A line with a slope of 45 degrees therefore represents a 100 per cent conception rate. The distance for November and December is much greater than for February and March, because far more cows were served in the first two months. The overall graph shows a serious fall in conception rate for cows served during late January and early February. This was because when the second clamp was opened the silage was much poorer and there was an overall fall in energy intake. Additional cereal feeding introduced in late February improved the conception rate of the cows served in March.

Minerals and trace elements

Dairy farmers spend millions of pounds each year on mineral and trace element supplements, with phosphorus probably coming top of the list. Specific and consistent associations between minerals and fertility are virtually impossible to prove. We have already seen the massive range of other non-nutritional factors which can affect fertility and which could confuse the results of feeding trials. Deficiencies of copper, manganese, cobalt, iodine, phosphorus and selenium have all been associated with poor conception rates and the calcium-to-phosphorus ratio in the diet is also said to be important. Details of the levels required and of the effects of deficiencies and excesses are given in Chapter Eleven.

Deficiency of vitamin A impairs fertility, and several workers have shown a relationship between B-carotene (a vitamin A precursion) and conception rates. The position with regard to vitamin E and selenium is less clear. Deficiency in rats causes sterility, but no relationship has ever been *proven* in dairy cows. If your herd has an inadequate vitamin E status however, then it is most sensible to provide additional supplementation. There is some evidence that inadequate vitamin E/selenium status leads to increased placental retention and endometritis.

The Repeat Breeder Cow

Over the years a good deal of effort has been expended in investigating the repeat breeder cow, that is, the cow which has been served five, six or even seven times and continues to 'return' to service every 21 days. However, table 8.3 shows that in a hundred-cow herd with a good conception rate (60 per cent), you would *expect* two cows to need five services before they conceived, whereas in a herd with a poor conception rate (40 per cent) thirteen 'normal' cows may need five services or more before conceiving. Many of the repeat breeder cows are therefore simply normal animals which, by chance, have not conceived. Having said this however, there will be a proportion of repeat breeders which do have a low-grade endometritis or maybe some scarring of the oviduct, or bursal adhesions, so it is well worth getting your vet to examine them when he comes on his regular visit.

Sometimes repeat breeders are given a 'holding injection' on the day of service. This is an injection of luteinising hormone (LH) or gonadotrophin releasing hormone (GnRH). These drugs ensure that the egg is released from the follicle (see page 206). They are said to give better synchronisation of ovulation with insemination and in so doing improve conception rates. The holding injection is sometimes followed up eight to ten days later by giving progesterone to boost the action of the corpus luteum, either as an injection, or as a small hormone implant. Although some seem convinced that these procedures work, there has never been any consistent or conclusive proof of their effectiveness, with some trials showing a significant benefit and other trials no effect at all.

ABORTION

The final hurdle in our components of the calving interval (see page 203 and table 8.2) is the maintenance of pregnancy to full term, so that a normal calf can be born. If early foetal death occurs, it is most likely that the foetus will be reabsorbed in the uterus and nothing else is seen. If the calf is expelled

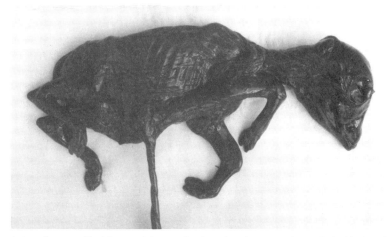

Plate 8.13   A mummified foetus. It is usually chocolate-brown and expelled with the placenta tightly wrapped around it.

from the uterus at any stage of pregnancy before full term, then this is called an *abortion*. The aborted calf may be fresh, or it may have died in the uterus weeks or even months before. In the second case sometimes all of the placental fluids are reabsorbed and the calf becomes dry and chocolate-brown in colour. This is known as a *mummified foetus* and an example is shown in plate 8.13. The age of the aborted calf can be estimated by the distance (in centimetres) from the crown of its head to its rump (or anus), using the formula:

age (days) $= 2.5 \times$ (crown to rump length $+ 21$).

With brucellosis almost eradicated, the average abortion rate for cattle in Britain in 1983 had fallen to approximately 2 per cent. This was based on the number of abortions reported and checked for brucellosis by the Ministry of Agriculture however, and so the actual abortion rate might have been somewhat higher. Some herds may experience a much higher rate than this, although it always seems worse when several cows abort over a short period of time. Most of the diseases causing abortion are dealt with in detail elsewhere in the book. They include infectious bovine rhinotracheitis (IBR), especially if the pustular vulvo-vaginitis form of the disease is present; bovine viral diarrhoea (BVD); leptospirosis; fungal infections (= mycotic abortion); salmonellosis, especially S. dublin and S. typhimurium, and any acute fever, for example, from summer mastitis. Toxins and poisons may also be involved.

Farmers tend to be more careful when handling heavily pregnant cows and while this is probably a good thing in order to avoid teat and leg damage, I suspect that fairly severe mishandling is necessary to cause abortion. Compared to the number of normal twins births, the incidence of aborted twins is relatively quite high and it is interesting to compare this with the mare, where the birth of normal, live twin foals is rare. Both the abortion rate and twinning rate are higher in cows than heifers.

Do not forget that the law obliges you to report all cases of abortion to the Divisional Veterinary Officer (maybe indirectly through your local vet), so that samples can be taken to eliminate the possibility of brucellosis.

PREVENTIVE MEDICINE AND HERD FERTILITY MANAGEMENT

Because preventive medicine programmes in dairy herds are usually based on a regular fertility visit, this is a good opportunity to introduce the subject. I like to define preventive medicine as '*the routine implementation of common-sense husbandry*'.

No new technical information is needed, but rather a different approach to disease control in general, that approach being towards prevention rather than treatment. For some conditions, for example blackleg, vaccination is the preventive measure and the disease can be completely eliminated, although infection remains in the soil and in the intestine of the animal. Most other conditions are far more complex however and the level of farm performance needs to be continually monitored if progess is to be made. Mastitis and fertility are good examples of this. Mastitis will never be eradicated and so preventive programmes must be devised to reduce the incidence of the condition to economically acceptable levels, such as those suggested on page 179. We can only assess the effectiveness of our preventive programmes if we actually record and monitor mastitis incidence, however, and I believe that this is one of the functions of your vet. Not only should he be advising you on the appropriate mastitis control measures for your herd, but he should also make sure that you are *recording* those cases of mastitis which do occur and that periodically the overall incidence of mastitis in your herd is assessed by an *analysis of the records*, so that you can compare your performance with other herds. This has been done already for subclinical mastitis using the Milk Marketing Board's cell count scheme, but it needs to be expanded to include clinical cases.

Herd fertility control should be tackled in a similar way. Your vet should be able to advise you on the type of records needed and make sure that a regular analysis of those records is carried out. You can then see if you need to put additional effort into fertility control. The concept of monitoring margin over concentrates and other criteria before making financial decisions has been well accepted and a similar approach is needed now for animal disease. Well-designed, computer-based systems are undoubtedly the best for monitoring fertility data, because they give the opportunity to analyse the data in depth should problems occur. Computerisation is quite expensive, so if you already have a manual system in operation which satisfies the requirements of recording and monitoring performance, then this may be quite adequate.

A good example of on-farm performance monitoring is the Cu-sum plot shown in figure 8.16. This is very simple and yet it gives a good check on conception rate. Fluctuations in fertility will undoubtedly occur: if possible the causes of these fluctuations should be identified, so that preventive measures can be introduced to prevent their recurrence. This is an area where computerisation has a great deal to offer. For example, we have seen already that poor conception rates may be due to a variety of factors and unless we have a fairly sophisticated means of analysing herd fertility data, it may be impossible to identify which of the factors is a problem in your particular herd. If you are choosing a computer system, make sure that it offers the facility of an in-depth analysis of data, as well as a routine monitoring. One day it may be important to know whether poor conception rates are correlated with a particular bull, or serving too soon after calving, or previous cases of endometritis, or the average interval between services, or the accuracy of heat detection, and so on. This is known as using records in a *diagnostic capacity*.

I have given several examples of what I think the vet ought to be doing in terms of preventive medicine programmes, so what part should the farmer be playing? First it is important that records are kept and that they are accurate. It is obviously pointless spending time monitoring performance if the basic records are incorrect. Second, you need to allow your vet to visit the farm on a regular basis, so that he knows what the problems are and how they have been tackled so far.

Perhaps I can briefly describe the system we have used for farms in our own practice to give an idea of what I mean. This is a non-computerised manual system which has proved successful for many years. Individual cow record cards for each herd are kept at the surgery and a few days before the routine visit is due a list is constructed of those cows which we think ought to be examined. There are three basic examinations carried out, namely:

- a post-calving examination to check that there is no residual endometritis. This is performed at between two and four weeks after calving because many discharges at less than two weeks post-calving will clear up without treatment. The examination simply consists of washing the vulva and then inserting a gloved hand into the vagina to check that the cervix is closed and that there is no gross evidence of pus in the cervical mucus. Some vets use a speculum and simply look at the cervix.

- cows not seen bulling by fifty days post-calving are examined to make sure they are cycling normally and that there are no cysts.
- pregnancy diagnosis is performed seven weeks after the last service date.

The list of cows has two important uses. Firstly it means that the farmer has to spend a few minutes going through his own records, deleting 'non-bulling' cows which have since been served, and cows due for pregnancy check which have returned to service, and secondly the list reminds him that the visit is due. The discipline of having to check through the herd records every two weeks in itself makes a big contribution to improving overall fertility. Problem cows are regularly identified and as such are watched much more carefully. For a routine visit system to be successful, I believe it should cause the minimum of disturbance to the cows and to the farm routine and, if possible, I like to carry out fertility examinations immediately after morning milking. Because your vet is checking cows on a routine basis, he can get an immediate idea of whether there is a problem with endometritis, or if too many normal cycling cows have not been seen on heat. This would then be verified by consulting the records. He is in a good position to suggest corrective measures. It may be that he will need to take samples, for example blood samples for a metabolic profile to check energy, protein or mineral status. Because he is attending on a routine basis, it is much easier to follow up at the next fortnightly visit with the results and any corrective measures needed. After a further two to four weeks the records may show if the necessary improvement was achieved.

In addition to carrying out fertility examinations, the routine visit is a good opportunity to check a few of the cows which have had troublesome feet, or maybe a group of weaned calves which are a bit loose and not growing as well as they ought. You may also want to talk about worm control in the young stock, or about a new animal health product which has been recently launched on the market. I think mastitis is such a complex subject that it is best to set aside an additional special discussion period at least once or twice a year. In our practice we like to visit just before afternoon milking. The records are examined to see what the current herd mastitis status is like and this in itself may give an idea of what to look for—there may be a high incidence of environmental cases for example, or possibly an excessive number (more than 20 per cent) of treated quarters have needed repeat treatment, suggesting a chronic staphylococcal problem. If it is the winter the cubicles are checked for comfort and cleanliness. Finally, in the parlour the milking routine is monitored, as are milking speeds and hygiene procedures such as teat dipping and udder washings, and a check for teat damage is made both before and after milking. The whole visit may take an hour or more, but it is an excellent opportunity for the herdsman to discuss mastitis problems and for the vet to check that none of the standard routine control measures are being overlooked. With mastitis costing an average of £21.00 for every cow in your herd, this is time and money well spent.

These are all aspects of preventive medicine. The overall concept is to reduce the effects of disease to economically acceptable levels by a regular assessment of performance as seen both in the records and in the cows themselves. It requires enthusiasm and trust on the part of both the farmer and his vet, but I am sure it is the way that veterinary services will progress in the future; that is, in the routine implementation of commonsense husbandry.

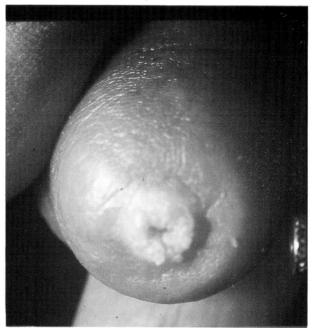

Colour plate 9   Early prolapse of teat sphincter from milking damage.

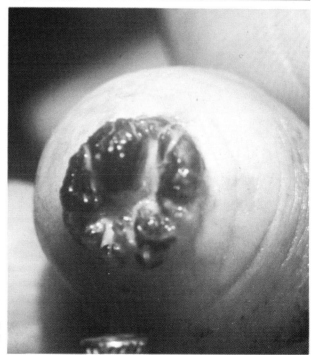

Colour plate 10 Advanced prolapse of teat sphincter.

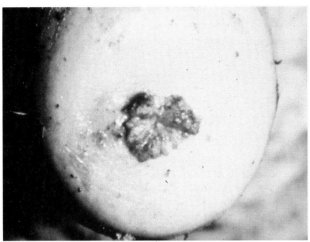

Colour plate 11 Typical black spot. The wound is obviously raw and inflamed.

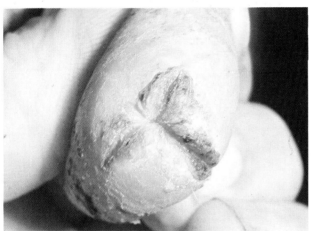

Colour plate 12 Teat slowly healing following blackspot.

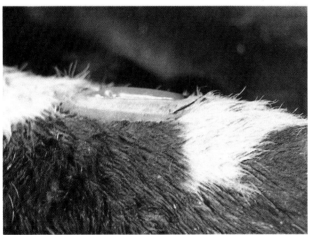

Colour plate 13 A kamar which has 'turned'. This is probably not a false positive because the cloth around the kamar is soiled, the rear edge of the marker is lifting and the cow's coat has been rubbed.

Chapter 9

LAMENESS—ITS CAUSES, TREATMENT AND PREVENTION

THERE ARE few conditions which lead to such a rapid weight loss as lameness and those of you with out-of-parlour computer feeders will appreciate that this is because an acutely lame cow virtually stops eating. In fact she may even reduce her concentrate intake some twelve hours or more before you see her hobbling. In 1978 our practice was one of forty-eight throughout Britain which recorded the details of every case of lameness treated, as part of a survey organised by the Institute for Research into Animal Disease at Compton. The survey showed that in that year 5.5 per cent of the cows in the national herd were treated by vets for lameness and of course this did not include the many other lame cows which would have received farmer treatment.

A second survey, this time at an abattoir, showed that three-quarters of all cows slaughtered had changes in their feet which could have produced lameness. In other words, the majority of cows are bred, housed, managed or fed to be potential lameness problems and we are lucky that the overall incidence is not much higher. The cost to the national dairy industry in terms of treatment, milk and bodyweight loss, and delays in conception was estimated to be £36 million at 1982 values—or on average £9.20 for every cow in the country, your herd included. The Compton survey showed that leg disorders accounted for only 12 per cent of the total cases (and these were mainly calving injuries) which meant that almost 90 per cent of lameness was associated with the foot. In the majority of cases (86 per cent) it was the hind feet which were affected, and in fact 64 per cent of all lameness was associated with the outer claws of the hind feet. Unfortunately more cows go lame during early and mid lactation than at any other time, and this is why the economic consequences are so great.

I would like to describe a few common leg problems first, then discuss conditions of the foot and finally deal with the causes and prevention of lameness, including a section on foot trimming.

LEG INJURIES AND ABNORMALITIES

One of my professors at veterinary school used to say that even if you think an

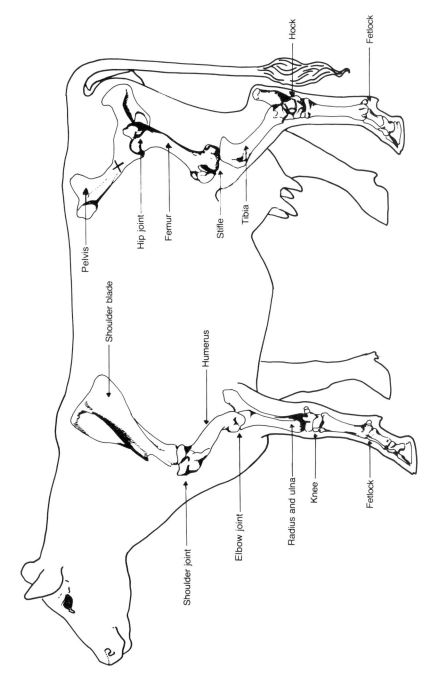

Figure 9.1 The bones and joints of the cow.

animal is lame in its head you should always examine its foot and I think this is an excellent piece of advice to pass on. Leg injuries do occur, however, and as you are driving the cow up to the crush to examine her foot, watch the way she walks: if the whole leg is stiff and being carried, or if it is hanging completely limp, then you may well be dealing with a leg injury. Figure 9.1 shows the names of the bones and joints in the front and hind legs. The correct technical terms will be used throughout the chapter, so be prepared to keep referring back to this diagram.

Knocked-Down Pin-Bone

The pin-bone is the front wing of the pelvis. It can be broken by cows pushing through doorways and other narrow entrances. Although the cow looks peculiar (plate 9.1a), with one side much lower than the other, it rarely causes any lameness and if the skin is not broken, no treatment is necessary. She will continue to lead a normal productive life.

Split 'H' Bones

The 'H' bone (sometimes written as 'aitch' bone) is the name given to the pelvis and so a cow which has 'split her Hs' has a broken pelvis. It occurs as a result of a cow 'doing the splits', either because she lost her grip on slippery concrete, or because of an injury when she was bulling, or perhaps following obturator nerve paralysis at calving (see page 121). Plate 9.1b shows a cow whose pelvis rotated on her spine as a result of a very tight calving. She

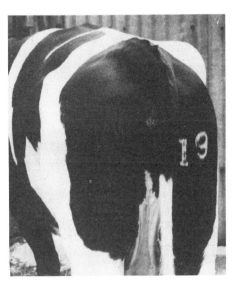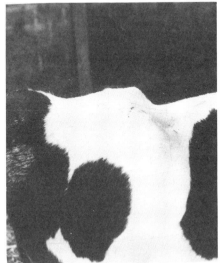

Plate 9.1   Pelvic injuries: (*left*) the knocked-down pin-bone did not affect this cow; (*right*) the pelvis rotated about this cow's spine at calving—she eventually lost the use of her legs.

eventually 'went down' and had to be sent off. Pelvic damage can also be the result of cows unsteady with milk fever being walked across a slippery yard.

There is no specific treatment, although your vet may prescribe drugs such as phenylbutazone which act as a painkiller and which also reduce the amount of bruising, inflammation and swelling which could otherwise put pressure on the nerves and result in their loss of function. Nerve damage at calving, lifting and moving recumbent cows and tying a rope around the hocks to prevent cows doing the splits are all described on pages 119–127. If you have a cow 'down' on a concrete yard it is most important that you move her, either out into a field or onto deep straw bedding. This is most easily done by rolling her onto her side on a gate and pulling the gate behind a tractor (plate 5.28). Taking her off the concrete will prevent any further injuries and it may give her enough confidence to get up and walk. Cows with minor fractures of the pelvis may recover, with time and rest, but they *must* be kept off slippery concrete. More severely injured cases have to be sent off.

Dislocated Hip

The normal position of the hip joint is shown in figure 9.1 Dislocation (sometimes called luxation or subluxation) means that the ball of the upper end of the femur has been forced out of its socket in the pelvis. The head of the femur then pushes forwards, and the ball normally rests on the edge of the pelvis, at the point marked X in figure 9.1, although occasionally it moves into other positions. It occurs as the result of a severe sprain or twisting of the leg and it is especially common in cows which have been on bulling and have fallen on slippery concrete while trying to mount other cows. This is exactly what happened to the cow in plate 9.2 and if you look carefully you can see the dislocated hip on her right side, producing a swelling under the skin. I find

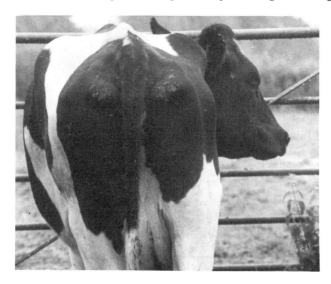

Plate 9.2   Dislocated hip: note the swelling over the right hip area. Hold your hand over the hip as she walks forward.

that the best way to appreciate this is to stand behind the cow with one hand over each hip joint and then let her walk slowly forwards. Very little movement is felt in the normal hip, whereas the dislocated end of the femur will force your hand out and slightly forwards as the cow tries to take weight on the affected leg.

If treatment is to be successful, it must be carried out soon after the injury, before the socket gets filled with blood and the joint becomes too loose. Your vet will sedate the cow and cast her onto her side, then he will extend the affected leg with ropes and pulleys as he tries to push the ball back into the socket. I have had a few successful cases, but many do not respond or the hip dislocates again as soon as the cow stands up. These cows may milk on for a while, but if they are already well past peak lactation, it may be better to sell them immediately, before excessive weight loss occurs.

Arthritis

The word means inflammation of the joint and the joints most commonly affected are the hip and stifle. I am sure you have all seen the smooth, glistening surfaces of a normal joint.

A cow with arthritis has little spicules of jagged bone protruding from the joint surface and you can imagine the pain caused as the surfaces rub across one another, especially with the weight of the cow pressing on them. Arthritis is most common in older cows, especially in winter. There is no long-term cure, but your vet may be able to suggest drugs such as phenylbutazone which will reduce the pain and inflammation in the joint. Moving her out of the cubicles and into loose housing where it is easier to get up and down will also help.

Calving Injuries

The most common are obturator nerve paralysis, in which the legs splay outwards, and peroneal nerve paralysis, in which the fetlock knuckles forwards. These were described on page 120 in Chapter Five, as was the use of the hoist, cow cushions and the general nursing of downer cows.

Rupture of Stifle Ligaments

There are several ligaments in the stifle joint holding it in place. Severe twisting of the leg can break one of the central ligaments. This results in excessive and abnormal movements within the joint and eventually the cow develops arthritis. There is no treatment.

Capped Knees and Hocks

Soft fluctuating fluid swellings over the front of the knee and at the side of the hock are quite common, especially in cubicle-housed cows. Plate 9.3 shows a typical example. The swelling is caused by continual bruising leading to excessive fluid production in the bursa, which is the name given to a type of

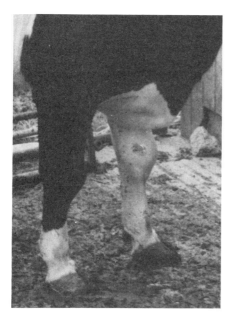

Plate 9.3 Swollen knees. The swelling is mild and would not need treatment.

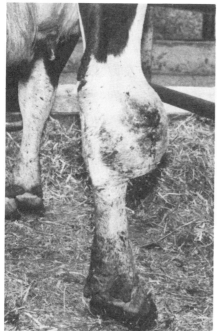
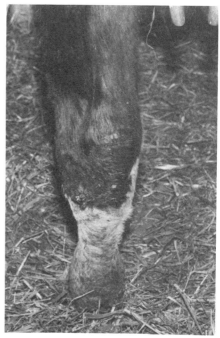

Plates 9.4 and 9.5 Plate 9.4 (left) shows a discharging abscess in the bursa over the hock. This should be compared with plate 9.5 (right) where the cellulitis produces more diffuse swelling and infection in the left hock.

shock absorber on the outside of the joint. The lesion is not painful and in the majority of cases it is best left alone and will slowly disappear after turn-out in the spring. Sometimes you may wish to drain off the excess fluid. To do this, clip the hair over the centre of the swelling, clean off the area very thoroughly, then insert a sterile needle. A light straw-coloured or sometimes reddish-brown liquid will flow out through the needle. Great care is needed, however, because of the risk of introducing infection and creating an abscess. If the swelling is large and gets damaged it may start to discharge on its own, as shown in plate 9.4. This now needs flushing out with water and antiseptic ointment put into the hole to keep it open and promote drainage.

Cellulitis (Infected Knees and Hocks)

This condition is also seen in cubicle-housed animals, and it is due to infection penetrating through the skin or even into the bursa over the joint. Rather than form a localised swelling, which we would call an abscess, the infection tracks up and down the leg and causes a more generalised enlargement, and this is known as *cellulitis*. This is clearly shown in plate 9.5. The affected animal will be holding its leg in pain, and there will be some rise in temperature. Treatment consists of giving antibiotics to eliminate the infection and anti-inflammatory drugs to reduce the pain and swelling. In severe cases this may have to be continued for a week or more.

Both capped knees and infections are caused by the same factors; that is, poor housing. Cubicle beds which are rough and have inadequate bedding, or where there is an excessively large or sharp lip at the rear, all predispose to bruising. In some cubicles, the design is such that the hock is knocked on a sharp edge of a wooden division when the cow stands up. This leads to the type of injury shown in plate 9.5. Cows which are lame from other causes also have difficulty getting up, and capped knees or infected hocks may develop secondary to the primary lameness.

Broken Legs

Fortunately this does not happen very often. The commonest point of fracture in cows is the top end of the femur, near the hip joint, and it is sometimes very difficult to distinguish between a dislocated hip and a fracture. Cows are so heavy that there is nothing strong enough to support the bones to allow healing. The young calf shown in plate 9.6 was luckier. He came in with a femur broken just above the stifle and, by using some metal bars for supports I was able to fit him with a plaster cast (plate 9.7) so that he eventually recovered.

Contracted Tendons

A proportion of calves are unable to stand at birth because their front legs are buckled over. Figure 9.1 shows the normal position for a front leg and plate 9.8 shows a calf which cannot straighten its fetlock joint because the

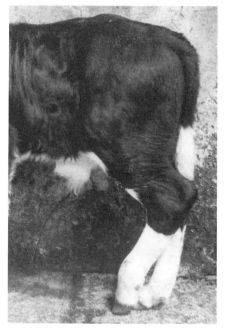 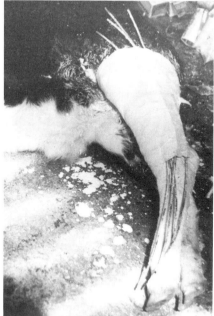

Plate 9.6 This calf has a broken left femur. Plate 9.7 Metal bars were used to strengthen the plaster cast.

flexor tendon running up the back of the leg is too short. The majority of calves slowly improve over two to three weeks and you can help them by providing plenty of room for movement and by lifting them up onto their front feet as often as possible. I knew of one calf which could not stand on its own until it was fourteen weeks old, but it eventually recovered. For more severe cases, keeping the leg extended with splints and elastoplast will help, and occasionally your vet may even have to cut one of the tendons to be able to extend the leg in the first place.

If the knee is also bent, the chances of recovery are much less. The calf in plate 9.9 had unfortunately been left until three months old before treatment and although I was able to cut through the tendons, straighten the leg and apply splints (plate 9.10), treatment was not successful.

LAMENESS IN THE FOOT

To appreciate the causes of foot lameness and their prevention, we need to understand the structure of the foot. Figure 9.2 shows a foot which has been cut in half. The hoof forms a casing around the foot. Inside we have the pedal bone (sometimes called the third *phalangeal* bone and equivalent to the last bone in our finger) and the pedal joint. Connected to this there is the second phalangeal bone, and then another joint, then the first phalangeal bone which

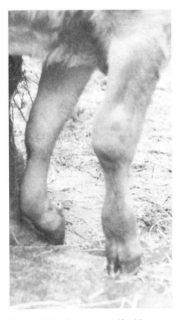

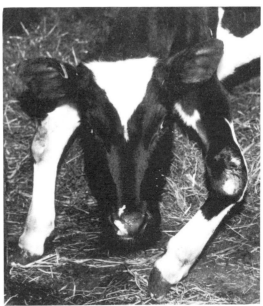

Plate 9.8   A young calf with typical contracted tendons.

Plate 9.9   More severe tendon contraction leading to inability to straighten the knees.

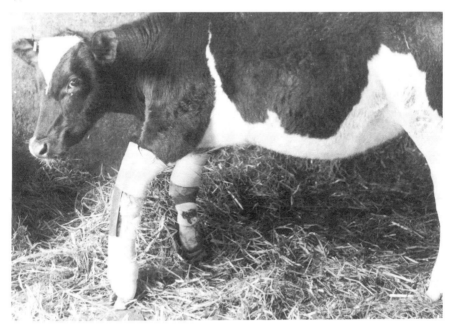

Plate 9.10   The legs were straightened by cutting the tendons and applying splints. Even then treatment was not successful.

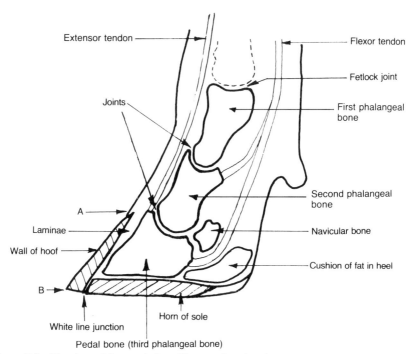

Figure 9.2   Structure of the cow's foot. Horn produced at the coronary band (A) takes approximately eighteen months before it comes into wear at the toe (B), although horn growth towards the heel is faster.

joints onto the main leg at the fetlock joint. These bones can also be seen in figure 9.1. Tendons run down the back and front of the foot to be attached to the pedal bone. The front one is called the extensor tendon, because it extends or straightens the leg, and the rear one the flexor tendon. The flexor tendon has to curve underneath the bottom of the foot and there is an extra bone at the bend which acts like a ball-bearing. This is called the *navicular* bone.

There are two types of horn in the hoof and they are produced at different sites. The horn of the wall of the hoof is produced by the skin just above it and this area of skin is known as the coronary band or coronet (point A, figure 9.2). The dead horn then slides down over the front of the foot on a very sensitive fibrous structure called the laminae. At the toe it moves at approximately one millimetre per week, which means that for a hoof 70 mm long it takes 1½ years for horn to pass from A to B (figure 9.2) and only when it reaches point B does it come into wear. This is one reason why changes in diet may take a long time to produce any dramatic improvement in foot condition. Hoof growth is much faster towards the heel and the horn produced there is much softer.

The other type of hoof is that produced by the laminae of the sole of the foot and this is called solar horn. To form a perfect case for the foot, horn

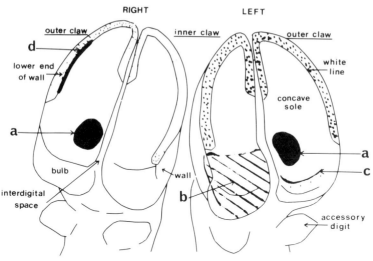

Sites of Lameness
(a) Sole ulcer
(b) Underrun heel
(c) Point at which pus escapes from an underrun sole
(d) White line penetration

Figure 9.3   The bottom of the foot, showing some of the common sites of lameness.

from the wall and from the sole must be sealed together and if you look carefully at the bottom of a cow's foot you can see the junction, known as the white line (figures 9.2 and 9.3). Many of the conditions leading to lameness in the foot involve the white line and the laminae, and they are described in the following section.

White Line Penetration

Inflammation of the laminae, the support structure for the hoof, can occur along both the wall and the sole and produces the condition of *laminitis*. We will return to the causes of laminitis later, but first let us examine its effects. The main effect of laminitis is that the white line junction between wall and sole becomes much weaker and if a cow stands on a small piece of stone, it is forced upwards into the weakened white line. This is shown in figure 9.4. What happens then is similar to a race. On the one hand the cow is growing hoof downwards, trying to shed the stone, but at the same time she may stand on another piece of gravel and force the stone further up. When the stone reaches the sensitive tissue, the race has been lost. Bacteria are bound to have been carried in with it and the warmth and food provided by the laminae allows them to multiply and produce pus. The pus increases in quantity, producing extreme pressure and this causes the pain which leads to lameness. Pus spreads along the line of least resistance, which in this case will be along the laminae, especially as they also provide nutrients for the bacteria. Most

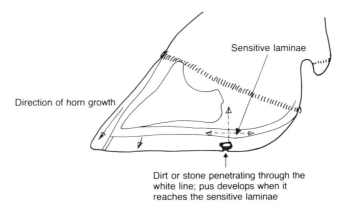

Figure 9.4   White line penetration. The dotted lines show how the pus spreads after infection has reached the sensitive laminae.

commonly the pus tracks up inside the wall of the hoof, but some will also spread across the sole. On occasions the whole of the sole may be underrun and pus will force its way out at the bulb of the heel (see figure 9.3) where the horn is softer. This releases the pressure and gives some alleviation to the lameness.

The condition is probably the most common of all types of foot lameness. It is called white line penetration, or sometimes a white line abscess and the treatment is to provide drainage for the pus. It is most important to remove all the underrun horn, so that there are no pockets of pus remaining. I sometimes use my finger nail to make sure that I have passed back to where the horn and laminae are no longer separated. When this has been done a dressing of antibiotic aerosol covered with a small wad of cotton wool can be applied and held in place by a roll of adhesive plaster (plate 9.11). This is left on for three to four days to give the new horn an opportunity to form and harden, but do not leave it too long as it may either cut into the skin or prevent proper drainage of the pus. If the latter occurs, it will lead to further under-running and the separation of more horn.

Sole Ulcers

The horn of the wall tends to be harder than solar horn and this is one reason why the weight of the cow should be taken on the shaded areas of the hoof as shown in figure 9.5. Some cows develop an excessive ledge of solar horn on the outer claw however (figure 9.6) which grows across to touch the inner claw. This ledge of horn now becomes the weight-bearing surface and the weight of the cow is transmitted to the *centre* of the sole, the point marked W in figure 9.6. Excessive weight at this point bruises the solar laminae: the horn which they then produce is of poor quality, often with clots of blood in it. This blood is a point of great weakness and is ideal for bacterial multiplication. When the soft and damaged horn reaches the surface of the foot, bacteria

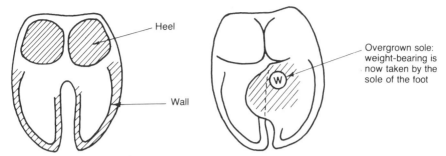

Figure 9.5   The shaded areas are the   Figure 9.6   Overgrowth of sole, leading
correct weight-bearing surfaces of the foot.   to ulcers.

enter and they can quickly grow down to the laminae. This produces pain and
lameness and the condition is known as a solar ulcer. There is an ulcer on
each claw in plate 9.19. When the ledge of horn in figure 9.6 is pared away
and the ulcer is exposed, a small lump of red proud flesh, about the size of
your little finger-nail, is often seen growing there.

A typical case is shown in plate 9.11. Bacteria are not necessarily involved
as primary agents in solar ulcers. Laminitis, excessive standing and other
factors leading to bruising and damage to the horn-forming tissue at this site
may cause ulcers in the absence of infection.

Sole ulcers are much more difficult to treat than a white line abscess. This is
because the abscess only causes separation of the horn from the laminae
which are producing it, whereas with a sole ulcer the laminae themselves have

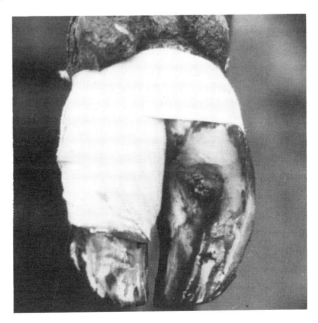

Plate 9.11   Typical lump
of proud flesh protruding
from an ulcer.

become damaged. The small lump of proud flesh is an indication of this. For treatment, first pare away all the excess ledge of horn and restore the correct weight-bearing surfaces shown in figure 9.5. Next, trim away infected and underrun horn around the perimeter of the ulcer. You should not be able to put your finger-nail between the edge of the hoof and the sensitive quick. If there is a large lump of proud flesh present in the centre you may wish to apply copper sulphate or some other astringent material to burn it back. Alternatively you could get your vet to amputate it. It is most important that the proud flesh is removed, as this will then allow the new horn to grow over the top. I would always recommend that the foot be re-examined four to six weeks later. The ledge of horn will probably have re-formed and will need to be pared back again, and there may be another small area of underrun sole and lump of proud flesh which will need removing. Some cows seem to have permanent ulcers and even when the affected claw is rested for two to three months by using a Technovit block (see page 255) they do not completely heal.

Punctured Sole and Pus

A variety of objects can penetrate the sole of the foot. Nails are the most common, but pieces of tin, metal or glass may be sharp enough and even teeth are by no means uncommon! Whatever the object, you can be sure that infection will be carried in with it and it is not sufficient simply to pull it out again. You must pare away the hoof around the penetration wound to make sure that there is no underrun sole and also to provide a hole large enough for the pus to drain out, rather than to track further into the foot. Whenever you make a hole deep into the horn it is most important that it is funnel-shaped to the outside (figure 9.7): a narrow hole may get impacted with dirt and this would prevent drainage of pus.

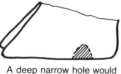
A deep narrow hole would become impacted with dirt

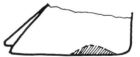
Make a funnel-shaped hole, even by taking away some of the wall, if it is near the edge of the hoof.

Figure 9.7   When paring a pus track, make sure that you leave ample allowance for drainage.

Deeper Infections

Whether you are dealing with a white line abscess, a sole ulcer or a punctured sole, prompt treatment to provide drainage for the pus is essential. If neglected, the pus may track deeper into the foot, causing either an infection of the flexor tendon, or of the navicular bone, or even of the pedal joint itself. The third condition is especially painful and even after you have provided

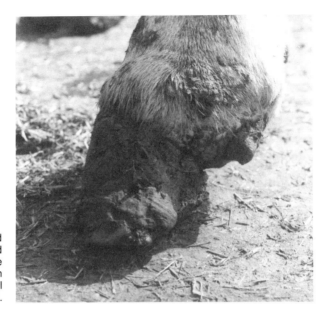

Plate 9.12   This cow had had her digit amputated two years before the photograph was taken and she was still walking well.

drainage for the pus in the normal way, you will find that the cow is still extremely lame. She will not put her foot to the ground and weight loss will be enormous. This is undoubtedly a case for veterinary treatment. Your vet will probably put the cow onto a long course of antibiotics (for example one to two weeks) and may even decide to amputate the infected digit. After a week or so to recover from the operation, cows with only one digit soon learn to compensate and can return to a useful productive life. The cow in plate 9.12 had an infected pedal joint, the result of an unusually deep sole ulcer. The digit had to be amputated, but she was walking well within three weeks and gave another two good lactations.

A slightly less radical alternative to amputation is the use of a *Technovit block*. This is about the only way to get the cow to rest her foot. The sound claw is thoroughly cleaned and a wooden block, 2.0–2.5 cm thick is fixed onto it by means of Technovit glue (plates 9.13 and 9.14). I usually encase the whole block in glue for added strength (plate 9.15). Even with over half a ton of cow walking about on it, the block may remain in place for two to three months and this gives the other claw plenty of time to heal. The technique is ideal for any of the deep infections mentioned above, and it can also be used if you have a particularly severe underrun sole or solar ulcer. In these two conditions relief is almost immediate and the block soon pays for itself in terms of weight gain and milk yield.

There is also a plastic boot available (plate 9.16) and some types have one claw more raised than the other. Although they are less expensive than Technovit blocks, they do not last as long and they tend to get mud impacted between the claws. If they are too tight they may chafe the skin at the back of the heel and if too loose they may fall off altogether.

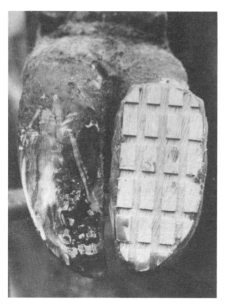

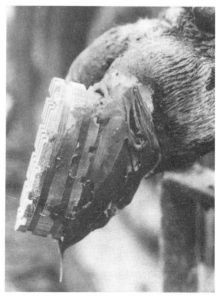

Plate 9.13 A wooden block is applied to the sound claw to raise the diseased claw from the ground.

Plate 9.14 Side view of Technovit block.

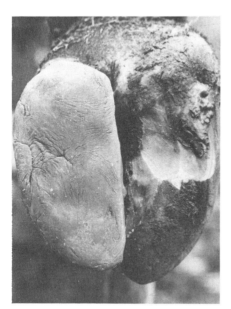

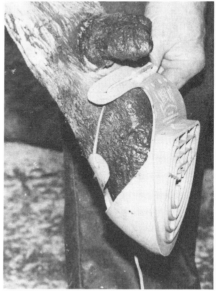

Plate 9.15 The whole block can be encased in Technovit glue for added strength.

Plate 9.16 A plastic shoe can be used as a temporary foot protection.

Underrun Heel

The heel consists of a pad of fat and fibrous tissue acting as a shock-absorber for the foot, and this is covered by a layer of much softer horn. It plays a very important role in weight-bearing. The horn surface should be smooth, but this is rarely the case in housed dairy cows. The protein-digesting enzymes and other corrosive factors in slurry eat into the heel and produce black pitted areas. Provided that they remain superficial these erosions are not important, but sometimes the cracks penetrate deeper into the sensitive tissues and an infection develops. Pus tracks along underneath the horn and hence the name underrun heel. Treatment is similar to the other conditions, namely, remove all the underrun horn and apply a dressing.

Underrun heels may alter the weight-bearing areas of the hoof, and this could predispose to other types of lameness.

Sandcracks

All the conditions mentioned so far have started at the sole of the foot. Sometimes the front wall of the hoof cracks, however, and a small particle of grit may enter. As the wall slowly moves down over the laminae the crack may become deeper and the grit may penetrate further until it reaches the sensitive tissues where of course it produces pus, pain and lameness. Treatment again consists of drainage: the sandcrack must be pared out with the curved end of the hoof-knife and you will certainly appreciate how hard the wall of the hoof is by the time you have finished!

Plate 9.17 shows a sandcrack which has been opened. Often there is only a very small speck of pus present, but this can still be enough to make the cow

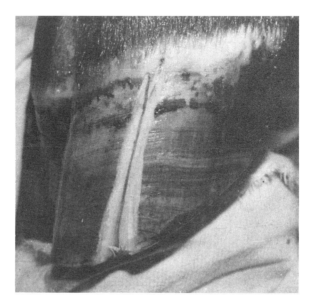

Plate 9.17   A typical sandcrack which has been pared out to release pus.

very lame. Sandcracks are seen more commonly in the summer when the hoof becomes very dry and brittle. Sometimes the whole hoof splits, from the coronet to the toe. This allows the two sides of the hoof to move slightly against one another, and such cases are much slower to heal. Occasionally proud flesh may develop in the sandcrack or the coronet itself may split and become infected. The proud flesh must be amputated and a pressure bandage applied to prevent regrowth, although these cases are often very slow to heal. A Technovit block could be used to rest the claw.

Bruised Soles

This is a condition seen especially in heifers during their first few months of lactation. At first you may not recognise it as lameness, because both hind feet are very sore and the heifer shuffles along very straight-legged. She will appear to have difficulty in standing up, almost as though she has arthritis, and she will probably lose weight rapidly.

When you examine the bottoms of her feet you will find that they are very soft: the sole can be pushed into the sensitive laminae with the point of your hoof-knife and this causes pain. If you start paring away the foot, looking for pus or an ulcer, you will find that you reach blood after taking off only a few thin shavings. You *must* stop at this stage. The only treatment is to take the heifers off concrete and put them into a straw yard, but it may still take six to ten weeks for them to recover. Young bulls running with a dairy herd on a concrete/cubicle system may suffer from the same syndrome, especially if they are overfat. The pressure on their hind feet when they are serving cows combined with laminitis due to overfeeding, are thought to be the two main contributory factors.

Fractured Pedal Bone

Sometimes the pedal bone inside the foot (figure 9.2) gets badly bruised, or even breaks, and this can cause an acute lameness. It is often the front foot which is affected, presumably because the cow was on bulling and came down heavily on the hard ground after mounting. In the early stages it is difficult to see anything causing the acute lameness, but after a few days the whole of the affected claw becomes hot. If it is the inside claw which is affected, the cow may stand with her front legs crossed, trying to put most weight on the outside claw and this is considered to be a characteristic position for cows with fractured pedal bones. The hoof provides an excellent 'plaster cast' and if a Technovit block is applied to the sound claw, relief may be almost instantaneous. In a few cases however, small spicules of bone grow along the fracture line, producing a type of arthritis and a permanent chronic lameness. Amputation of the digit is then the only cure.

Mud Fever

This is a condition more associated with horses, although I have seen it in cows which are out in very muddy conditions. The area of skin between the

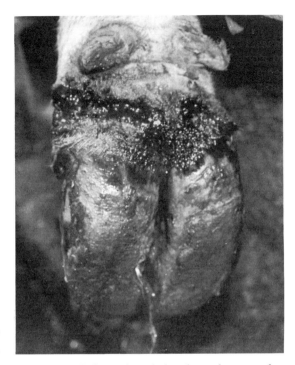

Plate 9.18   Severe cracking of the heel, typical of mud fever.

heel and the accessory digits becomes inflamed and develops deep cracks. The wound becomes infected and very sore. The cow in plate 9.18 was one of several cases which occurred in a herd during the very wet spring of 1983. For treatment, wash the wound with antiseptic and apply a greasy antiseptic ointment. Teat dips containing a high level of emollient are useful. Avoid foot-baths and, if possible, keep the cow's feet dry and away from muddy gateways for a week or two.

Foul-of-the-Foot

When you examine the foot of a lame cow, get into the habit of first running your finger along the skin cleft between the claws. It is surprising how often lameness is caused by a small stone or a piece of thorn or even a tooth impacted into the cleft. This is also the site of infection by the bacterium *Fusiformis necrophorus*, the cause of foul-of-the-foot. The interdigital cleft should be smooth and you should be able to run your finger along it easily. If the skin is broken, and especially if there is blood or pus present, then this is diagnostic of foul infection. The whole foot will also be swollen and if you stand behind the cow you can see the swelling forcing the claws apart. The pus between the claws has a rather putrid smell, and this is also considered to be a useful diagnostic feature. Take care however; there is often a foul smell in the interdigital cleft due to impaction with dirt, and unless the skin is broken and the foot is swollen do not diagnose foul on the basis of smell alone.

The most effective treatment is an injection of antibiotic and your vet will prescribe a suitable preparation. Sulphonamides can also be used and may be preferred. Foul is the commonest cause of lameness in young stock, both when grazing and when housed, and sometimes severe outbreaks occur with almost every animal in the group affected. Muddy conditions underfoot spread the infection and kale stumps or very hard and uneven soil (due to frost or dry weather) which damage the interdigital skin, help the bacteria to get established. If left untreated, the infection may penetrate the joint and one of the more radical measures described on page 254 will then be needed for treatment.

Interdigital Fibroma

The other condition which occurs in the interdigital space and which can be confused with foul is the presence of a large lump of fibrous tissue or gristle and this is known technically as an *interdigital fibroma*. A typical example is shown in plate 9.19. It develops from one of the folds of skin which are found each side of the interdigital space (see figure 9.3) and the condition is quite strongly inherited. It is more common in Herefords, although I know of a few Friesian herds where it is also quite a problem. It appears to be associated

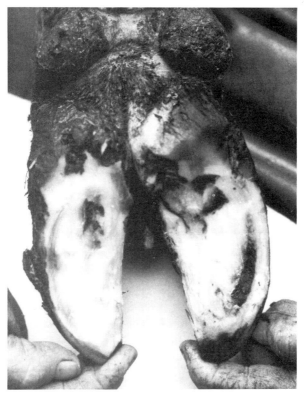

Plate 9.19 This foot has an ulcer on each sole, plus an interdigital fibroma.

with older and heavier animals, and is probably exacerbated by chronic irritation, possibly as a result of low-grade and long-standing foul infection. Another suggestion is that when the interdigital cleft is too narrow, dirt gets trapped, and the irritation this causes leads to proliferation of the skin fold.

Early cases can be treated by shaping the foot to increase the space in the interdigital area, and also treating for foul if the top of the fibroma has become infected. If there is a large lump present, then you need to get your vet to amputate it surgically. It is not a difficult operation. It can be performed with the cow standing in a crush and the foot in the normal position for hoof paring (see pages 266–8).

Some of the Causes of Lameness

I have left the causes and prevention of lameness until the end, because so many of the preventive measures are applicable to all the conditions we have discussed. Research workers have shown that soft horn differs from hard horn in that it has a lower content of sulphur and zinc and a higher water content (or, put another way, a lower dry matter content which means that it is less dense). Black hoof is also much harder than white. Laminitis leads to softening of the horn, because the inflamed laminae tend to produce horn faster; this also makes the claws overgrown. Laminitis is a painful condition; the cows' feet are throbbing and so they walk with an abnormal gait, throwing their feet outwards and this leads to uneven weight bearing and the ledge of horn shown in figure 9.6.

Laminitis can be produced by both physical and dietary factors. Physically, anything which increases the amount of bruising on the feet leads to laminitis, so rough, pitted concrete and gravel tracks should be avoided. In addition, there must be enough room for the cows to lie down and the cubicles must be large enough and comfortable enough to encourage the cows to take the weight off their feet. One of the worst outbreaks of laminitis and sole ulcers that I have ever seen followed the introduction of a herd from a strawyard into a new cubicle house. The cubicle beds had been made with tarmac, which in itself is comfortable, but they had been laid so that the front half of the

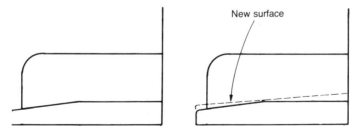

Figure 9.8   The cubicles on the left were uncomfortable because of the bump in the centre. They were altered as shown on the right and although this produced an excessively high kerb, the cows found them far more acceptable.

cubicle was level and the rear half had a steep slope, producing a bump in the centre, as shown in figure 9.8. The cubicles were obviously uncomfortable because very few cows were using them properly. The remainder of the herd were either lying in the passage, or standing with their front feet in the cubicle and their hind feet in the dunging area, or simply wandering around. The excessive bruising on their feet led to haemorrhage in the sole and the production of ulcers (as described on page 252). The cubicle beds were relaid, with an even 4 inch slope from front to rear, the cows used them better and eventually the lameness subsided. Those cows which had had severe ulcers took months to recover however, and many had to be culled.

Research workers have shown that cubicle dimensions, the design of the divisions and the comfort of the bed all have an effect on the length of time a cow spends lying down. Cubicles should be 1.2 metres wide and 2.2 metres long (approximately 4 ft by 7 ft) for large cows and if possible they should allow another 1.2 metres at the front for a 'lunge forward' space, that is an area that the cow can move her head forward into as she goes to stand up. The need for such a space is demonstrated in figure 9.9, which shows the sequence of movements a cow makes when standing up. I prefer to see the minimum of cubicle division and the type shown on plate 9.20(a) is good for comfort.

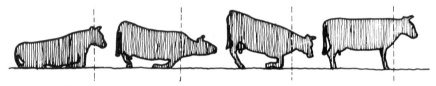

Figure 9.9   The cow stretches forward as she stands up.

Other useful designs are those which have a flexible lower rail provided by a rope or a suspended length of wood (plate 9.20(b)). Cubicles built with timber with sharp squared edges and consisting of a vertical rear upright and several horizontal dividing bars are particularly likely to cause bruising to hocks and pin-bones, and are therefore unlikely to be favoured by the cows. Cubicle bedding also has an effect on comfort. Table 9.1 shows the length of time that cows spent lying down in cubicles with varying types of floor surface. The advantage of the chopped straw or mat speaks for itself.

Table 9.1   In this trial it was found that cows preferred cubicles which were either deeply bedded with chopped straw, or those which had a thick cushioned mat.

Type of cubicle bed	Length of time cows spent resting each day
Bare concrete	7.2 hours
Insulated concrete screed	8.1 hours
Hard rubber mat	9.8 hours
Chopped straw on concrete	14.1 hours
Proprietary cow cushion	14.4 hours

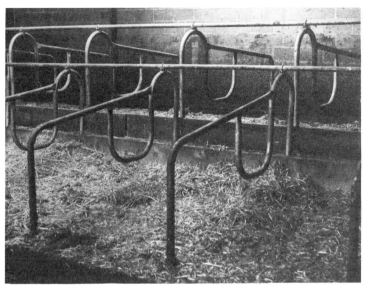

Plate 9.20   Two types of cubicle division—metal (A) and wooden (B).

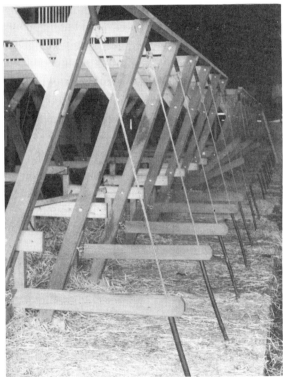

In addition to cubicle comfort, there must be enough space for the cows to move around. Overcrowding and lack of loafing areas mean that they do not walk about very much, their hooves are not worn down naturally and so the feet become overgrown. If cows stand still for long periods, especially in the wet and cold, the blood supply to the hoof is devitalised and this could lead to poor horn structure. A similar syndrome affected soldiers standing for long periods in muddy trenches during the First World War. Excessively sharp turns and uneven steps in cubicle passages and at the exit to the parlour have been suggested as leading to uneven wear on the foot, and even this may cause extra bruising and lead to lameness.

Be careful when laying new concrete. Select a round aggregate, rather than sharp flints and use a dry mix, avoiding excessive tamping, so that the small stones do not rise to the surface. New concrete is very caustic and has a corrosive action on feet so the surface should be thoroughly washed down or, even better, covered with straw or dung, before the cows are brought onto it.

Nutritionally laminitis is associated with diets which produce ruminal acidosis, that is very acid conditions in the rumen. This can occur when there is insufficient long fibre in the ration and as a good 'rule of thumb' guide you should aim for a diet of not more than 70 per cent compound feed, containing at least 5 kg of long fibre (or provide 1 per cent of bodyweight as forage dry matter). Diets based on high-quality precision-chop silage or maize silage may predispose to acidosis and in such cases I would recommend providing access to 2–3 kg of hay or straw each day as long fibre. It is surprising how readily the cows will eat this. Feeding large quantities of concentrate in the parlour twice daily leads to periods of acidosis for one to two hours after the concentrate has been eaten and in some cows this may be severe enough to virtually stop all ruminal movements. The problem can be overcome in part by the incorporation of 1½–2 per cent sodium bicarbonate in the feed as a buffer, but it would be better to aim for more regular concentrate feeds throughout the day, for example, using out-of-parlour feeders. Prevention of acidosis also helps to maintain butterfat levels in the milk. A further description of acidosis is given in Chapter Six, page 154.

High-protein feeds have been incriminated as a cause of laminitis, especially if the amount of degradable protein in the diet is high. Silages with an abnormal level (e.g. above 20 per cent) of free ammonia nitrogen (sometimes called non-protein nitrogen) could be dangerous in this respect although its main effect would be to decrease palatability. Overeating in any form, or any toxic condition, for example from an acute metritis or associated with photosensitisation may lead to laminitis in an individual animal. It is the composition of the diet and not simply the overall energy intake achieved by the cows which affects the incidence of laminitis. Table 9.2 shows two groups of cows, one of which (a) was fed a high-fibre diet and the other (b) a low-fibre and high-concentrate diet. Both rations had the same crude protein content and both groups of cows achieved a similar total daily energy intake, although the high-fibre group clearly needed a greater dry matter intake to do so.

The higher incidence of both laminitis and sole ulcers in the low-fibre group is most striking, although it was found that precalving feeding had no

Table 9.2   Cows fed a high concentrate/low fibre ration are much more likely to develop laminitis and sole ulcers, even though the total daily ME intake of the two groups was very similar.

	ME (MJ/kg)	CP (g/kg)	No. of cows per group	No. showing clinical laminitis	No. showing sole ulcers
Diet A high fibre	10.8	158	26	2 (8%)	2 (8%)
Diet B low-fibre	11.1	157	25	17 (68%)	16 (64%)

(from Livesey C. T. and Fleming F. L. (1984) *Vet. Record 114* 510)

significant effect. Despite regular foot trimming, the low-fibre group also developed far more solar overgrowths of the type shown in figure 9.6.

In addition to laminitis, very wet conditions underfoot may also lead to softening of the horn and so it is important to keep cubicle passages clean, to avoid muddy gateways and, if possible, provide concrete tracks through fields. Slurry is doubly important because it also contains protein-digesting enzymes and other factors which are corrosive to the hoof.

Certain families of cows seem to be more affected by lameness than others and I have always felt that some of the very heavy standard British Friesians are especially prone. Factors such as straight hocks, very curved fetlocks which almost touch the ground and the angle at which the sole of the hoof contacts the floor, have all been suggested as factors predisposing to lameness. Dry cows in late pregnancy have additional weight to carry; in early lactation cows may be overfat and if their udders are big they will walk splay-legged, producing uneven foot wear. All these factors are additional reasons why lameness is more common in cows at peak yield. Not only is the cow physically at a stage when she is more susceptible, but she has also been subjected to recent changes in housing, feeding and management, all of which might exacerbate the incidence of lameness. It is essential that these changes should be made *slowly* if problems are to be avoided.

PREVENTING AND REDUCING LAMENESS

Many of the ways of preventing lameness will be the reverse of the causes we have described already, that is, avoiding laminitis by correct feeding and by making sure that the feet do not get excessively bruised. Cubicle design is probably the single most important feature in reducing bruising of the solar horn. Soft horn has a lower zinc content and if faced with a massive outbreak of lameness it may be worth supplementing the ration with 3.0 grams of zinc oxide per cow per day. Trials in France and Greece have shown beneficial results, although no experimental work has been carried out in Britain so far and there is some risk that overuse of zinc will induce a copper deficiency. Increasing the level of biotin (a B vitamin) in the ration may improve the rate of healing of sole ulcers. Biotin is certainly considered to be beneficial to hoof conditions in pigs and horses.

Keeping the feet dry will harden the horn, so removing urine and slurry has a double benefit in that both are also corrosive. Remember that normal horn should contain about 15 per cent moisture, but this may almost double if the feet are continually in wet conditions. Cubicle passages should be scraped twice daily and cubicle beds kept clean. The sprinkling of slaked lime used in cubicles for E. coli mastitis prevention is probably also beneficial to the feet in that it is bound to dry and harden the hoof.

Foot Bathing

Foot bathing is an excellent preventive measure, and I would recommend that cows are walked through the footbath twice a week during the winter months. A 5 per cent solution of formalin is most common, although you can also use a 2.5 per cent copper sulphate solution, or even a dry mix of one part copper sulphate to nine parts of slaked lime. Any of these will act as a good disinfectant for the foot, reducing the incidence of infections such as foul and underrun heel, and they may also promote the healing of ulcers. Some say that the drying action of formalin has a hardening effect on the hoof and this would certainly be the case with the dry mix. I like to see two footbaths, separated by a raised strip of concrete. The dimensions are shown in figure 9.10, and a typical design in plate 9.21. The first bath contains water to clean the feet, then excess moisture can drain off while the cow is walking on the central section of raised concrete before she enters the formalin. Trials have shown that formalin can be very dirty before it loses its effect, and one mixture should be enough for four baths for a hundred cows, although it depends on how dirty the feet are and whether an initial foot wash is being used.

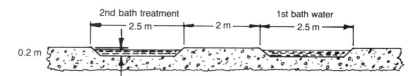

Figure 9.10   The dimensions of the footbath.

Foot Trimming

Foot trimming needs to be carried out on a regular basis and so you must ensure that facilities are available to make it easy. I prefer to have the cow in an ordinary crush and to lift and hold the foot as shown in plate 9.22. Tie one end of a rope around her hock in a slip knot. Pass the other end over the second side bar of the crush, back under the hock and then over the second

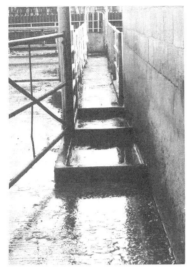

Plate 9.21 A double foot bath conveniently situated at one end of a race. There is no central strip of concrete as appears on figure 9.10.

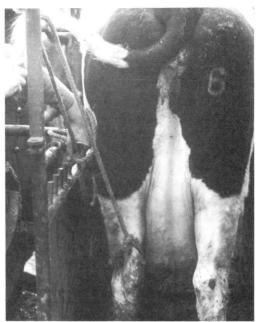

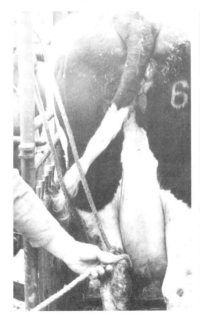

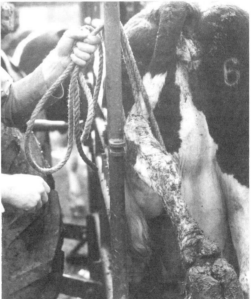

Plate 9.22 (a, b, c) Lifting a cow's foot. There is a slip knot around the hock. The rope is then passed up over the side bar of the crush, back under the hock again and finally back up to the bar of the crush, beside the first loop, to give a double lift. The foot is then secured by a second rope tying the fetlock to the vertical at the rear of the crush.

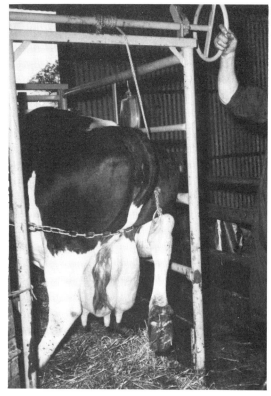

Plate 9.23   A simple winding gear for lifting the cow's leg.

side bar again. Attach a second, shorter rope to the fetlock, then pull on both ropes together. The cow will kick backwards and you will be able to tighten the first rope and thus lift the leg until the hock is firmly fixed to the side bar of the crush. Use the short rope to tie the cow's foot to the vertical bar at the rear of the crush. You now have the foot firmly secured with the sole facing upwards towards you. You can sometimes rest the front wall of the hoof on your knee for extra support and I find that this is the ideal position for firm but controlled work with the hoof knife. Plate 9.23 shows a simple winding gear which can be used to lift the foot into a similar position.

I have used specialist foot crushes either with belts under the cow's belly or a rotating table (plate 9.24) but for most work I find them either slower or the foot is at a less accessible angle for using the hoof knife. The only exception to this is working on front feet. Here a belly belt is an advantage, because it stops the cow kicking and if you also modify your crush by welding on an additional bar as shown in plate 9.25, or using a length of wood as a support for the cow's knee (plate 9.26), tackling front feet becomes a little less arduous. Thank goodness that most lameness occurs in the hind feet!

The only equipment I use is a hoof knife and hoof clippers (plate 9.27), although others include a surform and chisel. I much prefer a double-edged

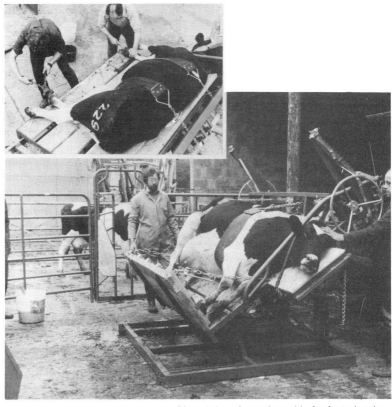

Plate 9.24　A rotating table for foot trimming.

Plate 9.25 (left)　Modification of crush for dealing with front feet.

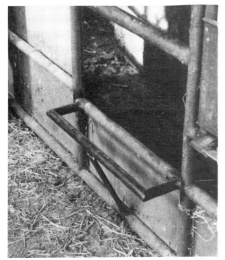

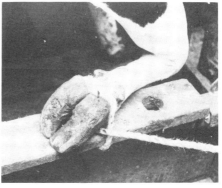

Plate 9.26　An alternative wooden support for holding front feet.

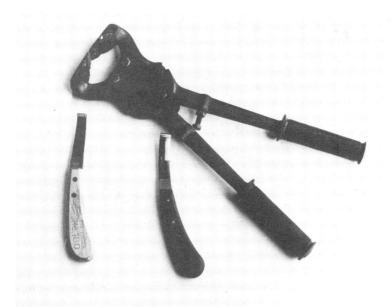

Plate 9.27   Hoof clippers and hoof knife: the double-edged knife is on the right.

knife because it is far more versatile. Whether you are examining a lame cow for ulcers or pus, or whether you are simply doing routine foot paring, it is essential that the hoof is removed in thin shavings, using the flat edge of the knife. I like to use both hands, as shown in plate 9.28, because I find this gives extra purchase, but still maintains good control over the knife. If you scrape the solar horn with the curved tip of the knife you produce furrows and this can sometimes obscure the small black line which might have led you down to the site of an abscess.

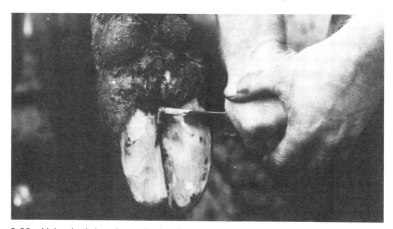

Plate 9.28   Using both hands on the hoof knife increases the strength and control of paring.

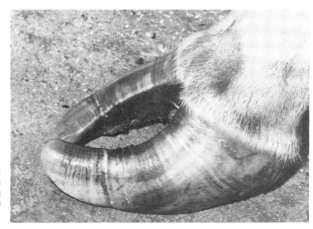

Plate 9.29 An overgrown claw. Note the rings on the hoof which are considered to be an indication of laminitis.

First clean the foot with a brush and water and then use the knife to remove any ledge of overgrown horn (figure 9.6) so that you have formed a reasonable interdigital space. Next take the hoof clippers to cut back the toe. Plate 9.29 shows a typical overgrown claw. The rings running over the surface of the hoof are considered to be a sign of laminitis. Plate 9.30 shows the action of the hoof clippers. Some say that the length of the toe should always be

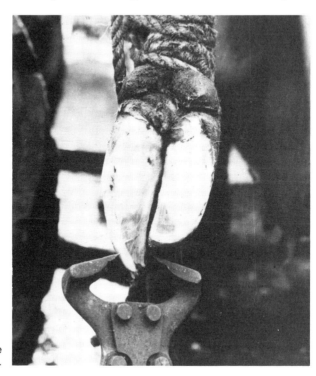

Plate 9.30 Using the hoof clippers.

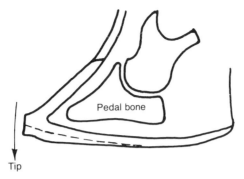

Tip

Figure 9.11   After cutting the toe square it may be necessary to trim along the dotted line to tip the foot forward.

7.0 cm (distance A to B in figure 9.2), but I find that in a proportion of cows with badly overgrown and flat feet, cutting back this much would draw blood. You are now left with a cow with a square-ended toe (figure 9.11). The final stage of foot trimming is to shape the foot so that the weight-bearing surfaces return to normal (shown in figure 9.5) and the foot is tipped forwards to prevent rapid regrowth of the toe (trim along the dotted line in figure 9.11). When you have finished, you should be able to lay your knife over the surface of the foot and check that it touches only the shaded areas shown in figure 9.5. The outer claw usually needs more trimming than the inner claw and this will help to bring the hooves equally into wear and the leg upright, as shown in figure 9.12. Badly overgrown and misshapen feet can be very difficult to trim. There is always the risk of over-paring and producing acute lameness from soft soles, as described on page 258. It may be necessary to reshape feet over two or three trimming sessions to regain reasonable weight-bearing surfaces.

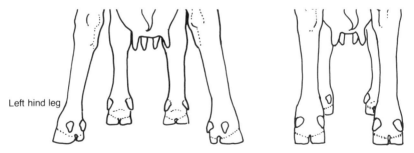

Left hind leg

Figure 9.12   The cow on the left has overgrown lateral claws. Careful paring will help to regain the normal standing posture shown on the right.

If possible, I would thoroughly recommend that you attend one of the excellent foot-trimming courses run by the Agricultural Training Board, or at least obtain some of their literature. Although I have tried to describe the procedure, there is nothing to match seeing it done and trying for yourself.

Ideally, feet need to be examined on three occasions. First, as soon as the

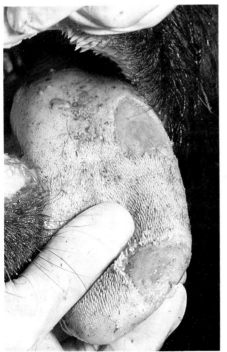

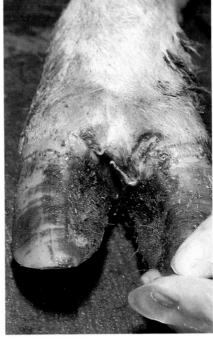

Colour plate 14 Foot and mouth. The appearance of tongue and hoof lesions after the fluid-filled vesicles have burst.

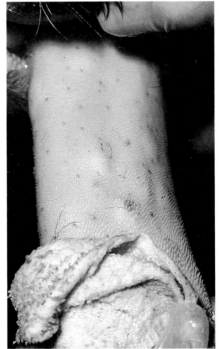

Colour plate 15 Foot and mouth. There may be so many vesicles present in the early stages that the skin of the tongue simply falls off in your hand.

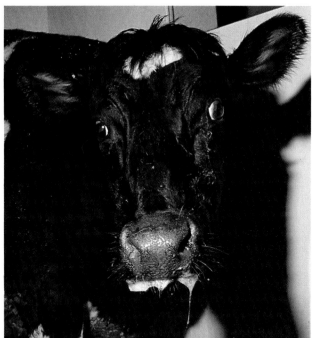

Colour plate 16   Foot and mouth. Affected animals are lame and they drool badly because their tongues are so sore.

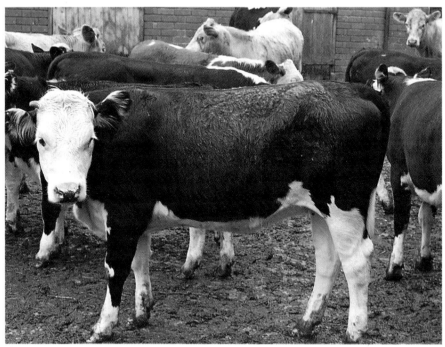

Colour plate 17   This animal shows a 'rusty' coat but it was not affected by copper deficiency, nor was it in any poorer condition than the remainder of the group in the background.

cow goes lame: delays in treatment could lead to deeper infections and a much more protracted recovery. Second, whenever they are seriously overgrown: this is especially true for the ledge of solar horn (figure 9.6) which can lead to sole ulcers. If you watch your cows walking out of the parlour you can often see this ledge—it may be present without any elongated toe, or other abnormalities, so you have to look fairly carefully. Third, I think it is an excellent idea to examine the feet of every cow at drying-off. Most cases of lameness occur in early lactation, and at drying-off you may be able to remove the piece of gravel or trim the ulcers which could otherwise cause problems later. In addition, if you *do* happen to over-trim, leaving thin soles or even drawing blood, the dry cow is less likely to develop bruising because she does not have to walk in for milking twice a day. If you cannot manage every cow at drying-off, then at least trim the cows with overgrown feet and those which had ulcers during the previous lactation.

Routine foot trimming is a very important part of the prevention of lameness and combined with foot bathing, attention to diet and provision of a suitable environment, there is no reason why your herd should suffer severe losses. Unfortunately the management practices involved in purpose-built concrete and cubicle systems, feeding for high yields and reducing the available labour, all tend to be contrary to this and I suspect that lameness will continue to be a significant problem in the foreseeable future.

Chapter 10

NOTIFIABLE DISEASES AND SALMONELLOSIS

MOST OF the legal powers conferred onto the Ministry of Agriculture are contained in the *Diseases of Animals Act, 1950*, which has now been incorporated into the *Animal Health Act, 1981*. This enables the Ministry to record and control the movements of livestock, to regulate imports, to enforce quarantine and to establish and finance national disease eradication programmes. It is the Orders made under this Act which makes it a legal requirement for all owners of livestock to keep detailed records of the movements of their animals, to identify cattle by means of an ear-tag, to report all cases of abortion and sudden death in cattle, and to dip their sheep at certain times of the year. There are many other regulations of a similar nature. The Act also states that any person in charge of an animal suspected of suffering from a *Notifiable Disease* must report it immediately to the police or to an inspector of the Ministry. Diseases are classed as notifiable when regulations have been made to control their entry into the country or to eradicate them.

Current examples include:

Anthrax	Brucellosis
Foot and Mouth	Warble Fly
Tuberculosis	Enzootic Bovine Leucosis

The *Zoonosis Order, 1975* requires that certain *zoonotic* diseases, that is diseases which are transmissible from animals to man, must also be reported to the Ministry of Agriculture. At present this includes only salmonellosis and brucellosis.

Anthrax

Anthrax is an infection caused by the bacterium *Bacillus anthracis*. In cattle it causes an acute septicaemic illness, resulting in very rapid death. I have only once been called to a live affected animal. It was extremely ill, swaying on its legs and died before I could treat it. In the typical case, after death dark blood often runs from the nose, mouth and possibly the anus and vulva. As it is a notifiable disease, any animal found dead without an obvious cause must be reported to the Ministry of Agriculture. At no expense to the owner of the animal, the Ministry will send a local veterinary inspector to take samples and

275

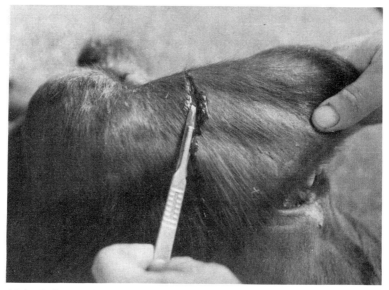

Plate 10.1   Anthrax testing: a cut is made through the ear vein to obtain a blood sample.

test for anthrax. A small cut is made in an ear vein (plate 10.1), a swab is taken and one side of a microscope slide is coated with a film of blood. This is taken back to the laboratory, a special stain is added to the blood film and the slide is examined microscopically for the presence of anthrax bacteria. The carcase must not be moved or interfered with in any way until the results of the tests are available.

The spores of anthrax are extremely resistant (see page 2) and they are infectious to man and other animals. If anthrax is confirmed, the carcase must be destroyed on the farm by burning it together with any soil, bedding or any other material contaminated with the animal's blood or faeces.

The disease is now relatively rare, with the total confirmed cases numbering approximately ten to twelve per year. The most common source of anthrax is in the imported meat and bone meal which is incorporated into animal feedingstuffs, and in 1977 there was a minor epidemic (139 cases) originating from this source. Disease can occur in man, either as 'boils' arising from an infected scratch, or as pneumonia if the spores are inhaled. The latter used to be known as 'Wool-sorter's Disease', because dockers unloading hides and fleeces were occasionally exposed to skins which had been taken from anthrax carcases. Anyone at risk is now treated with penicillin or given anthrax vaccine.

Foot and Mouth Disease

This is a highly infectious virus disease which can spread very rapidly to other cloven-hoofed animals (pigs, sheep and goats) and to adjacent farms. The virus produces large 'vesicles', that is fluid-filled blisters, some 2–4 cm in diameter. These are most commonly seen on the tongue and between the claws of the feet, although they may also occur on the teats. The blisters soon burst, leading to the areas of exposed raw and painful tissue shown in colour plate 14. You should imprint these pictures carefully in your mind in case you are unfortunate enough to see such cases in the future. There may be so many vesicles present that if the tongue is grasped in the early stages almost all of its covering may fall off in your hand (as shown in colour plate 15). This makes affected animals drool (colour plate 16) and they also become very uncomfortable on their feet, stepping from one to another and possibly kicking or shaking their legs. They will also be running a high temperature which puts them off their food and causes a drop in milk. If the disease were allowed to progress, affected animals would lose weight rapidly and milk production would suffer, but many would survive.

Sources of infection
Because Great Britain has an eradication policy for the control of the disease, determining possible sources of infection is extremely important. Imported live animals represent the greatest potential danger and so the countries of origin are strictly monitored. After arrival animals are quarantined and submitted to regular veterinary inspections. Imported carcases and other animal products can also carry infection. Again, the countries of origin are carefully defined, as is the hygiene at their processing plants. For example, only boneless meat may be imported, because if any infected animals were slaughtered the virus is most likely to die in meat which has 'set', whereas it can survive for much longer periods in bones. Infection from imported meat reaches farms via waste foods being fed to pigs, and there are strict regulations relating to the storage of swill and to ensure that it is cooked in approved equipment for at least one hour prior to feeding. The virus is so infectious that air-borne spread is also a possibility. Many of the outbreaks of Foot and Mouth have started along the south and east coasts of England where migrating birds may have carried infection from the Continent. The outbreak which occurred on the Isle of Wight in 1981 was thought to have been carried by the wind alone and there is considerable meteorological data to support this. By a careful examination of the direction and speed of the wind, and of the prevailing temperature and humidity, it is now possible to predict mathematically the climatic conditions which might enable Foot and Mouth virus to blow across from Europe. This provides a useful forecast of when extra vigilance is required.

Control of Foot and Mouth
This is based on identification and slaughter of infected herds, plus restrictions on the movement of all livestock within a ten-mile radius, known as the *infected area*. Much larger *controlled areas* may be established if disease is thought to be spreading. Slaughtered carcases, plus bedding and other infected material, must either be burnt or buried under six feet of earth. The farm must be thoroughly disinfected and cannot be restocked for a further six weeks. Because of the rapid spread of infection, early identification of disease

is vital and I would remind readers that it is their *legal obligation* to report even *suspected* cases of Foot and Mouth to the Divisional Veterinary Officer immediately. Failure to do so has in the past resulted in prosecution of stock owners, with quite heavy penalties being imposed.

Following the 1967–8 outbreak of Foot and Mouth, one of the worst on record and one which lasted for over three months, stocks of vaccine were accumulated to carry out a 'ring vaccination' of animals around an infected area, should the disease ever get totally out of control. There are at least five good reasons why it is hoped that these measures will never be used. First, once Britain becomes an infected country, it will lose many of its export markets. Second, because there are a variety of different strains of Foot and Mouth, the vaccine in use may not be totally effective. Third, vaccinated animals can become 'carriers', shedding infection to other stock. Fourth, some of the outbreaks on the Continent have been associated with inadequate vaccine inactivation, so that vaccination has actually been spreading the disease. Finally, and by no means least important, to give full protection, vaccination would have to be carried out each year, and in the long term this would be much more expensive than the current slaughter policy.

Brucellosis

Brucellosis is caused by an infection by the bacterium *Brucella abortus*. Its preferred sites in the body for growth are the uterus, udder, testicles and joints, although the uterus is by far the most important. Infection can only become established in animals of breeding age and although it is usually

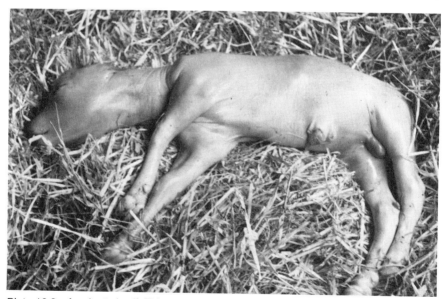

Plate 10.2   An aborted calf. This was approximately 6 months pregnant.

contracted by licking aborted calves or eating contaminated pasture, it can also be spread by an infected cow swishing her contaminated tail and flicking droplets of brucella bacteria onto the eyes or noses of 'clean' animals. Inside the cow brucella grows in the placenta, especially on the cotyledons (see page 96) leading to damage and loss of function. This then causes death of the calf and subsequent abortion, most commonly at the seventh or eighth month of pregnancy (plate 10.2 shows a foetus aborted at about six months of pregnancy). A few cows may abort for two to three years in succession and many others may shed infection for two weeks or more after subsequent normal calvings. Following abortion, infected cows frequently develop a chronic uterine infection. This endometritis leads to difficulties and delays in getting them back into calf. It also causes a uterine discharge, so that aborted cows may remain important sources of infection for several weeks.

Disease can spread very rapidly in a non-infected herd and abortion 'storms', with a major part of the herd aborting, were once common. This led to a tremendous loss of calves and of milk in the first year and to production problems in the future because of the difficulty of getting cows back into calf again. The financial consequences were often disastrous. As dry cows are usually run together in a group, if one animal aborts there is a strong chance that infection will quickly spread to the others. This is because of the inquisitive nature of cows and the likelihood of their licking or sniffing the aborted foetus.

Other forms of brucellosis
In man, infection is known as *undulant fever*, because it causes intermittent bouts of 'flu-like symptoms, with aching joints, severe lethargy and depression. Because the brucella bacteria grow *inside* the body cells (most bacteria live in the tissue fluid between cells) they are very difficult to kill with antibiotics and a course of treatment for six to twelve months may be necessary. Farmers, vets and slaughtermen are most at risk. Although milk can carry brucella, it is not a common feature of infected cows and in any case the bacteria are destroyed by pasteurisation. Humans are usually infected by splashes from handling contaminated cows, the classic case being a heavily infected retained placenta following abortion.

Brucellosis can also occur in horses and dogs where it may cause chronic joint or tendon infections, for example fistulous withers in horses. Bulls may develop brucellosis in the testicles and could spread infection during service, although most infected bulls become sterile and would therefore be culled.

Control of brucellosis
In 1967 a voluntary register of non-infected herds was started and eradication began in 1971. Good progress was made and by 1983 Great Britain was virtually free of the disease. Initially all calves between three and six months old were vaccinated with a live 'Strain 19' vaccine and in more severely affected herds the killed '45/20' product was used in adult animals. Although a few carriers could persist, vaccination dramatically reduced the incidence of abortion storms and therefore decreased the spread of infection within herds.

This policy was combined with a 'test and remove' regime. All breeding stock were subjected to blood tests at intervals of four months. Infected animals were identified and removed on each occasion. Milk ring tests, carried out by the Milk Marketing Board on bulk milk supplies from each farm, gave further assistance in detecting infected herds.

The early identification of infected cows is vital, especially as vaccination was discontinued in most parts of the country in 1979. This means that the national herd is now highly susceptible. For this reason, farmers have a *legal obligation* to report all cases of abortion or premature calving to their local Divisional Veterinary Officer. Affected animals should be isolated to prevent possible spread of infection to others and samples of blood, milk and placenta and/or uterine discharge will be taken and tested for brucellosis. If you wish the laboratory to check for other causes of abortion, including leptospirosis, then ideally the whole foetus and part of the placenta should be submitted as fresh as possible. Causes of abortion are discussed on page 236.

Warble Flies

There are two species of warble fly, *Hypoderma bovis* and *Hypoderma lineatum*. They have very similar life cycles which are shown in figures 10.1 and 10.2. Adult flies lay their eggs on the skin of the animal's abdomen and

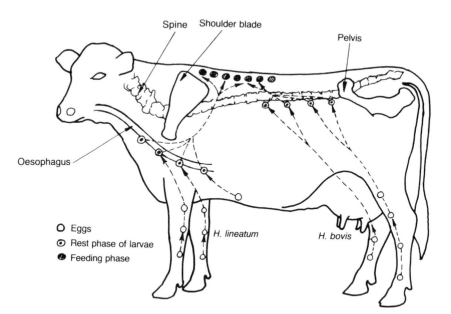

Figure 10.1   Life cycle of the warble fly. *Hypoderma lineatum* lays its eggs on the animal's front legs and its larvae have a rest phase in the oesophagus, whereas H. bovis lays its eggs on the hindquarters and the larvae 'rest' adjacent to the spine. Both types of larvae arrive under the skin of the back from January onwards where they undergo a feeding phase before falling to the ground to pupate.

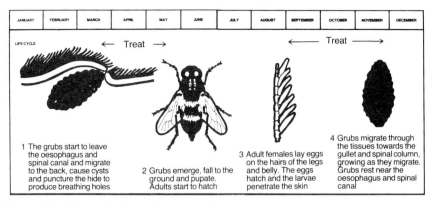

| JANUARY | FEBRUARY | MARCH | APRIL | MAY | JUNE | JULY | AUGUST | SEPTEMBER | OCTOBER | NOVEMBER | DECEMBER |

LIFE CYCLE   ← Treat →   ←——— Treat ———→

1 The grubs start to leave the oesophagus and spinal canal and migrate to the back, cause cysts and puncture the hide to produce breathing holes

2 Grubs emerge, fall to the ground and pupate. Adults start to hatch

3 Adult females lay eggs on the hairs of the legs and belly. The eggs hatch and the larvae penetrate the skin

4 Grubs migrate through the tissues towards the gullet and spinal column, growing as they migrate. Grubs rest near the oesophagus and spinal canal

Figure 10.2   The warble fly treatment periods.

legs during May to August, with H. lineata attacking primarily the front legs and H. bovis the hindquarters of the animal. The eggs hatch into small larvae which burrow through the skin and into the tissues. They then migrate upwards through the other organs, some having a 'rest' stage in the oesophagus (H. lineata) or around the spine (H. bovis) before arriving under the skin of the back from January onwards. There they make small breathing holes through the skin (plate 10.3) and the larva stays in one place, feeds and begins its slow transition towards the pupa stage. From the end of March to May the warbles may be seen as lumps under the skin of the back (plate 10.3). Eventually they emerge as large white fleshy grubs, falling to the

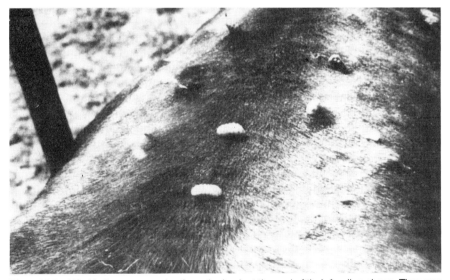

Plate 10.3   Warble larvae emerging from the back at the end of their feeding phase. They now fall to the ground and pupate into adult flies.

ground to finish their development into adult flies in four to six weeks. This is called the pupation stage.

Damage caused by warbles

This is of four kinds. Firstly the noise of the adult fly frightens cattle and herds of dairy cows may become restless and start 'gadding'. This obviously depresses milk production and growth and can lead to physical injury, especially to the udder and teats. Secondly the presence of large numbers of warbles under the skin in the spring is very uncomfortable and this also reduces production. Third the air-holes made by the warbles render this part of the hide useless for leather and the back is the most valuable part of the hide. Finally, occasional larvae migrating through the body enter the spine and cause paralysis, although this is more common when treatment is applied incorrectly.

Treatment and control

Traditionally the animal's back was scrubbed with derris to kill the emerging larvae; this has now been superseded by the organo-phosphorus pour-on preparations (see page 14). These are about 98 per cent effective if applied during the autumn (figure 10.2) but less efficient for spring treatments. Pour-on preparations cannot be used between 20 November and 15 March. Although the vast majority of larvae migrating through the spine cause no damage, if they are killed by organo-phosphorus compounds when at this site, they can stimulate a hypersensitivity reaction by the animal. This causes inflammation, swelling and pressure on the spine and may lead to paralysis of the hind legs. Several cases of treatment outside the recommended time periods have resulted in animals having to be sent for slaughter. It is interesting to note that ivermectin (see table 1.3) which is also effective against warbles, can be used at *any time* during the winter and as such is an extremely useful drug to administer to cattle which are being housed later in the year, for example in December, because it kills lice, mange, warbles, lungworms and intestinal worms, including the inhibited stages of type II Ostertagia larvae.

In 1978 legislation was introduced to make it compulsory to dress all obvious warble-infested cattle the following spring and this was accompanied by a vigorous advertising campaign to encourage voluntary autumn treatments, since these are more effective. There is now a *legal obligation* for stock-owners and others, to report all *suspected* cases of warble-fly infestation. There are movement restrictions and compulsory treatment regulations for individually affected animals and a compulsory herd inspection and treatment at the owner's expense if these regulations are infringed. In the first five years of eradication, the incidence of infested cattle was reduced from 34 per cent (1979) to 0.02 per cent (1983) with Anglesey having a significant pocket of infection, but provided that the impetus is maintained, eradication should be feasible.

Enzootic Bovine Leucosis (EBL)

This is a virus infection of cattle which produces tumours in the lymph nodes. Affected animals develop hard swellings under the skin, approximately the size of a flattened grape-fruit and the skin moves freely over them. One such animal is shown in plate 10.4. Weight loss is quite marked. Other clinical signs may be seen, for example chronic bloat due to an enlarged lymph node in the chest compressing the oesophagus, or roaring breathing from pressure on the trachea. There is no treatment and affected animals slowly die. A word of caution however—there are other causes of tumour development in the lymph nodes apart from EBL and blood samples need to be taken to confirm the presence of the disease.

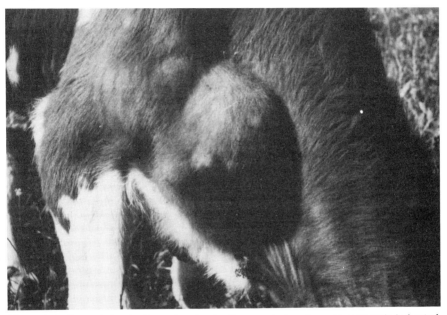

Plate 10.4   Enzootic bovine leucosis, showing the massively enlarged lymph node in front of the shoulder. (Photo: Dr Roberts, Weybridge.)

Transmission of infection

Calves are born free of disease but become infected via the colostrum during the first few hours of life. In infected animals the virus is found only in the lymphocytes. Lymphocytes are one of the types of white blood cells and are the main constituent of lymph nodes. The DNA of the virus actually becomes incorporated into the nucleus of the lymphocyte cell, and in so doing it alters its chromosome pattern and therefore the genetic content of the lymphocyte. This is a 'natural' form of genetic engineering. Transmission to in-contact animals can only occur following transfer of infected blood cells and this could occur via blood-sucking insects, contaminated injection needles or even sputum, as sputum contains white blood cells. Only 0.0005 ml of blood would be needed, an amount far too small to be seen with the naked eye. Even so, the risk of spread from one animal to another by physical contact is very low and by far the most important method of transmission is from the cow to the calf by colostrum. This means that provided infected animals can be identified and removed, control and eradication should be easy.

Control of EBL

The disease was made notifiable in 1977 and in the following year imported cattle and their progeny, a total of nine thousand animals were blood-sampled. Evidence of infection was found in sixty-seven Canadian Holstein animals and in two others but even then only 20 per cent of the calves from the infected cows were carrying EBL. A register of EBL-free herds was established in January 1982, based on two consecutive clear blood tests, and even previously infected herds were rendered EBL-free extremely easily. Because of the low rate of transmission of infection and the accuracy of the blood test, it is likely that EBL will soon be eliminated from Great Britain.

Tuberculosis

This is caused by a bacterial infection and was once one of the major diseases of cattle, especially milking cows tied in byres in close contact with one another. It was estimated that well over one-third of all such animals were infected. Many developed tuberculosis in the udder. This led to infected milk and hence to human tuberculosis, known as *consumption*. Tuberculosis in man, especially children, was extremely common. Some four thousand children each year were said to be infected, many dying and others remaining debilitated for life. This however was due primarily to the poor standards of housing and hygiene at the time which permitted a greater spread of infection within the community, although animal reservoirs of infection did play a part.

It is now very unlikely that clinical tuberculosis will ever be seen, although it should always be considered in cows with gross thickening of the udder, or in cows which progressively go thin and cough up blood and pus.

Eradication of tuberculosis

A voluntary scheme to establish a register of 'free' herds was started in 1935 and by 1950 there was a sufficient pool of clean stock to introduce compulsory eradication. This was generally very successful and by 1960 the whole country had reached the Attested Herd status. Testing is based on the 'comparative double intradermal test'. Two sites, one above the other, are located on the side of the neck by means of a scissor mark (plate 10.5). The skin thickness at each point is measured using a pair of special calipers (plate 10.6) and then a small volume (0.1 ml) of tuberculin is injected (plate 10.7). The injection is made into the skin and not under it, that is intradermally and not sub-cutaneously. Tuberculin is an extract of tuberculosis bacteria and if an animal has been previously exposed to TB it reacts to tuberculin by producing a nodule at that point. The test is a 'comparative' measurement, with injections of avian and bovine tuberculin being necessary. This is because there are

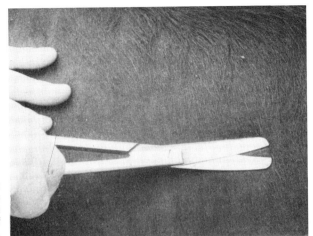

Plate 10.5 Tuberculin testing. Two sites on the side of the neck are identified by means of scissor marks.

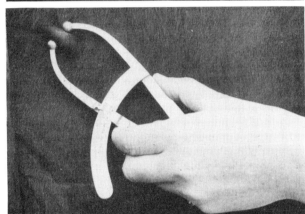

Plate 10.6 Tuberculin testing. The thickness of the skin at this point is measured using calipers.

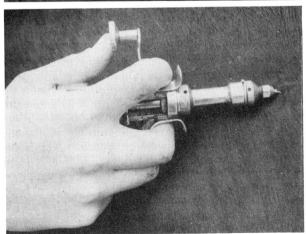

Plate 10.7 Tuberculin testing. A small volume of tuberculin is injected, avian at the upper site, bovine at the lower.

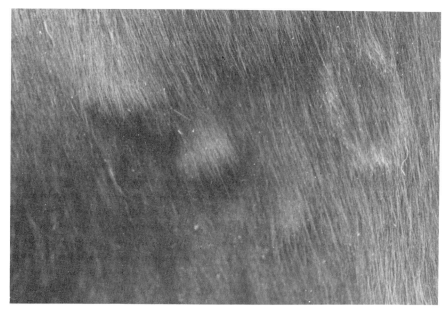

Plate 10.8   A chain of skin TB nodules. These may give a reaction which interferes with the test.

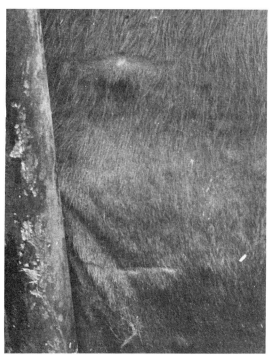

Plate 10.9   Tuberculin testing. The size of the avian and bovine nodules are measured 72 hours after injection.

conditions other than bovine tuberculosis which can give a reaction to bovine tuberculin. These include avian TB and skin TB, neither of which are harmful to cattle or man, and *Mycobacterium phleii*, an infection found on certain grasses. Plate 10.8 shows a cow with typical skin TB nodules running down the side of her neck. They may also be seen on the lower limbs of cows. Reactor animals are identified by the increase in thickness at the avian site compared with that at the bovine (lower) injection site (plate 10.9). A large bovine reaction and a small avian indicates trouble.

Tuberculosis in badgers
In 1970, despite the falling incidence of cattle reactors in most areas of the country, the level of infection in parts of Gloucestershire, Avon and a few other counties remained unchanged at around 0.1 per cent. This was associated with the high incidence of TB in badgers in these areas. It is almost certain that cattle infected the badgers initially, but in areas of heavy badger density, and where they are living in close confinement, tuberculosis is rife. The Cotswold hills provided an ideal habitat and in the mid-1970s 27 per cent of badgers examined in this area were found to be infected. Compared with cattle, badgers have relatively little resistance to TB. Once infected, disease spreads rapidly and they excrete large numbers of bacteria in their urine, faeces and saliva.

There are thought to be two main methods of transmitting infection to cattle, pasture contamination and contamination of feedingstuffs. The former is especially common because badgers have a specific 'latrine' area on pasture some distance away from their woodland sett and of course cattle will sniff and lick any unusual objects including badger urine and faeces. Badly affected badgers become weak and are no longer able to dig and forage for their food. This drives them towards farm buildings for easier access to feedingstuffs and hence TB contamination of cattle feedingstuffs can occur.

Control of TB in badgers was originally carried out by gassing infected setts with cyanide, but in 1982 trapping was introduced because it was said that death following exposure to cyanide was inhumane. In the long term the elimination of infected setts must be beneficial to badgers as well as to cattle and to man.

Occasionally infection has been seen in foxes and rats, but only at a very low incidence and in no case were these animals shedding any tuberculosis bacteria, so they could not act as a source of disease for cattle. Badgers are therefore the only known species of wildlife maintaining a reservoir of infection which can be transmitted to cattle.

Salmonellosis

Many aspects of disease caused by salmonella have been covered already, for example in the young, bucket-fed calf (page 37) and in the weaned animal (page 45). This section deals with the disease in the adult cow and discusses some of the possible sources and the human health aspects.

There are many different strains of salmonella (almost 2000 in total) called *serotypes*. In the 1960s the commonest serotype in cattle was *S. dublin*, but from mid-1970 onwards *S. typhimurium* became much more common and, in addition, a whole range of 'exotic' strains were encountered, with names like:

S. agona	*S. newport*
S. virchow	*S. enteriditis*
S. heidelberg	*S. seftenburg*

and many others. S. dublin is found almost entirely in cattle and the source of infection must therefore be direct or indirect contact with other cattle. S. typhimurium and the exotics, on the other hand, are much more wide-spread. Infection occurs in a whole range of animals, including man, which means that the possible sources of infection are much more variable.

Clinical signs and treatment
Salmonella particularly affects the intestine and *scouring* is therefore the most frequent clinical sign in animals of all ages. There is a profuse diarrhoea, sometimes with blood, and often mixed with large pieces of 'fleshy mucus'. This is the damaged lining of the gut being shed. Lactating cows completely stop milking, their eyes become dull and sunken due to dehydration, and they run a very high temperature. The dung will contain millions of salmonella bacteria and hence *isolation* is vital to reduce the risk of infecting other cows. Ideally use a loose-box with no drainage to the outside and particularly avoid surface drains which run across an open yard.

Next phone your veterinary surgeon. He will take samples to check for salmonella and will advise you on the likely spread of disease on your farm. Treatment will be necessary: kaolin and chlorodyne physically help to reduce scouring and intravenous fluids may be needed in severely dehydrated animals.

The use of antibiotics in the treatment of salmonellosis has been called into question on two counts. Firstly because of the risk of antibiotic-resistant strains spreading into the human population and secondly because antibiotics prolong excretion rates and produce more carrier animals. However, I consider that antibiotics are justified on both economic and welfare grounds. A septicaemic animal with a high temperature cannot be left to die and provided that an adequate dose of the correct antibiotic is administered for a reasonable period of time to a cow in isolation, the risk to the human population is low.

Infection with salmonella does not always cause scouring. Abortion, especially from mid-pregnancy onwards, may be the only clinical sign seen, although salmonella can be recovered in very large numbers from the after-birth. S. dublin especially may be involved and sometimes abortion may precede an attack of acute diarrhoea and death. S. dublin may also cause pneumonia, joint ill or even meningitis with nervous signs, and cattle of any age may be affected. I have also seen S. typhimurium isolated from an aborted cow showing no other symptoms and with no further cases occurring in the herd. This makes it very difficult when advising farmers what action they ought to take following the confirmation of salmonellosis in their herd.

Progress of a herd outbreak

Disease due to S. typhimurium and the exotics appears to be much more common in the autumn and this is thought to be because warmth and humidity predispose to the survival and spread of the organism. The isolation of salmonella from one cow, whether she is scouring or following an abortion, should certainly cause alarm and lead to increased vigilance, but possibly no other immediate action is needed, apart from treatment and separating her from the remainder of the herd. Ideally, faecal swabs should be taken from her until at least two consecutive negative results have been obtained. The cow can then be released from isolation

However, if disease starts to spread, careful control measures will be needed. The precise details will depend on the management and design of your unit and the action necessary should be discussed with your vet. However, as a general rule, calves from infected cows should be given ample colostrum and then penned individually to prevent the spread of infection. Nutritional stress, for example a sudden change in diet for either the cows or calves should be avoided, because stress can precipitate an outbreak of disease. Separation of the different age groups of cattle is important, and any measures to prevent faecal contamination of food should be taken.

Salmonellosis often strikes batch-calving herds, with disease being seen as a severe scouring just after calving or following abortion. In such herds control measures should include:

- Calve each animal in isolation in a clean box. With the stress of calving, a cow which has been carrying salmonella may start shedding infection in her dung. Ideally every cow should remain isolated until faecal swabs are negative, even if she is not scouring.
- Consider swabbing the whole herd at intervals of one to two weeks and then running infected and non-infected cows as separate groups. However, there are problems in identifying carrier animals by means of faecal swabs. (The reasons were given on pages 38 and 45.)
- Ensure that slurry from the infected yard does not contaminate the 'clean' group. This will be very difficult around milking time, so milk the infected group last. Chickens and other animals which could carry faecal infection onto silage, hay and other feedstuffs ought to be shut in until the outbreak subsides.
- Dose for liver fluke in areas where infection is a possibility, since moderate fluke infestations will increase the likelihood of disease from S. dublin.
- Vaccination. There is a good live vaccine available against S. dublin which can be given to calves soon after birth, or before they enter an area of known risk. The same vaccine gives reasonable immunity against S. typhimurium and although the period of protection is rather short (three to four weeks), this may be sufficient to control the worst of an outbreak. Some vets have given the live vaccine to adult cows in the face of an

outbreak without adverse reactions, although others say that it is dangerous to administer vaccine to an animal which is already incubating the disease. Killed vaccines are probably of limited value.

Sources of infection

The most common source of infection in calves is undoubtedly other calves which have been obtained via markets or through dealers' premises. The reasons for this are given on page 37 and clearly calves which repeatedly pass through such premises present an even greater risk. In 1982 proposals were made to restrict the number of occasions that calves could be exposed for sale to once every four to six weeks. If this is implemented, it would have a significant effect on reducing the overall incidence of salmonellosis.

Often disease outbreaks in dairy herds are not associated with recent purchases and other sources of infection need to be identified. The exotic salmonella species may be found in imported feedstuffs, especially fishmeal. Current importations are routinely screened at the docks and in 1982–3 approximately 17 per cent of 131 samples of fish, meat, and bonemeals tested by the Ministry were positive. Unfortunately no legislation existed for impounding such imports and by the time that the laboratory culture results were available, many consignments had already been incorporated into feedingstuffs and were being fed to livestock. At least the monitoring is able to identify commonly infected sources however. For example one type of South American fishmeal featured prominently in the results. Pelleting and other heat treatments destroy many of the salmonellae during processing, so that the number of contaminated finished feeds will be very much lower than 17 per cent.

Home-produced animal protein food, for example, from chicken offal, was also once a high risk, but the *Protein Processing Order* (1981) made it compulsory for all such material to be heat treated before its incorporation into feedingstuffs and this should no longer present any risk. The legislation would be considerably strengthened if compulsory powers of sampling were included, however.

Sewage is a further possible source of salmonella, from both human and animal origin. Human carriers are not uncommon and seagulls or other birds feeding on effluent discharged directly into estuaries, or from inadequately supervised septic outflows, have been shown to contaminate grazing land. Sewage sludge is a possible source, although there are strict codes of practice governing its use and the subsequent grazing of treated land, and most of the salmonellae die from desiccation within a few days of being spread onto the pasture, especially in the summer. Some may persist for a considerable time, however, particularly those protected in the moist environment of a dung pat. Although survival periods of up to six months have been recorded for both S. dublin and S. newport, it is doubtful whether there would then be a sufficiently large dose to lead to disease, since experiments feeding a hundred thousand S. dublin bacteria daily to healthy cattle failed to produce any symptoms. It does indicate a further possible source however and pasture contamination may be important in producing carrier animals which could develop disease following stress at a later date. During periods of flooding, salmonellae may be deposited directly onto pasture and be ingested by grazing animals. The importance of hygiene and disposal of faeces during an outbreak of disease cannot be overstressed.

Many wild animals have been shown to be carriers of salmonella and they can contaminate animal feed. Salmonella-infected rats mice or birds can contaminate stored feedingstuffs and it would be impossible to tell if infection came in with the original imported fishmeal or whether it was due to subsequent contamination either on the farm or at the mill. Clearly vermin control is important in this context.

Dogs or foxes could drag an aborted foetus or its placenta from an adjacent field, or they may simply carry infection on their feet. This is why the placenta and foetus should always be carefully disposed of by burning or burying. One of the major problems in trying to identify the source of salmonella during an outbreak is that exposure to infection may have occurred some considerable time in the past. It is only under subsequent stress that disease then develops, and by that stage the original source of infection may have long since gone.

Salmonellosis in man
With the increase in incidence in animals, there has been a corresponding rise in human infections of S. typhimurium and the exotics; infection with S. dublin is very rare. Symptoms are seen as 'food poisoning', with fever, severe abdominal pain, vomiting and diarrhoea. The elderly and very young children are particularly susceptible and deaths may occur. As with cattle, symptomless human carriers can develop and these people could be a risk to livestock, either directly or through inadequate sewage treatment.

The reverse, that is the spread of salmonella from animals to man, occurs most commonly through improperly cooked meat, improperly stored food or through drinking unpasteurised milk. For example, in Scotland, where 'raw' milk consumption was once common, there were 1,090 confirmed human cases of salmonellosis between 1980 and 1982, including eight deaths. In 1983 legislation was introduced to enforce pasteurisation (heat treatment) of all milk prior to sale and it is expected that similar legislation will eventually follow in England.

Chapter 11

MINERALS, VITAMINS, TRACE ELEMENTS AND WATER

MINERALS

CATTLE REQUIRE a dietary supply of at least fifteen different minerals for proper growth and production. Some, such as calcium, phosphorus, magnesium, potassium and sodium are needed in quite large amounts and these are known as the major minerals. Others are required in only minute quantities, usually expressed as ppm, parts per million, and these are called the *trace elements*. Table 11.1 shows the average mineral content of samples of temporary leys analysed by ADAS laboratories over a three-year period. This is compared to the requirements of an adult Friesian cow giving 20 litres per day.

Table 11.1 **The adequacy of mineral content of grazing for dairy cattle. All figures are given on a dry-matter basis.**

Element	Average values in temporary leys	Dietary requirements for a cow giving 20 l/day	% of samples which were below requirements
Calcium	0.63%	0.52%	33% < 0.5%
Phosphorus	0.37%	0.42%	61% < 0.4%
Magnesium	0.16%	0.15%	40% < 0.15%
Potassium	2.75%	0.7%	1% < 1.0%
Sodium	0.21%	0.14%	48% < 0.1%
Manganese	85 ppm	80 ppm	58% < 80 ppm
Zinc	38 ppm	50 ppm	93% < 50 ppm
Copper	8 ppm	10 ppm	81% < 10 ppm
Cobalt	0.12 ppm	0.1 ppm	52% < 0.1 ppm
Iodine	0.20 ppm	0.8 ppm	100% < 0.8 ppm
Selenium	0.07 ppm	0.1 ppm	—

Source: Mr G. Alderman, ADAS.

It can be seen that an average pasture (first column in table 11.1) contains insufficient phosphorus, zinc, copper and iodine to meet the needs of 20 litres production (expressed in the second column of table 11.1). The *average* mineral content of pasture consists of the mean of a very wide range of individual values, however. Soil type and geographical location can have a marked effect. Very acid soils tend to reduce the availability of all minerals to plants. In addition, temporary leys tend to be lower in minerals than permanent pastures and this is especially so if they have been heavily fertilised and growth is lush—which is exactly the stage at which cows would be grazing without supplementary feeding. On the other hand, mixed swards, for example with clover or other legumes, generally have higher mineral contents.

All of these factors lead to an enormous variation in the mineral content of pastures and the third column in table 11.1 shows the proportion of the pastures analysed which did not meet the cow's requirements. Taking calcium as an example, the table shows that although the average calcium content of the leys was 0.63 per cent and this would satisfy the cow's requirements (0.52 per cent), 33 per cent of the individual samples contained less than 0.52 per cent calcium and were therefore inadequate. In the case of phosphorus, the average mineral content (0.37 per cent) was less than the cow's requirements (0.42 per cent). This accounted for only 61 per cent of the individual values, however; or put another way, 39 per cent of pastures were adequate despite the fact that the average pasture level provided less than the requirements.

The table shows that there is a real need for mineral supplementation when the cows are grazing—and yet this is often not provided. Another survey looked at conserved forages in a similar manner. It was found that all the samples of hay analysed contained sufficient calcium for maintenance, but some 20 per cent were deficient in magnesium and over 90 per cent of hays and silage were deficient in phosphorus. The latter was especially common if the forage was very mature. Cereal-based rations, on the other hand, contain quite high levels of natural phosphorus and low levels of calcium and this helps to counteract the imbalance in the maintenance ration.

Mineral and trace element supplements are of course added to proprietary 'cow cake' to try to ensure dietary adequacy over a wide range of basic rations. The manufacturers will be assuming that you are feeding concentrate for almost all production, however, and if the overall diet contains malt residue, brewer's grains, sugarbeet pulp or some other by-product, then additional minerals may well be necessary. Although it can be a costly exercise to have each component of the ration checked for its mineral and trace element content every year, this would be the ideal situation and I would certainly recommend that at least the forage is analysed every few years. You will then build up a picture of the mineral status of your own farm and supplementation can be provided much more precisely. The money wasted from the haphazard and over-use of mineral supplements could well be equal to the loss of productivity due to inadequate supplementation!

So far only deficiency has been mentioned. The classic signs and symptoms of deficiency may be fairly specific, and there is a tendency for farmers to think that if they cannot see any of these changes then minerals are not a problem. This is a fallacy however, because mineral *imbalance* can also occur, when an excess of one element interferes with the action of another. Typical examples would be high levels of molybdenum, sulphur or iron interfering with copper metabolism, and the importance of the Ca:P ratio in the diet. The symptoms of such imbalances can be very vague, for example lack of thrift, depressed production or poor fertility, and the condition would be much more difficult to diagnose. There could still be a significant economic effect however. Avoiding excessive supplementation and providing each mineral at the correct level is almost as important as counteracting deficiencies.

Some of the more important mineral deficiencies have been covered already, for example magnesium in Chapter Six and vitamin E/selenium in Chapter Three. This chapter discusses the animal's requirements and some of the deficiency symptoms which may be seen. The information is summarised in tabular form in Table 11.2. Because any one mineral may be involved in a variety of metabolic processes, deficiency signs can vary considerably from one animal to another and it is often difficult to recognise a deficiency on clinical grounds alone. Blood, liver or even bone samples will probably be needed for laboratory testing. In addition, many deficiencies render the animal more susceptible to disease, for example to ringworm or calf pneumonia, and there is always a danger that the secondary disease is treated but the primary mineral deficiency is overlooked.

Calcium

Calcium accounts for one-third of the constituents of teeth and bones and in fact 99 per cent of all the calcium in the body is found in the animal's skeleton. Calcium also has important metabolic functions in the soft tissues. For example, it is involved in blood-clotting mechanisms and in the transmission of nerve and muscle impulses. Blood levels of calcium normally remain very stable and are maintained in this state by an interaction of vitamin D and parathyroid hormone (see page 142). The general term of *homeostasis* is given to the sequence of processes which maintain the various body systems in equilibrium. Milk fever is due to a breakdown of homeostasis. The cow is not suffering from an overall deficiency in calcium, she simply cannot mobilise her reserves sufficiently rapidly to cope with the sudden increase in short-term demand. This concept is explained in more detail on page 139. Blood calcium levels also show very little variation with dietary intake and are therefore a poor indicator for the metabolic profile test (see page 138).

Forages contain ample calcium for maintenance but as milk production has a very high requirement (2.8 g calcium per litre—table 11.2), high-yielding cows on grazing alone may fall into 'negative calcium balance' (table 11.1) and have to withdraw calcium from the reserves in their skeleton. Provided that this can be restored during later lactation and in the dry period, it is probably of limited importance and does not seem to harm the cow. Cereal grains are rich in phosphorus but low in calcium and if high-yielding cows are fed a diet based on straw and grain, additional calcium supplementation would definitely be needed.

If young growing cattle are affected by a combined calcium and vitamin D deficiency, then symptoms of poor growth, lameness, stiffness, bone fractures

Table 11.2　A summary of the mineral and trace element requirements of cattle, including the more important deficiency signs.

Element	Minimum Requirements For Adult Friesian			Deficiency Signs	Comments
	Maintenance	M+preg.	milk/per litre		
Calcium[1]	21 g	42 g	2.8 g	Milk fever = short-term imbalance	Short-term deficiencies occur in high-yielding cows at peak, but may cause no problems.
Phosphorus[1]	28 g	39 g	1.7 g	When severe, licking bones & soil. Ca:P imbalance may impair fertility	Low levels on some pastures, in kale and in sugar beet. Supplementation required.
Magnesium[1]	9 g	12 g	0.6 g	Grass staggers	Continual daily intake required. Falls in spring and autumn, and with high K fertilisers.
Sodium[1+2]	9 g	12 g	0.6 g	Licking, drinking urine, then poor growth and production	Deficiency can occur if milking from grass alone in summer. Ample salt in minerals and concs.
Potassium	3.5 g/kg DM			Never seen	All plants contain very high levels.
Copper	10 mg/kg[3,4] 15 mg/kg DM for preg. and growth			Coat colour, anaemia, poor growth and production	May be primary soil deficiency or induced by excess Mo, S, or Fe.
Cobalt	0.1 mg/kg DM			Anaemia and weight loss	Needed to form vit. B_{12}. Some soils deficient.
Iodine	0.2 mg/kg DM 0.8 mg/kg DM for preg. and lact.			Reduced milk prod; stillborn calves; increased retained placenta	May be primary soil deficiency or induced by goitrogens, e.g. kale.

Manganese	80 mg/kg DM[5]	May lead to impaired fertility	Some pastures are low.
Zinc	50 mg/kg DM	Dry scaly skin. Poor hoof strength and lameness	Some UK pastures are low.
Iron	30 mg/kg DM	Anaemia in milk-fed calves Never seen in grazing animals	All plants contain very high levels.
Selenium	0.1 mg/kg DM	Muscular dystrophy in calves and possibly increased retained placenta	Many UK soils are deficient.
Vitamin E	Depends on Se intake	As for selenium	High intakes will compensate for selenium deficiency.
Vitamin A	85 i.u./kg b.wt.	Night blindness, poor appetite, fainting, bone defects in calves	Seen only with poor-quality feeds in winter.
Vitamin D	10 i.u./kg b.wt.	Bone irregularities and other signs of rickets in growing calves	Problems in housed cattle only. vit. D is synthesised in the skin by sunlight.
B Vitamins		See Cobalt (B_{12}) and CCN[6] (thiamine)	All B vitamins are synthesised in the rumen. Deficiency can only be induced.
Vitamin C	NIL	Not seen	Produced in the animal's tissues.

1. Figures taken from M/A publication LGR21.
2. This is the sodium requirement. For salt, multiply by 2.5.
3. All levels are expressed as the amount required in the dry matter of the final ration. Units are mg/kg = pp = g/ton.
4. If induced deficiencies are present (e.g. high Mo, S or Fe), minimum dietary requirements may be very much higher.
5. Some sources quote much lower requirements than this.
6. A full description of CCN is given on page 60.

and other signs of *rickets* would be seen. This can occur in the winter in calves which are on diets of very poor hay and unmineralised barley, and especially if they are housed in dimly lit buildings, because light is needed to produce vitamin D in their skin.

In dairy cows excess calcium may also present a problem. This can occur with over-enthusiastic mineral supplementation, or on diets involving large amounts of kale, sugarbeet, or delactosed whey, all of which are very high in calcium. Calcium interferes with the uptake of manganese, zinc and phosphorus from the intestine and if these elements were originally present in the diet at only marginal levels, increasing the calcium intake can produce a deficiency.

Phosphorus

Phosphorus is the other major component of bones and the combined calcium (36 per cent) and phosphorus (17 per cent) contents account for over half (53 per cent) of the total bone ash. Phosphorus is also an extremely important element in the soft tissues. It is involved in the structure of membranes, in the formation of a suitable framework for nuclear division and other cell functions, and in the all-important transfer of chemical energy for metabolic reactions.

Phosphorus deficiency occurs in many parts of the world and in the British Isles additional supplementation is usually provided at grazing. Milking cows on grazing alone could be deficient even if they were only producing 10–15 litres a day (see tables 11.1 and 11.2) and blood phosphorus levels may fall because homeostatic mechanisms are less precise than for calcium. However, as with calcium, there are considerable reserves available in the skeleton and there is some doubt regarding the importance of a temporary shortfall of intake over requirements. Some feeds, for example kale and sugarbeet, are notoriously high in calcium and low in phosphorus, with a calcium:phosphorus ratio of around 10:1. It is best to aim for a ratio of between 1:1 and 2.5:1 calcium:phosphorus in the overall ration. Certain silages, especially those made from lush leys, may also be phosphorus-deficient. Protein supplements, cereals and their by-products (e.g. brewer's grains), tend to be high in phosphorus and low in calcium and are therefore very useful as 'balancers'. Alternatively you could feed a 'reverse ratio' mineral, that is one which contains a higher content of phosphorus than calcium.

Symptoms of severe deficiency would be similar to those of calcium rickets, although weight loss and lethargy are likely to be much more pronounced, and affected animals develop a craving for chewing bones and other phosphorus-rich materials. The temporary phosphorus deficit incurred by grazing or silage-fed cows may result in impaired fertility. There are experiments which show that phosphorus intakes below 18 g/day may reduce conception rates, and below 10 g/day fertility is seriously impaired. Opinions tend to be divided on this subject, however, and my own approach would be to say that when a herd fertility problem exists it is very difficult to be sure which factor or combination of factors is involved and it is therefore most logical to correct all dietary abnormalities when trying to improve the situation. This concept is discussed in greater detail on page 233.

In the majority of situations, additional phosphorus can be fed in the dairy cake and the manufacturers will willingly provide you with a 'special mix'. This is the best method because you can be sure that it is the higher-yielding cows, which need the additional phosphorus for milk production, that are then receiving the largest intakes. Alternative methods are to adjust the basic ration by feeding cereal products, possibly with added minerals, or to provide minerals on free access. I do not believe the theory that, when faced with a multiple choice, cows will only eat those minerals which they need. If this were the case, hypomagnesaemia would never occur. On a free access, free choice system, some cows will eat far more than their requirements of a mineral, simply because they enjoy its taste, while others will not bother to take any (see pages 148 and 307). It is pointless allowing the cows to consume massive amounts of a high-phosphorus mineral. Provide the daily intake which you have calculated will generously balance their phosphorus requirements and allow no more than this.

If possible, ask about the source of the phosphorus supplements being used. Certain types of rock phosphorus once contained high levels of *fluorine*, an element which can be toxic to cattle, leading to teeth and bone deformities. Sources are now carefully monitored however, and it is unlikely that such products would find their way onto the market.

Magnesium

Magnesium is the third of the major elements and, like calcium and phosphorus, it is important in the structure of the skeleton as well as having many metabolic functions. Magnesium deficiency and hypomagnesaemia are described in detail on page 145.

Sodium

Sodium is generally provided as sodium chloride, that is, common salt. As cattle enjoy its strong flavour it is used as a constituent of free-access minerals, to encourage the animals to eat them. Most free-access minerals contain between 20 and 30 per cent salt. Severe deficiency, leading to depressed growth and milk production, is unlikely, although periods of temporary deficiency may occur in grazing cows especially towards the end of a dry summer, when they develop a craving for drinking urine and licking objects. Modern intensive swards will have a lower sodium content than permanent pasture, especially if high levels of potash fertiliser have been applied. Table 11.1 shows that almost half the spring leys contain insufficient sodium for maintenance plus 20 litres.

Potassium

Potassium is such an abundant element in plant material that deficiency will never occur. In fact the urine of cattle contains very high levels from excess potassium which is being excreted from the body. The main importance of potassium is that it interferes with magnesium uptake by plants. As there are high levels in slurry, cows should not be allowed to graze slurry-fertilised pastures in the spring because of the increased risk of hypomagnesaemia.

Copper

Copper deficiency is seen in many parts of the United Kingdom and is a widespread problem in the rest of the world. Table 11.1 shows that over three-quarters of leys contained insufficient copper for milk production. Copper deficiency may be either *primary*, that is the pasture simply does not contain sufficient copper, or *secondary*, that is some other element is interfering with copper uptake. The best example of secondary copper deficiency is found in the teart pastures of Somerset, where high levels of molybdenum and/or sulphur interfere with copper absorption. Pasture levels of 2.0 mg/kg molybdenum can produce a deficiency, even though copper levels appear adequate, and sometimes levels up to 100 mg/kg molybdenum are found. A ratio of less than 3:1, copper:molybdenum, is undesirable and even at this ratio very high sulphur intakes (e.g. 3–5 mg/kg DM) may still cause deficiency. Sulphur forms an important linkage bond in the construction of protein molecules, and this is why proteins contain quite high levels of sulphur. A more mature pasture with a lower protein content will therefore have a lower sulphur level, and this makes its copper more easily absorbed. On the other hand, lush spring leys not only have a lower initial copper level, but their high protein content gives them increased sulphur, and this interferes with their already marginal status. Other factors such as excess zinc, iron and lead and excessively low or high soil pH may also have a detrimental effect on copper absorption.

Recent experiments have shown that animals with a low blood copper alone (primary copper deficiency) do not show any clinical signs. If a trace of molybdenum is then added to their ration, however, deficiency signs (coat colour changes, loss of wool crimp in sheep etc.) appear very rapidly. This has led to the proposition that the function of copper is to prevent molybdenum poisoning. Elements such as sulphur and iron interfere with this action of copper, and hence if they are present in the ration in significant quantities signs of molybdenum poisoning may be seen.

Copper is needed in the body for the formation of haemoglobin, in the processes of energy transfer, for hair and wool production and in the shaping of bones during growth. Deficiency signs are associated with these processes and are therefore very varied. Affected cattle will be stunted, anaemic and generally unthrifty. Many will be scouring, especially if molybdenum interference with uptake is involved. Milk production will be affected. In young calves the only symptom seen may be lameness and this is due to swelling of the ends of the bones near the joints. The calves may be in good condition, although they will be small in stature for their age and their coat colour may have a 'rusty' appearance, a feature which is most easily seen in black animals. The classic symptom is considered to be loss of hair pigment from around the eyes, leading to a 'spectacled' appearance, but I have never been convinced of this in the cases of copper deficiency which I have seen. A word of caution: loss of coat colour can be a feature of many other conditions, for example poor growth due to inadequate nutrition, some previous illness from which the animal is still recovering, or simply bleaching of the normal winter coat which is being shed in the spring (colour plate 17). In my experience, lack of coat colour and 'rustiness' are far more common than copper deficiency. In adult cattle, and others affected by molybdenum and/or sulphur-induced deficiency, scouring and weight loss are the most prominent features, although the scouring may subside if the animals are brought indoors. Copper deficiency may lead to reduced conception rates and poor oestrus behaviour and although there is some dispute over the importance of this under UK conditions, it is most sensible to ensure that adequate supplementation is provided. Much of the variation in results of experiments has probably been because insufficient attention was paid to molybdenum, sulphur and iron levels.

Diagnosis of copper deficiency
Analysis of the ration for copper, molybdenum and sulphur levels will indicate if deficiency is a possibility and why it is occurring, but the best method is to take samples from the animal. Blood is most commonly used, although in the early stages of copper deficiency blood levels remain high at the expense of liver stores and it is not until deficiency is quite well advanced and liver stores have been exhausted that blood copper values fall. The most reliable method of diagnosis is therefore to take liver samples from cull cows, animals being sold for slaughter, or even get your vet to take a biopsy, that is a small piece of liver from a live animal. Bloods are best taken from late pregnant heifers which have not been receiving supplementary feeding, because the copper requirements for growth and pregnancy are higher than for maintenance and milk production (see table 11.2).

Methods of supplementation
Dairy cakes generally provide sufficient copper for milking cows, although circumstances exist when it is necessary to have a special 'high-copper' mix. You may need a veterinary prescription for this. Copper is stored in the liver, and this, plus the introduction of several slow-release preparations, means that *copper injections* can be used. This is a very simple and positive way of ensuring that every animal gets its correct dose and there is no risk that molybdenum or other elements can interfere with copper absorption. Ideally give one injection three to four weeks before calving, so that calves are born stronger with better copper reserves. Although colostrum has a high copper content, levels rapidly fall and milk soon becomes insufficient to meet the needs of the growing calf. The interval needed between copper injections will depend on the severity of the deficiency and your vet will have to monitor samples to work out a programme for your herd. A common frequency would be once every three or four months.

Other methods of supplementation include application of copper salts to pasture, or to the soil; the use of slow-dissolving pellets suspended in a container in the drinking water (Aquatrace, see page 58) or the use of copper oxide wire, sometimes known as copper needles. These are given by mouth in a gelatin capsule. The capsule bypasses the rumen but is dissolved by enzymes in the abomasum. The small fragments of copper oxide penetrate into and remain in the wall of the abomasum and the copper is then slowly absorbed over a period of four to six months. Finally a glass bolus (Cosecure—Coopers Ltd) has been introduced containing copper, cobalt and selenium. This is given by mouth and then slowly dissolves in the reticulum over the next twelve months.

Cobalt

Cobalt deficiency occurs in small but well-defined areas of the United Kingdom, particularly those associated with the old red sandstone and granite soils of Devon, Cornwall and Derbyshire. Deficiency is widespread in North and South America and Australia. Cobalt is a vital component of vitamin B_{12}, which is synthesised by the bacteria in the rumen. B_{12} is needed by the micro-organisms to digest cellulose. The excess vitamin is then absorbed by the cow and it plays an essential role in her energy metabolism. The changes in cobalt deficiency are an inability of the animal to utilise the energy in its diet, a syndrome sometimes referred to as 'pine'.

Sheep seem to be more susceptible than cattle. In both species the symptoms are poor growth, anaemia and increased susceptibility to infection. There is some evidence that dairy cows suffer reduced milk yields and infertility. Clinical signs such as these can occur from a wide variety of causes however, including inadequate nutrition and parasitism, and cobalt deficiency should never be diagnosed on the basis of clinical signs alone. Occasionally vitamin B_{12} deficiency arises from chronic digestive upsets, leading to depressed ruminal synthesis.

If you suspect that you have a problem your vet will take blood samples to check vitamin B_{12} levels and will probably analyse hay and silage for their cobalt content. Supplementation by adding cobalt sulphate to the soil is quite successful. Cobalt bullets and glass boluses can also be used or cobalt can be added to the drinking water using an Aquatrace dispenser. Because cobalt is required by the ruminal micro-organisms, the animal must receive a regular supply by mouth: supplementation by injection (apart from giving vitamin B_{12}) would not be effective. The amount needed each day (see tables 11.1 and 11.2) is extremely small—only 20 mg for an adult cow—and provided that cobalt minerals are available, deficiency is unlikely. Cobalt is an expensive element however, and may not be present in some of the cheaper products. The analysis of a mineral should always be checked before purchase. Improving marginal hill pasture by the application of lime tends to reduce the availability of cobalt to the plants and can worsen a deficiency.

Iodine

Iodine is required by the cow to produce the thyroid hormone, *thyroxine*, which acts as a general metabolic stimulator for all body processes. Iodine deficiency thus leads to a lack of thyroxine and normal body functions simply proceed more slowly: milk production and growth rates are retarded, reproductive activity is suppressed and there will be an increase in the number of stillborn or weakly calves, possibly with more retained cleansings. The thyroid gland, which is situated in the throat area, works hard to compensate for a deficiency of iodine and this often leads to an increase in the size of the gland, a condition known as *goitre*. To confirm the diagnosis your vet will want to take blood samples from a group of young pregnant animals which have not received concentrate and he will also want to dissect out, weigh and examine the thyroid glands from stillborn calves.

Iodine deficiency may be primary, when the soil and plants are deficient in the element, or it may be a consequence of feeding *goitrogenous* diets. Examples of the latter include kale, turnips and raw soya beans. These foods prevent thyroxine production and should only be fed in moderate amounts. For example kale intakes of greater than 20 kg/day fed for long periods have been shown to affect fertility.

Dairy concentrates generally contain sufficient iodine, but if additional supplementation is required, free access to iodised salt is a simple and effective source. Tables 11.1 and 11.2 show that all pastures contain inadequate iodine for pregnant and lactating cows, so if they are not receiving concentrates, supplementation is essential. This is likely to be important when dry cows are on autumn grazing, in order to avoid stillborn calves. Young growing stock have a lower iodine requirement (table 11.2).

Manganese

Manganese is an element which is often discussed in relation to reproductive problems in dairy herds, especially where poor conception rates and failure to show heat are involved. There is certainly a wide variation in the manganese contents of pasture in the UK and some people have produced results showing an improvement in fertility following manganese supplementation. Others would dispute this. Dairy concentrates normally contain sufficient additional manganese to make up any deficit, but in the spring and early summer, when no concentrates are being fed, over half of the diets are likely to be deficient (table 11.1). Deficiency could also arise in the winter if the ration consisted of a high proportion of by-products such as sugarbeet pulp or malt residue. It has been suggested that an overall content of 80 ppm manganese in the dry matter (see table 11.2) is sufficient to avoid fertility problems, and as the mineral is very cheap it would be foolish not to provide this. However, other sources quote a much lower manganese requirement.

Zinc

Zinc is similar to manganese in that many pastures do not contain sufficient to meet the requirements of lactating cows (table 11.1). Deficiency in pigs causes skin problems and a similar *parakeratosis* which responds to zinc treatment has been reported in calves. Affected animals have a dry, crusty, scaly skin, especially over the head and shoulders, but sometimes the whole body is affected. This should not be confused with ringworm or lice, where the scaling effect is much less. Dosing with 15 g zinc oxide once a week will help recovery.

For many years zinc ointment has been used as a stimulant for healing. More recently, dietary supplementation has been shown to improve foot conditions in sheep and cattle, especially where the interdigital skin between the claws is involved. Soft horn has a lower zinc content than hard horn and supplementing with 30 g zinc oxide per cow per week may be beneficial in severe outbreaks of lameness. When testing procedures have been simplified, routine screening of zinc blood levels in dairy cows may show that deficiency is more common than was once thought. In a very limited survey carried out in our own practice several herds with low blood levels were found. Very high calcium intakes may induce a zinc deficiency. Care should be taken with zinc supplementation, however, since excessive zinc levels can induce a copper deficiency.

Iron

Iron, like potassium, is unlikely ever to be deficient in cattle diets. There are high levels in most plants, and as animals normally consume significant quantities of soil when grazing, overall intakes are boosted even further because soil is very rich in iron. For example, grazing cattle probably eat around 150 g soil daily, but this may increase to 1.5 kg if the grass is very sparse. The importance of iron is that in excess it reduces the availability of copper. This is an interesting point. At one time it was almost traditional that minerals should be either red or green and these colours were achieved by the addition of high levels of iron salts. Minerals with iron levels greater than 1,250 ppm should be avoided. Heavy soil contamination of silage will lead to high iron, lead and zinc levels and may therefore induce copper deficiency. This can occur when silage is made over very rough ground; on inadequately rolled swards; during wet weather; or from pasture which has been recently flooded or trampled.

Selenium

Selenium functions in association with *vitamin E*. Deficiency in the United Kingdom is quite common. The average value in pastures is insufficient for lactating cattle (table 11.1) and the trend towards high fat concentrates will increase the overall requirements of the animal because vitamin E is involved in the metabolism of fat. The symptoms seen are those of white muscle disease in young calves (see page 56) and possibly increased retention of the placenta (see page 127). These conditions have been covered in detail elsewhere in the book.

Ways of Improving Trace Element Status

Several different methods of supplementation were described with the individual trace elements. The purpose of this section is to take an overall look at the advantages and disadvantages of the various supplementation systems and these can be divided into three categories, namely:

1. Methods of altering the trace element content of the soil and herbage;
2. Oral supplementation, that is by mouth;
3. Supplementation by parenteral methods, that is, by injection.

Soil and herbage
The type of soil in a particular area affects not only its trace element content but also the type of plant which grows there and the rate of uptake of minerals and trace elements by those plants. It is for precisely these reasons that there is a wide geographical variation in the deficiency areas. Various treatments can affect the uptake of mineral by the plants. The effects of liming are well known and are clearly demonstrated in figure 11.1. The uptake of all elements, apart from iron, is decreased in acid soils and hence liming will invariably have a beneficial effect.

Artificial fertilisers have three actions on this soil/plant relationship. First, some fertilisers, for example ammonium sulphate, will acidify the soil, and this leads to a reduced mineral uptake by the plants. Second, fertilisers produce faster plant growth, often with a higher protein level, and this tends to decrease its mineral and trace element contents. Third, the elements contained in the fertiliser either intentionally (for example, phosphate) or as contaminants (for example fluorine) may react with natural minerals and trace elements and reduce their uptake. Heavy use of artificial fertilisers therefore generally decreases the mineral and trace element levels of plants.

Trace elements can be applied directly to the soil in an attempt to boost levels in plants. This works well with cobalt, but for copper such large applications are needed that it is not economic. Manganese has been applied to soil and pasture and while it may boost herbage growth in deficient plants, it has little effect on the overall manganese content of the pasture and is therefore of no value for animal supplementation.

Oral supplementation
Giving trace elements by mouth is probably the cheapest and most efficient way of counteracting deficiency, especially if it is a primary rather than an induced deficiency, and this must be the method of choice if cereals or concentrates are being fed. Animals must either be given a regular daily supply, for example using Aquatrace in the drinking water (page 58), or a method of providing a single large dose in a slow-release form must be found. Examples of the latter include 'bullets' for cobalts, selenium and magnesium supplementation (see plate 6.4), a glass bolus containing a mixture of copper, cobalt and selenium, and copper oxide wire which lodges in the abomasum

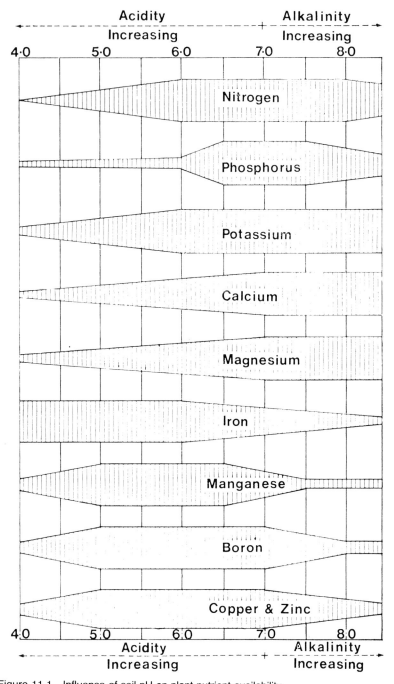

Figure 11.1   Influence of soil pH on plant nutrient availability.

and is then slowly dissolved over the following six to twelve months. Magnesium can be dusted onto pasture to give a regular daily supply and although this works well, it entails a fairly high labour input.

Minerals can be offered on a free-access basis, and while this is a simple system, individual intakes can be very variable. For example, one trial showed that cows ate an intake varying from 0 to 500 g/day of one particular mineral, with less than half the cows taking in sufficient to meet their requirements. Free-access is not a reliable method of supplementation therefore.

Parenteral supplementation

The word 'parenteral' means that the trace element is injected or implanted directly into the animal's body ('parenteral' can also be applied to drug administration). This is undoubtedly the preferred route for the treatment of animals clinically ill from deficiency, since it can produce an immediate improvement in trace element status. It also has the advantage that there are no interactions to consider which might compete with plant uptake or intestinal absorption and that a precise and controlled dose can be given to each animal. Unfortunately it is difficult to produce preparations which can give a single large dose, capable of slow release over a period of time. Injectable products for copper and selenium supplementation are now available and certainly for copper they provide a reasonably cheap and efficient preventive method. One disadvantage of parenteral administration is the risk of toxicity from overdose, since the animal cannot regulate its intake and absorption.

VITAMINS

Only the fat-soluble vitamins A, D and E have any real importance in ruminant diseases.

Vitamin A

Cattle obtain their vitamin A from *carotene* which is the yellow pigment present in abundance in all green plants. Provided the animals are grazing or are receiving well-made forage, deficiency will not occur. Drying, bleaching and weathering of grass will reduce carotene levels however and there is relatively little in cereal grains. Overheating of hay and prolonged storage also reduces the vitamin A content. Cattle fed on poor-quality hay in winter or on a straw and cereal diet will need additional supplementation and levels of 10.0 million i.u./ton are usually recommended. Provided that the feeding of the dry cows is adequate, colostrum will be rich in vitamin A and give the calf the reserves it will need during its suckling period. This is often not the case however, and winter-born calves may be deficient, leading to an increased susceptibility to scouring, pneumonia and other diseases.

Deficiency of vitamin A produces a variety of symptoms. There is decreased appetite leading to reduced growth and, even in the early stages, night vision is impaired. Reproductive function may be affected and there may be an increase in the number of stillborn calves. This could be especially relevant when the dry cows are being fed only very poor quality fodder. Fainting fits may also be seen: the calf collapses as if in a deep sleep, but a few minutes later it gets up and walks away quite normally. In the later stages of deficiency bone growth becomes affected. This can cause pressure on the nerve to the eye and eventually leads to total blindness. Most of the changes (apart from total blindness) are reversed when the deficient animal is injected with vitamin A. Vitamin A assists in maintaining the membranes of the body in a healthy state and deficient animals are more susceptible to disease, especially ringworm, calf pneumonia and scouring.

A diagnosis of vitamin A deficiency is made from an investigation of the history of the animals, especially their diet, and from an analysis of blood and/or liver samples.

Vitamin D

Vitamin D is involved with the absorption of calcium and phosphorus from the intestine, the deposition of the minerals in bone and the maintenance of normal blood levels. It acts in conjunction with parathyroid hormone. There is relatively little vitamin D in plants, and cattle obtain the majority of their requirements by synthesising the vitamin in the skin under the influence of ultra-violet light from the sun. Milk contains only low levels, and calves on whole-milk diets may develop a deficiency. However, deficiency is most likely to occur in young growing cattle in dimly lit buildings during the winter, especially when only poor-quality hay is being fed. The symptoms are those of *rickets*: growth rates are reduced, the legs may be bent and have abnormal swellings and many animals show stiffness and lameness. The teeth may be pitted and out of line and the jawbone deformed. Treatment is by injecting vitamin D and by correcting the ration, which may include oral supplementation with vitamin D.

Vitamin K

Vitamin K is involved in blood-clotting mechanisms. It is synthesised by the ruminal micro-organisms and there are also ample supplies in leafy forages. Primary deficiency does not occur therefore, although deficiency may be induced by poisoning with *dicoumarols*, compounds which prevent the action of vitamin K. Sources of dicoumarol include Warfarin rat poison and mouldy clover hay. The latter is sometimes known as sweet clover poisoning. Symptoms are associated with a failure of the blood clotting mechanism and include bleeding excessively from cuts, the appearance of large red haemorrhagic areas on the membranes of the mouth, eyes or nose and often abdominal pain and lameness. The latter is due to haemorrhage into the joints. The treatment is to give vitamin K by mouth or by injection and to try to identify and remove the source of the poison.

B Vitamins

The B vitamins are all synthesised by the micro-organisms in the rumen and the excess is absorbed by the cow. They are also present in ample quantities in milk, so primary dietary deficiency is never seen. Induced deficiencies can occur however, for example with CCN (page 60) where there is a factor preventing the action of thiamine (vitamin B_1) and with cobalt deficiency which leads to inadequate vitamin B_{12}. There is some suggestion that supplementation with biotin (vitamin B_6) may improve the quality of the hoof structure.

Vitamin C

Vitamin C is produced in the tissues of all farm livestock. A dietary supply is therefore not necessary and deficiency is never seen.

DRINKING WATER

Without an adequate supply of water, animals are unable to fully utilise their food, and this is something which can easily be overlooked. Water requirements will of course vary with the level of milk production, with the amount of moisture already present in the food (that is, its dry matter content) and, especially during the summer, with the temperature, humidity and wind speed. The variation can be from as little as 10 litres per day when wet spring grass is being eaten in dull weather, to as much as 65 litres per day when the cows are grazing dry pasture in the scorching late summer weather. Despite this, the daily pattern of drinking is surprisingly constant in both summer and

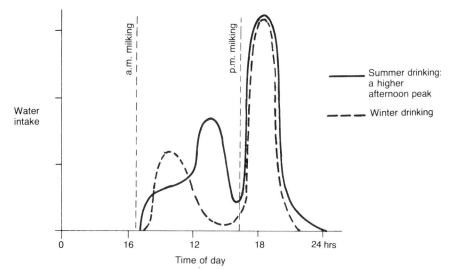

Figure 11.2   Daily drinking patterns of cows in summer and winter.

winter. This is shown in Figure 11.2. There is a rise in intake around midday and a considerably greater peak soon after evening milking, when up to 50 per cent of the total daily intake may be drunk in three consecutive hours. This short peak of drinking activity has important implications in terms of the supply provided. Because all the cows want to drink at the same time, it is essential that you have sufficient space to allow adequate access, that there is ample reserve capacity in your trough and that the supply pipe is of sufficient bore to carry water at the rate at which the cows are drinking it. As cows can drink at a rate of up to 14 litres per minute, and as there may be several cows drinking at any one time, an enormous rate of supply would be needed, so a large-capacity tank is by far the best idea. Circular troughs holding 1,600 litres, and which allow fifteen cows to drink at any one time, are now available. Building a concrete apron around the trough improves cow comfort, increases access and reduces foot problems. Cows are reluctant to walk more than about 250 metres to drink, so water troughs must be placed close to grazing areas.

As milk is 87 per cent water, thirsty cows will have depressed yields. Thirst also reduces food intake and this can cause a further fall in milk production and even bodyweight loss.

Water can also be a problem for sick animals. If they are too weak to reach the trough, or unable to compete with the other cattle when they get there, dehydration soon sets in. Even low levels of dehydration will make the animal feel lethargic and depress its appetite, and this is bound to retard recovery. Sick animals, cows or calves, are therefore best penned individually so that food and water can be made easily accessible and their intakes monitored.

Chapter 12

MISCELLANEOUS DIGESTIVE, RESPIRATORY AND OTHER CONDITIONS

IN THE earlier chapters we dealt with diseases affecting one particular age group of cattle. These tended to be mainly of an infectious or metabolic nature. There are many other conditions which can occur on a 'one-off' basis however, affecting only an individual animal but in any age group. Some of these conditions will be described now, starting with those associated with the digestive tract. The anatomy of the digestive system is shown in Chapter Two in figures 2.1 and 2.4 and plate 2.2, and you may need to refer back to these diagrams.

THE DIGESTIVE TRACT

The Teeth

Cattle have front teeth, or incisors, only in their lower jaw (figure 12.1). They pull grass into their mouth using their tongue and then cut it off by closing the incisors against the upper gums. Calves are born with eight temporary incisors and these are replaced at a later date by permanent teeth. As in children, it is the central pair of incisors which is replaced first and the number of permanent teeth present at any one time can be used to age the animal. The approximate ages of eruption are given in table 12.1.

Table 12.1 The approximate age at which the permanent incisors erupt

Incisor teeth	Age of eruption
Central pair	1 year 9 months
Second pair	2 years 3 months
Third pair	2 years 9 months
Outside pair	3 years 3 months

311

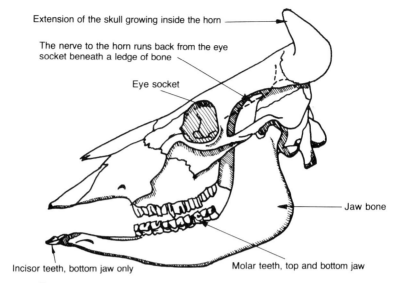

Extension of the skull growing inside the horn

The nerve to the horn runs back from the eye socket beneath a ledge of bone

Eye socket

Jaw bone

Incisor teeth, bottom jaw only

Molar teeth, top and bottom jaw

Figure 12.1 The skull of the cow. Note that there are front (incisor) teeth in the lower jaw only.

The teeth come into wear approximately three months after eruption, so that a heifer is 3½ years old before she is using her full set of permanent incisors. The table also shows that a two-year-old calver will have to change almost all her teeth during her first lactation and this is bound to cause problems with feeding.

There are three temporary molars, or grinding teeth, on each side of the upper and lower jaws. These are replaced by six permanent molars, so that the adult cow has a total complement of thirty-two teeth (four sets of six molars plus eight incisors). The permanent teeth grow throughout adult life and the incisors change from a spade shape in a young cow to small square pegs in the aged animal (figure 12.2).

Tooth abscesses and toothache do occur in cows and in my experience it is the incisors which are the most commonly affected. As you might expect, cattle with toothache are slow to eat their food, they drool and may lose

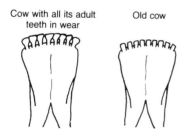

Cow with all its adult teeth in wear

Old cow

Figure 12.2 The teeth change from a spade shape to small pegs in the old cow.

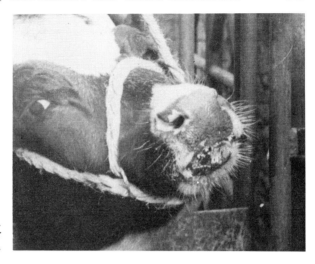

Plate 12.1   Tooth abscess.
Note the very swollen lower
lip. The animal is drooling.

weight. Always look inside the mouth of a drooling animal. Sometimes the
tooth has to be removed, but at other times it can be treated and your vet will
advise you on the most appropriate course of action. The animal in plate 12.1
had to have one of its incisors removed because of an abscess in the root, but
it eventually made a full recovery.

Lumpy Jaw

This is an infection of the jaw-bone caused by the bacterium *Actinomyces
bovis*. The lower jaw on one side may very slowly develop a swelling. If you
examine it carefully you can feel that the swelling is extremely hard and that it
is firmly attached to, and even part of, the bone. As the condition progresses,
the roots of the molar tooth become displaced, eating and chewing the cud
are painful and the cow begins to drool and lose weight. At this stage
treatment is hopeless, although some say that injecting antibiotic (penicillin
and streptomycin) into the lump in the early stages may effect a cure. Severe
knocks and bruising can cause a similar reaction in the jaw-bone, but these
will eventually heal, so you need to get your vet to examine it carefully before
deciding to cull the animal.

Wooden Tongue

This is sometimes confused with lumpy jaw. It is caused by a different
organism, the bacterium *Actinobacillus lignieresii* which invades the soft
tissues of the mouth. The tongue is the favourite site, although sometimes the
cheek or oesophagus may be affected and I knew one farm where animals
developed large, discharging lumps in their skin at almost any site over the
body. As the infection progresses, the tongue becomes hard and swollen. The
animal is reluctant to eat, it drools and loses weight and often there is a
secondary swelling in the throat as shown in plate 12.2.

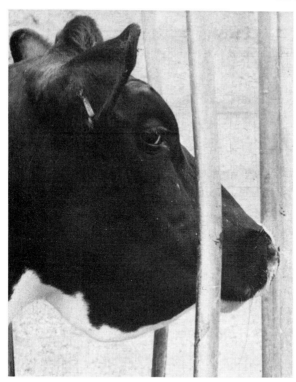

Plate 12.2   Wooden tongue. Although this cow has a secondary swelling in the throat, it does not always occur.

Treatment

Unlike lumpy jaw, wooden tongue responds to treatment very well. Traditionally iodine is used, giving an initial 'loading' dose of sodium iodide intravenously, followed by potassium iodide by mouth. Antibiotics are also effective.

Prevention

Both conditions gain entry via abrasions in the mouth, lumpy jaw perhaps beside a loose tooth. Both organisms are found in the soil and outbreaks of disease may be associated with feeding potatoes or other foods heavily contaminated with earth and small stones, the stones leading to the abrasions which allow the entry of infection.

Jaw Abscesses

This is a common condition in cattle of all ages, and leads to a hard swelling at the angle of the jaw bone. The lesion is clearly seen in the cow in plate 12.3. Infection most probably originated from a penetration wound at the back of the pharynx (figure 2.1), in other words from inside the mouth, but the pus then accumulates under the skin. Sometimes the abscess bursts on its own, but usually it has to be lanced, drained and flushed with antiseptic solution. Antibiotic cover may be needed.

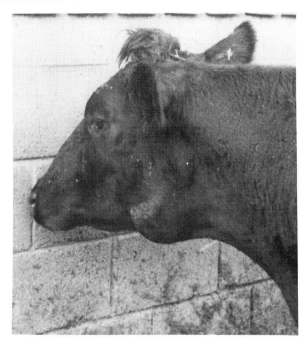

Plate 12.3   Typical site of jaw abscess. Infection most probably entered from a penetrating wound at the back of the mouth.

Choke

Moving away from the mouth and down into the oesophagus, the main problem here is an obstruction and the animal is said to have *choke*. Potatoes and apples are most commonly involved and it is said that they are especially dangerous if they are eaten from raised troughs. This is because when the animal eats from the ground, food is more likely to be chewed into small pieces before it is swallowed.

Clinical signs
The first indication that there is something wrong may simply be that one animal is standing apart from the others, with its head stretched forwards and its mouth slightly open. It may go up to feed, but then turn away again. If the blockage is severe, saliva produced in the mouth cannot be swallowed and so the animal will be drooling. On the other hand, gas cannot escape from the rumen and bloat develops. If left untreated, there is a risk of death either from severe bloat or from infection due to an erosion of the oesophagus at the point of obstruction.

Treatment
Saliva and digestive juices from the mouth sometimes dissolve enough of the potato or apple for the remainder of it to be swallowed and some people say that the best treatment is to insert a trocar and cannula (plate 12.7 and figure 2.3) into the rumen to alleviate bloat and then leave the animal to recover on its own.

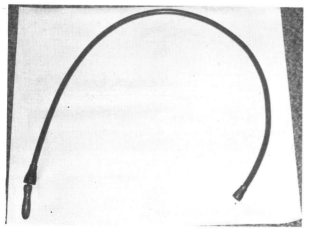

Plate 12.4   A probang. It consists of a length of nylon tubing with a metal lump at one end. The handle on the left is attached to a cane which runs through the centre of the tube to give added rigidity.

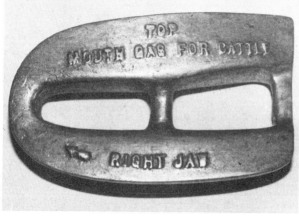

Plates 12.5 and 12.6 A mouth gag, showing how the molar teeth fit into its grooves so the mouth is held open.

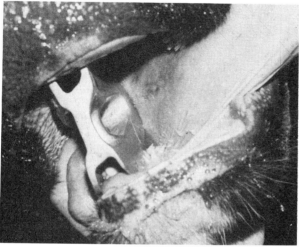

Alternatively you can try to push the obstruction down into the rumen using a probang. This is a long length of pliable nylon tubing with an enlarged metal lump at one end (plate 12.4). The handle is attached to a long cane which runs through the centre of the tube to give added rigidity. The animal's mouth is held open using a metal gag (plates 12.5 and 12.6) inserted between the teeth and the probang is carefully pushed down the oesophagus. If you push too hard there is a danger that you will rupture the wall of the oesophagus, so this is a job which is best left to your vet.

The best treatment, but sometimes not possible, is to work the potato up the oesophagus from outside then, with a gag in position, push your hand down the animal's throat and pull the potato out.

Bloat

Gas is produced by the micro-organisms in the rumen as part of the normal fermentation of food; following a meal the rate of gas production may be as much as 30 litres per hour. If it cannot escape, it makes the rumen swell and this we call bloat. The rumen is situated on the *left* side of the animal, so that bloat is first seen as a swelling in the left flank, as can be seen in the calf in plate 2.13. In more advanced cases, however, both sides will be distended. The animal is obviously in discomfort by now and it stands stiffly, with its legs spread wide apart. It may be drooling or frothing at the mouth and if you were to examine it carefully you would find that the heart was beating extremely rapidly. Eventually the pressure inside the rumen becomes so great that the animal goes down onto its side and death soon follows, either from heart failure or because liquid rumen contents have been forced up into the throat and inhaled into the trachea.

Causes of bloat

To appreciate how bloat develops it is important to understand how the normal rumen functions. There are approximately two waves of rumen muscle contraction each minute. In the first wave the lower sac of the rumen and the reticulum contract: this mixes the food, and any liquid sludge which has finished its digestion is transferred into the omasum, the third stomach (see figure 12.3). During the second wave of muscular contraction, the upper sac of the rumen compresses the gas, forcing it towards the reticular end of the oesophagus, which then opens to allow the gas to escape into the mouth. Fibrous food is transferred back to the mouth for further chewing by the same process, known as *eructation* and we say that the cow is 'chewing her cud'. An essential part of any examination for health is to stand back and watch the cow to see if her rumen is functioning correctly. It is easy to see the left flank moving in and out as the rumen contracts twice each minute, and eructation with regurgitation is clearly audible.

Bloat occurs when something interferes with the natural processes of gas release. This can occur in three ways. First a lack of ruminal contractions, second an obstruction in the oesophagus and third the presence of froth or foam in the rumen.

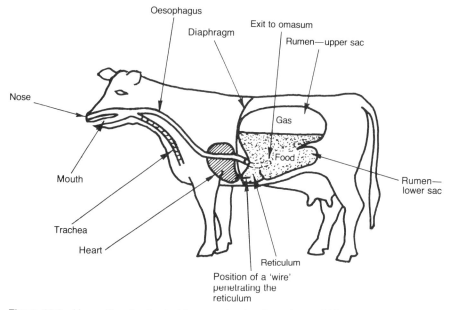

Figure 12.3   Upper digestive tract of the cow showing the point at which a wire penetrates the reticulum and its close proximity to the heart.

Cessation of ruminal contractions. This is technically called ruminal 'atony'. It occurs most commonly in the weaned calf and the symptoms and treatment were discussed in Chapter Three. Atony is also seen as part of the vagus indigestion complex in adult cows, where the nerve supply to the rumen has been damaged and it may be secondary to other conditions such as a wire, overeating or other digestive upsets.

Obstruction in the oesophagus. Choke is the commonest obstruction, although abscesses or even tumours on the outside of the oesophagus (for example from enzootic bovine leucosis) can cause a partial blockage. Actinobacillosis (wooden tongue infection) of the lower end of the oesophagus has also been reported.

Frothy bloat. Normally free gas collects as a single bubble in the upper part of the rumen (figure 12.3) until it is expelled. However, under certain conditions, as the gas is released from the semi-solid fermenting food in the bottom of the rumen it forms a froth or foam. This foam can be very stable, so much so that the gas it contains cannot be expelled by the normal mechanisms of ruminal contraction, so although the rumen is contracting and there is no obstruction in the oesophagus, a severe and often fatal bloat develops. Certain pastures are particularly prone to producing frothy bloat. For example, alfalfa is a problem overseas and animals may become bloated and die only ten to fifteen minutes after they have started grazing. In Britain, clovers, lush leys and even kale may be involved. It seems to be the stage of growth rather than the species of plant or weight of crop which is important. If you find that you are getting several blown cows in a particular field, simply take them away for two to three weeks. After this period the same pasture may be quite safe to graze again, even though the crop may then be even heavier.

Treatment
Whatever is causing the bloat, the prime objective of treatment must be to relieve the pressure of the gas before it leads to heart failure. You may not know which type of bloat you are dealing with, so, provided that the animal is only moderately affected, first take it out of the field if it is grazing, and give it a bloat drench. Your vet will supply you with a suitable preparation and it is something which you should always have in stock, 'just in case'. If you do not have any, then 500 ml (one pint) of linseed oil works well for a cow. If she is unable to swallow the drench, then you know you are dealing with an obstruction and you need to call for veterinary assistance. Bloat drenches (including linseed oil) act by dispersing the foam. Free gas can then be expelled in the normal way. You may even hear the cow belch within a few minutes of giving the drench and then you know that all is well.

It is important to keep a bloated animal on its feet for as long as possible and traditionally this is why they were walked for long periods. Once the cow lies down you have an extreme emergency on your hands because death follows quite quickly. Try to get her to stand up again so that you can give her a bloat drench. If this is not possible, or if it has not worked, you must release the gas, preferably using a trocar and cannula. The trocar, which has a handle at one end and a sharp metal point at the other (plate 12.7), fits inside the cannula. It will need to be held in both hands like a dagger and brought down

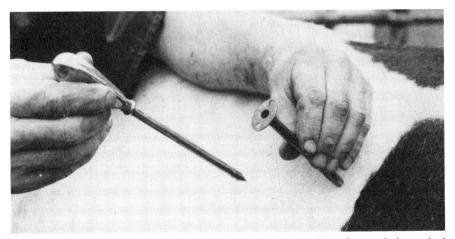

Plate 12.7   A trocar and cannula. The trocar fits inside the cannula as they are being pushed through the skin into the rumen. Once in place, the trocar is removed and the gas can then escape through the cannula.

with tremendous force to penetrate the skin of the cow. Once in the rumen, remove the trocar so that gas can escape through the cannula. If you do not have a trocar and cannula, then a large carving knife with a wide blade can be used. Push the knife into the rumen then turn the blade through 90 degrees and hold it transversely across the original cut, so that the gas can escape. The correct position to puncture and deflate a cow is shown in figure 2.3. It is on the *left* side, 5 cm behind the last rib and 15 cm down from the spine.

I should stress that releasing the gas in this way should only be done as an extreme measure and only when the cow is recumbent. There is a serious risk of peritonitis and other complications which could be fatal to the cow, especially if a carving knife is used. In either case, you should call your vet to advise you on how to dress the wound and to give any other antibiotic treatment necessary to prevent peritonitis.

An alternative way of releasing the gas is to pass a stomach tube. Hold the cow's teeth apart using a gag (plate 12.5) and push a length of fairly soft 20 mm plastic tubing into the throat. As you feel her swallow, push the pipe slightly further and then down into the oesophagus. If this produces a cough, or if you can feel air rushing in and out of the end of the pipe as the animal breathes, you know that you are in the trachea and you must start again. I find stomach tubing works well in younger cattle, but it is less successful in adults, partly because the end of the pipe gets caught in the food and liquid at the bottom of the rumen (figure 12.3) and so the gas still cannot escape. Whether you are using a trocar and cannula or a stomach tube, if frothy bloat is present the foam will probably be so stable that it will not pass out and this is why a froth-dispersing drench should always be given first.

Prevention

Cows grazing lush pasture should always be given access to hay or palatable straw before turnout. Not only does this reduce the incidence of bloat, but it also helps to maintain butterfat, reduces the incidence of hypomagnesaemia and helps to prevent ruminal impaction, the 'cold cow' syndrome (see page 322). If you are forced to graze bloat-producing pastures, they can either be sprayed daily with mineral oils, or a better alternative is to add the chemical *paloxalone* either to the drinking-water, using a proportioner similar to that shown in figure 6.4, or even include it in the concentrate. The drinking-water route is preferred, because supplementation can be installed very quickly and all cows must drink, whereas many of them may not be receiving concentrate when they are grazing lush pasture. Paloxalone can also be used very effectively as a bloat drench, that is, for treatment.

Overeating Syndrome

Another condition which primarily involves the rumen and which can affect cattle of all ages is the overeating syndrome. This is most commonly seen when a door to a concentrate or grain store has been blown open, or possibly some sacks of concentrate have been left within reach of the cows. Sometimes a group of calves is accidentally given double their normal ration and a few gorge themselves. Once in the rumen the grain is rapidly fermented by the bacteria. This produces very acid conditions (lactic acid) and, if severe, contractions cease and the whole of the contents of the rumen turn sour. The rumen wall then becomes inflamed (a rumenitis) making it more easy for toxins to be absorbed. It is the effects of these toxins, producing liver damage, a generalised metabolic acidosis, and then shock which can eventually lead to the death of the animal. The condition is also referred to on page 154.

Clinical signs
The clinical signs depend very much on the amount of cereal eaten and the time lapse since the animal gorged itself. If you are lucky, rumen contractions will continue and eighteen to twenty-four hours after overeating the cow will develop a profuse, foul-smelling scour, containing whole particles of undigested grain. The beige-yellow colour, semi-solid consistency and foul smell of the faeces is almost diagnostic of overeating. There will be a drop in yield and the cow will be off her food for a few days, but apart from this there will be no other adverse effects.

If contractions cease and acidosis and toxaemia set in, then the syndrome is much more severe. The cow becomes very dull, her eyes sink and she may appear blind and start to stagger. In the early stages she may be almost constipated, although the faeces which are passed later will be typically foul-smelling and pale yellow in colour. When she becomes recumbent, stops drinking and grunts with every breath, the chances of recovery are very poor.

Treatment
Provided the rumen is still working, I tend to treat cases medically. Sulphadimidine by mouth (250 ml of a 33 per cent solution) is very useful because not only does it stop the rapid bacterial fermentation, but being very caustic it also neutralises the acid in the rumen. One of the main groups of bacteria which proliferate are the lactobacilli, so penicillin could be used as an alternative to sulphadimidine. Sodium bicarbonate (at least 250 g four times daily) can also be used as a neutralising agent, and large doses of water (10–15 litres or more) help to reduce the concentration of lactic acid and thus prevents fluid from being withdrawn from the circulation. Calcium given intravenously or subcutaneously will stimulate ruminal contractions and both calcium and B vitamins assist the liver to metabolise the toxins absorbed from the rumen. Severely affected cows do in fact have a mild hypocalcaemia. Thiamine is a particularly important B vitamin to use, because there are often thiaminases present which destroy thiamine. You must then watch your cow very carefully for the next twenty-four hours. If she deteriorates and no cudding or any other signs associated with ruminal movements can be detected, your vet will probably have to empty the rumen. This can be done surgically, by cutting a large hole in the left side (a rumenotomy) and removing the contents by hand. Alternatively, a large tight-fitting plastic tube can be passed into the rumen via the oesophagus, or through the skin, and the toxic products and concentrate 'sludge' washed out with water. This

procedure is quite stressful to the animal however and she would need careful nursing afterwards.

The 'Cold Cow' Syndrome

Following turn-out to lush spring grazing, some cows develop a digestive upset which leads to a type of shock reaction. The symptoms vary considerably, but usually include dullness, off food and a drop in milk production. Ruminal movements are poor, the dung has a partially digested appearance and it will probably be rather loose. The nose and skin of the animal feel cold and hence the name 'cold cow' syndrome. Some cows are unsteady in their movements, almost as if they are drunk, and with a high pasture intake you are bound to suspect hypomagnesaemia. Most cows recover following symptomatic treatment, but it may be a while before milk yield returns to normal. Various theories have been put forward regarding the possible cause and these include fungal toxins in the grass and the rapid fermentation of pasture with a very high sugar content. Personally I think that a contributory factor may also be a sudden intake of cold and very wet grass reducing the rate of fermentation by the ruminal bacteria. The rumen contents then turn sour, leading to stomach pain, the absorption of toxic products and scouring due to the passage of only partially digested food.

Rumen Impaction

In some ways impaction is similar to the cold cow syndrome. The cow gorges itself on very dry or fibrous food, which becomes impacted as a hard, fibrous mass in the rumen. The symptoms are also similar, but generally much less severe. One dose of 500 g epsom salts by mouth usually produces a cure, although on two occasions I have seen deaths from ruminal impaction, when very hungry animals have gained access to unlimited quantities of straw.

Wire = Traumatic Reticulitis

This is one of the classic causes of stomach pain in the cow and it can also lead to other complications. Fragments of metal wire, copper flex, pig netting or even sharp bristles from a broom, which are accidentally taken in with the food, tend to drop into the reticulum. As the reticulum contracts, the sharp pointed object may penetrate its wall and with further contractions the object can slowly work its way through to the peritoneal cavity, where the infection it has carried with it sets up a localised peritonitis. The position the wire normally penetrates is shown in figure 12.3. Affected cows usually suffer a sharp drop in yield, they are off their food, dull, stand with their back slightly arched and they may be reluctant to move. They will have a raised temperature and will be slightly blown. The cow in plate 12.8 shows the typical stance of a wire. She has her head and ears forwards, depicting pain, and she is reluctant to move. She is not blown, however. Grunting is a classic sign.

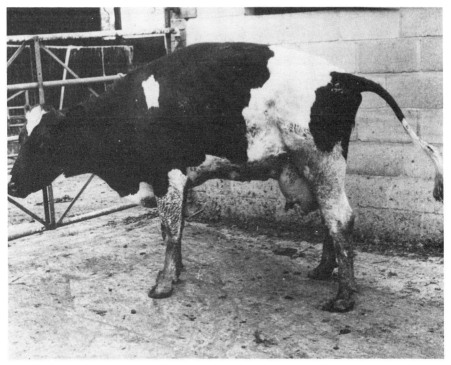

Plate 12.8   A cow with a wire. Her head and ears are forward, suggesting pain. She was reluctant to move.

Earlier (on page 317) we saw that there were two phases of ruminal movements, so stand back and watch your cow. The left flank will move slightly as the first wave of contraction passes through the rumen and the cow belches immediately afterwards. This was activity in the upper ruminal sac. You then see another ruminal contraction, but without a belch, and at the same time the cow may grunt with pain. This second contraction is the mixing phase and as it passes through the lower ruminal sac and then the reticulum, the wire moves slightly causing pain and the cow grunts. This is an excellent diagnostic feature and is known as the Williams reflex. Another test for a wire is to squeeze her back. As you pinch the skin she dips her spine. This stretches the reticulum and causes pain, which again elicits a grunt. The next time you squeeze her back she knows what will happen and will probably remain with her spine horizontal. The 'pain grunt' can also be evoked by lifting the reticular area, either by raising your knee underneath her stomach or by a pole held by two people one each side of the cow.

Diagnosing a wire is certainly not an easy task and you are bound to want veterinary advice. The best treatment is to remove the wire by surgery. If this is not done, there is a magnet available (plate 12.9) covered by a plastic case approximately 10 cm long and 3 cm in diameter, which can be given by mouth

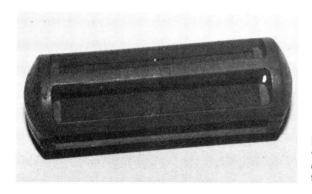

Plate 12.9   Magnet, covered with a plastic frame, which can be given by mouth to treat a cow with a wire.

and which pulls the wire back into the reticulum. If left untreated there is a risk that the cow may die, either from a more generalised peritonitis, or because the wire works forward to penetrate the heart, which is very close to the reticulum (see figure 12.3). Whichever treatment is used, antibiotic therapy will be necessary to counteract peritonitis.

Displaced Abomasum

The abomasum is the fourth and last stomach of the ruminant (plate 2.2). It resembles the true stomach in man, in that it is the site of digestion by enzymes produced by the animal. It normally lies along the right side of the cow, just under the abdominal wall, as shown in figure 12.4, and it is held in

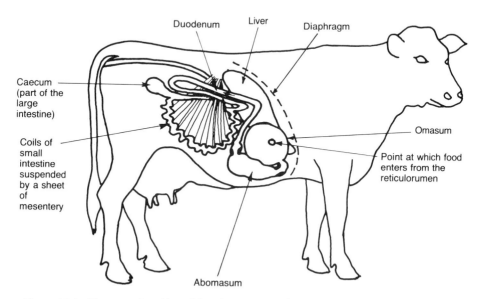

Figure 12.4   The normal position of the abomasum on the right flank.

this position by attachments to the duodenum at one end and to the omasum at the other. However sometimes these attachments weaken and the abomasum passes underneath the rumen and up to the left flank, and lies between the skin and the upper sac of the rumen (figure 12.3). This is a displaced abomasum. Gas accumulates and cannot escape because the duodenum is stretched under the rumen. If you listen carefully, you may be able to hear the gas and liquid making resonant splashing sounds under the left flank. This is what your vet will be trying to detect with his stethoscope.

Clinical signs
Probably the first thing you will see is a sudden drop in yield and the cow off her food, especially her concentrates. In this respect the clinical signs are very similar to acetonaemia. After a few days a proportion of cows do in fact develop acetonaemia as a secondary symptom. Their dung tends to be very hard and they soon lose weight. The left flank over the rumen becomes distended due to the presence of the abomasum, and the cow looks slightly blown. It is not necessarily an acute condition however and affected cows can live for several weeks. In mild cases the abomasum may even return to the correct position on its own, but the majority become displaced again a few

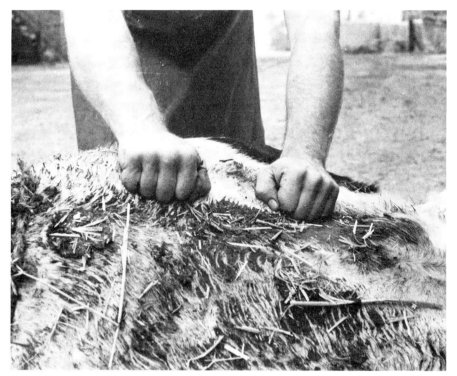

Plate 12.10 Correcting a displaced abomasum. With the cow lying on her back, the abomasum can be pushed from left to right over the top of the rumen.

days later. Acute cases do occur, when the abomasum ulcerates or even ruptures and causes death.

Treatment

There are two main types of treatment and your vet will probably have his own preferences. By far the most successful is to open the cow surgically on her right flank and pull the abomasum back underneath the rumen into its correct position. It can then be sutured in place, thus preventing further displacement.

Surgery is expensive however, and carries a degree of risk and I like first to try to replace the abomasum by rolling the cow. If she is sedated and then laid on her back, the abomasum can be pushed from left to right over the top of the rumen by a pummelling action with the fists (plate 12.10). It is always possible to replace the abomasum in this way, but unfortunately more than half the cases recur a few days later and still have to be treated surgically. Even so, I consider that this simple approach is worthwhile for the few cows which do recover and only a few days have been lost if the abomasum does displace again.

Causes and prevention

The abomasum is suspended by attachments to the duodenum at one end and the omasum at the other (see figure 12.4), so that as it contracts during normal digestion it pulls itself into the correct position. Displacement occurs when these abomasal contractions are weak or absent, or sometimes when a bubble of free gas accumulates. This can happen in cows receiving high concentrate intakes in early lactation, especially if the fibre content of the ration is low. In such animals food which has not undergone its full ruminal digestion may pass into the abomasum, and with its high content of ruminal volatile fatty acids there is both a decrease in abomasal movement and a rise in abomasal gas production. The presence of sand in the abomasum, weighing it down, and a lack of rumen fill (again with high concentrate/low fibre diets) are both said to be contributory causes. Prevention of abomasal displacement is therefore by careful attention to the diet.

Abomasal Torsion

Sometimes the abomasum remains in its normal position but twists over on itself. This blocks the exit to the duodenum and again gas and fluid accumulate, but this time under the right flank. Cows with abomasal torsion tend to be much more seriously ill and would die within a few days if left unattended. Surgery is the only treatment.

Abomasal Ulcer

Stomach ulcers are of course common in man and they also occur periodically in dairy cows. Most of the cases which I have seen have been in early spring, when the cows are grazing lush grass with a high nitrogen content. The initial symptoms are mild abdominal pain, a drop in yield and loss of appetite. There will be a slight increase in temperature. Many ulcers bleed profusely however, and when the blood is passed the dung turns to a dark, black, tar-like scour. Badly affected cows will need a blood transfusion and some animals die, either from excessive blood loss or by perforation of the ulcer leading to peritonitis. Less severe cases can be treated medically using kaolin and astringents (e.g. 120 g copper sulphate) given by mouth to try to arrest the bleeding, and iron injections to assist with re-forming blood.

Intestinal Obstruction (Stoppage)

The intestine is suspended from the animal's spine by the mesentery, and resembles a small piece of tubing running around the outside of a fan (figure 12.4). Sometimes the whole mesentery twists over on itself (a twisted gut). This cuts off the blood supply to the intestine and causes a blockage. It may be that only one segment of the intestine is twisted, or that a length of intestine has been telescoped into the piece behind, a condition known as *intussusception*, shown diagrammatically in figure 12.5. The symptoms of a

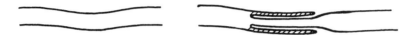

Figure 12.5   An intussusception: a segment of intestine telescopes into the piece behind. This constricts the blood flow and leads to a stoppage.

stoppage are essentially the same, whatever the cause. Initially the animal is dull. She picks at her food or stops eating altogether. She will probably show signs of colic, that is abdominal pain, by kicking at her flanks, looking at her sides or maybe getting up and lying down repeatedly, in obvious discomfort. There may be some dry dung passed in the early stages, possibly covered with mucus, but later the rectum becomes sticky and empty. Her temperature will probably be below normal and her pulse very fast. If left she will develop peritonitis and die. I have rarely had any success with surgical correction. Prompt casualty slaughter is probably the best treatment.

A word of caution however: cows and young stock can develop colic simply from a spasm in the gut, that is from excessive muscle contractions. This would give symptoms very similar to the initial stages of a stoppage, but it is a colic which responds rapidly to treatment with muscle relaxants, so make sure that you get your vet to examine the animal before sending her off. This temporary syndrome is particularly common in young stock.

Dilation and Torsion of the Caecum

The caecum is a blind-ended sac which is part of the large bowel (figure 12.4). It lies under the right flank high up towards the spine, and torsion and dilation can occur in the same way as with the abomasum. The symptoms are also similar though generally less severe. Surgery is the only treatment.

Johne's Disease

Johne's Disease is an infection caused by *Mycobacterium johneii*. The bacterium is related to tuberculosis and this is why Johne's is sometimes called *Paratuberculosis*. Infection is taken in by mouth and produces a thickening of the lower part of the small intestine and the upper large intestine, although lesions can sometimes extend down as far as the rectum. The thickening interferes with the function of the gut, particularly the absorption of water and nutrients. Disease is usually seen following the stress of calving. The cow develops a profuse watery diarrhoea which characteristically froths when it hits the ground. Symptomatic treatment with kaolin, chlorodyne or astringents such as sulphadimidine or copper sulphate may temporarily alleviate the scour, but it soon returns. The other prominent feature of Johne's Disease is a massive weight loss. This continues until the cow is so thin and emaciated that she cannot stand and she dies from an inability to absorb the nutrients from her food. No animals should ever be allowed to reach this stage of course, and I imagine that once your vet has confirmed his diagnosis with a blood or dung sample, he would recommend casualty slaughter. Johne's Disease is a good example of bacteria which live inside cells and are therefore protected from the action of antibiotics. Tuberculosis and brucellosis are similar.

Although typical Johne's Disease is by no means as severe a problem as it used to be, there is now good evidence that it can persist in a subclinical form in some of our cows for eight to ten years or more and it may still be a cause of chronic poor growth and disappointing production. These cows will be intermittent excretors of infection and will perpetuate the disease within a herd.

Control of Johne's

Although calves up to six months of age are the only animals in which infection can become established, because the incubation period is *two years* or more, disease will not be seen until after the first or second calving at least. The stress of calving precipitates the onset of scouring and at this stage the dung will contain massive numbers of Johne's bacteria. Important control measures are therefore to remove the calf from its mother immediately after birth; to avoid further faecal contamination of its environment; to identify and cull infected animals as soon as possible, and to make sure that feed and drinking water have not been infected. Probably the two major reasons why Johne's is now less common are that calves are removed from their dams soon after birth and that clean water troughs have replaced drinking from dirty farm ponds.

In herds where Johne's is a problem, vaccination can be carried out. A special licence must be obtained from the Ministry of Agriculture, because the vaccine may interfere with the interpretation of the Tuberculosis Test. Calves are vaccinated during the first four weeks of life, by means of a subcutaneous injection into the dewlap between the front legs. Check that a hard nodule has formed. This indicates that there has been a good vaccine 'take'. As it takes two to three weeks for the vaccine to become effective and as it will not protect against a very heavy challenge of infection, vaccination should always be combined with the hygiene and management measures described above.

Liver Fluke

The liver plays a vital part in dealing with the products of digestion and so I have included liver fluke in this section. Fluke is caused by a small parasite called *Fasciola hepatica* and hence you sometimes see the disease described as *fascioliasis*. It is an important condition in both sheep and cattle and is especially common in the warm and wet areas of the country.

Life cycle

The life cycle of the fluke is shown in figure 12.6. Taking the adult egg-laying fluke in the liver as our starting point, fluke eggs may be shed in the dung throughout the winter, but it is only when the weather becomes warm (above 10°C) and wet that they begin to hatch. Hatching releases the miracidia and these swim around in a film of moisture until they contact and penetrate the snail *Lymnaea truncatula*. There is a multiplication phase inside the snail, so that one fluke miracidium entering the snail can lead to the release of over a

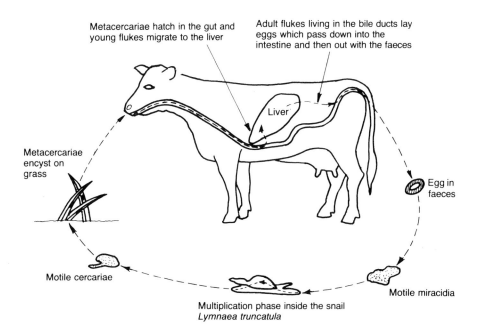

Figure 12.6   The life cycle of the liver fluke, *Fasciola hepatica*.

thousand fluke cercariae from the snail. Cercariae swim onto blades of grass and encyst to form resistant structures, the metacercariae. After infected pasture has been eaten by cattle, the metacercariae hatch in the intestine to produce immature flukes. These migrate to and then burrow across the liver, continually feeding as they pass through its substance, until they reach the bile ducts. In the bile ducts they complete their final stage of development to adult egg-laying flukes. The eggs pass down to the gall-bladder, into the intestine and then out in the faeces, thus starting another cycle.

Compared with other parasites like husk or the stomach worm Ostertagia, liver fluke has a fairly long life cycle as shown in table 12.2. The stage inside the cow, from eating the metacercariae until eggs are seen in the faeces, takes around three months and even under favourable conditions, the stage outside the animal, that is the hatching of the eggs, development through the snail and production of metacercariae, takes at least another two months. By favourable conditions I mean a temperature above 10°C and plenty of wet weather. It is said that if there are eleven weeks of continuous wet weather, including the four weeks of June, this will produce ideal conditions for fluke. Hatching of the fluke eggs *and* the development of the snails are both stimulated by warmth and humidity, so if June and July are wet, all the fluke eggs which have been passed from December of the previous year onwards and which have overwintered on the pasture, hatch at the same time as the snail population increases. This leads to a massive production of cercariae with a subsequent heavy infestation of metacercariae on the pasture. The metacercariae may be eaten by cattle from September onwards, but as adult flukes take three months to develop, there may be no significant disease seen until December or January. If, on the other hand, the summer months are either very dry or very cold, fewer fluke eggs hatch and there are fewer snails around anyway, so far fewer metacercariae encyst on the grass. This is the basis of the 'Fluke Forecast' issued by the Ministry of Agriculture. It is a very useful warning to farmers of when there is likely to be a high incidence of fluke and when treatments are necessary.

Table 12.2   Time spans in the fluke life cycle

Ingested metacercariae to immature flukes in liver	= 4 weeks ⎫	3 months
Immature flukes pass through liver feeding	= 6 weeks ⎬	inside the
Flukes mature in bile ducts and produce eggs	= 2 weeks ⎭	animal
Egg to miracidium to snail to cercaria to metacercaria	= 2 months *minimum* outside	the animal

So far we have been talking about what is known as the 'summer infection' of snails. If September and October are warm and wet, then a second wave of fluke eggs may hatch and these same weather conditions would also lead to an increase in the number of active available snails. By the time that the snail has become infected, however, the coldest weather will almost certainly have arrived and the snail then becomes dormant until the spring. As soon as weather conditions permit, snail activity starts again and metacercariae are deposited on the pasture. This is known as the 'winter infection' of snails.

Occurrence of Disease

Fluke populations can therefore survive the winter in three ways. First as adult flukes in the livers of infected animals and, if outwintered, these will be continually passing fluke eggs which all hatch at approximately the same time to produce the summer infection of snails. Second, flukes can over-winter as resistant metacercariae on pasture and third they can persist as cercariae in dormant snails, the result of the 'winter infection'.

Summer infection of the snails is by far the most common, producing pasture infestation with metacercariae in the autumn, so that disease can be seen from December onwards, but usually not until January and February. However, as metacercariae can persist on grass over the winter and as snails can carry cercariae until the following year, it is possible to get outbreaks of fluke in the spring or even in the summer. Cattle slowly build up an immunity to fluke and they seal them off in their bile ducts by laying down a thick, fibrous barrier, reinforced with calcium. This produces the classic 'pipe-stem' liver seen on post-mortem. The immunity limits the life span of the adult flukes to approximately 1½ years, so continual reinfestation of dairy cows is needed to maintain fluke populations.

Clinical signs

Although immature flukes cause some damage during their migration, the main effect in cattle is due to their blood-sucking activities in the bile ducts. There is no 'acute fluke' type of disease as is seen in sheep. The blood loss

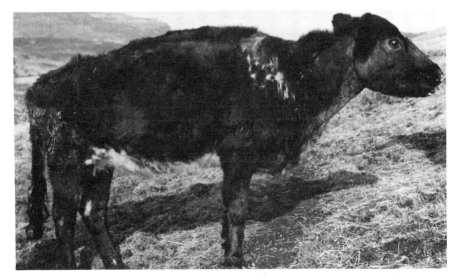

Plate 12.11 Suckler cow with a heavy fluke infestation. Note the very poor condition and 'bottle jaw'.

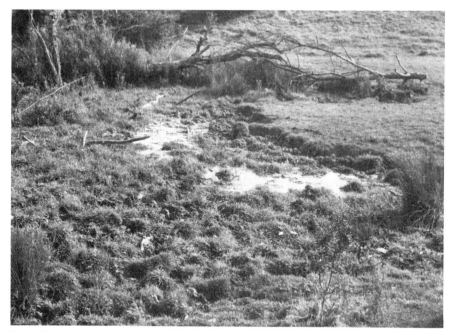

Plate 12.12   A typical wet area which produced fluke infestation in both sheep and cattle.

leads to anaemia and affected cattle look in poor condition, with rough staring coats and they are generally unthrifty. Occasionally they develop a 'bottle jaw' appearance, due to the accumulation of fluid (known as dropsy or oedema fluid) under the skin of the chin, although again this symptom is much more commonly seen in sheep. In dairy cows quite low fluke burdens will depress solids-not-fat in milk and heavier infestations can lead to reduced yields. I have seen beef suckler cows so badly infected that many went down after calving and never recovered. A typical 'severe fluke' cow with a bottle jaw is shown in plate 12.11, and plate 12.12 shows a wet area which produced fluke infestation in both sheep and cattle. Scouring is not a common feature of fluke and outbreaks of scouring in animals in poor condition in February or March are more likely to be due to type II Ostertagia (see Chapter Four). Liver fluke may increase the susceptibility of cows to *Salmonella dublin* infection.

Treatment and control
Only the drug oxyclozanide ('Zanil', ICI Ltd) is currently licensed for use in milking cows, and on fluke farms the dairy herd should be drenched twice during the winter period; for example, once in late December and then again in early February. The second dosing needs to be at least 2½ months after housing, so that all the metacercariae which were eaten during the autumn have reached adult stage and are then susceptible to the drug. If there is only a low risk of infestation, the first dose can be omitted. Outwintered cows and

heifers which could have been eating infected pasture throughout the winter ought to receive a further dose in March or April.

Some of the newer drugs such as nitroxynil ('Trodax'), rafoxanide ('Flukanide'), or triclabendazole ('Fasinex') kill flukes at a much earlier stage of their life cycle and are very good to use in young stock and non-lactating animals. One dose four weeks after housing should be adequate in the majority of cases.

The other aspect of the control of liver fluke is either to remove the snail habitats by drainage, or simply to fence them off. Cattle can then neither graze in these areas and become infected, nor dung there to deposit fluke eggs to infect snails with miracidia. *Lymnaea truncatula* snails prefer to live in a moist environment. They like the puddles beside streams and ponds (plate 12.12), or even hoof-marks in the mud if the ground is very wet. They do not like very acid soils such as peat bogs, so the application of lime to increase soil pH may lead to an outbreak of liver fluke. Under adverse conditions such as the cold in winter, or a very dry summer, snails become dormant and do not allow flukes to multiply.

RESPIRATION AND THE BLOOD

Turning away from the digestive tract, some miscellaneous conditions associated with respiration, the blood, the kidneys and the bladder will now be described.

Fog Fever

Fog fever is the name given to a syndrome of severe respiratory distress in cattle. It is mainly seen in the autumn, especially in September and October and affects cattle which are two years old or more. Suckler cows are particularly prone, although I have also seen outbreaks in milking cows. Disease occurs one to two weeks after the cattle have been moved onto a lush autumn aftermath and this is especially so if their previous grazing was a very sparse and dry pasture. Many theories have been suggested as to a possible cause, for example an allergy to lungworm larvae or to fungal toxins on pasture, but recent research has shown that the syndrome is due to *anaphylaxis*, sometimes called a *hypersensitivity* reaction. This is the name given to an overactivity of the normal immune defences of the animal, as described in Chapter One (page 6). Lush autumn grazing, particularly if it has a high nitrogen content, contains increased levels of the amino-acid L-tryptophan. In the rumen this is converted to the chemical 3-methyl indole, a toxin which is absorbed into the bloodstream and leads to a hypersensitivity reaction, the most prominent effects of which are seen in the lungs.

Clinical signs of fog fever

The syndrome is very sudden in onset. One or more of the cattle may be seen standing listlessly in the field, not grazing and characteristically their breathing is accompanied by forced grunts. The toxin 3-methyl indole leads to congestion of the lungs and many of the small alveoli burst. (The alveoli are shown in figure 4.6.) Although the cow can breathe in without any problems, the loss of elasticity in the broken alveoli means that she has great difficulty in breathing out, and if you stand and watch her carefully you will see that she grunts as her flanks and chest move inwards, trying to *expel* air from the lungs. In this respect fog fever resembles human asthma but differs from cows with severe pneumonia which would show difficulty both when breathing in (inspiration) and when breathing out (expiration). The burst alveoli allow air to infiltrate between the lung tissues and to pass deeper into the body, and in long-standing cases I have even seen cows with air crackling under the skin of their backs. Although this looks peculiar, it is no cause for alarm and provided the animal recovers, it will slowly disperse. Badly affected animals stand with their necks stretched forwards, mouths open and froth around their lips. They cannot eat or drink and eventually they die, simply because they cannot get sufficient air.

Prevention and treatment

Making a more gradual change from bare summer grazing to lush autumn aftermaths, for example by strip-grazing, is considered to help reduce the severity of outbreaks and feeding hay or straw at this time may also be worthwhile. Treatment is quite complex, and the drugs used will depend on how bad the animal is and how long it has been affected. Your vet may use antihistamines, corticosteroids or other anti-inflammatory drugs to try to reduce the toxic effects of 3-methyl indole and he will almost certainly give antibiotics to prevent a secondary bacterial pneumonia developing in the congested lungs. Respiratory stimulants may be needed if the cow is very ill. One drug which is effective in both treatment and prevention is monensin. Monensin is also used as a growth promoter in beef rations and is effective against coccidiosis in chickens. Fed at the rate of 200 mg/cow/day this prevents the conversion of L-tryptophan into 3-methyl indole in the rumen and if given at the start of an outbreak it will certainly stop the syndrome deteriorating and may prevent further cases from occurring. Even though only a few animals may be showing clinical symptoms, it is likely that the majority are subclinically affected. Fortunately the dose of 200 mg monensin/day is the same as that recommended as a growth promoter for grazing cattle, so you can simply purchase a few sacks of standard ration and start feeding it immediately. Even if all these treatments are given there will still be a proportion of animals in which the lung changes are so severe that death is inevitable. Affected cattle may have great difficulty in breathing, so it is important not to walk them too far or too quickly. It may even be necessary to pen them into the corner of the offending field and carry hay and water rather than risk moving them.

Blaine

This is another allergic or hypersensitivity condition with a sudden onset, although the chemical which causes the allergy has not been identified. Animals of all ages can be affected, but with most cases being seen in cows and heifers over twelve months old. The eyelids, lips and sometimes the vulva become swollen with oedema or 'dropsy' fluid. A good test for this is to squeeze the tissue gently between your finger and thumb. You can make quite a significant depression and when you remove your hand the finger-marks remain. Sometimes the allergy is so severe that the whole head and neck is affected and this may interfere with breathing.

Mild cases disperse without treatment, but if severe, antihistamines and cortisone can be used to alleviate the symptoms and diuretics, drugs which remove fluid from the body, may help to decrease the swelling. In some areas the syndrome is also known as 'ting'.

Tick-Borne Diseases

There are two major species of cattle ticks in the British Isles, namely *Ixodes ricinus* and *Haemaphysalis punctata*. Ixodes is by far the most common and it is found throughout Scotland, Wales, North and South-West England and in a few areas of Dorset and the South-East. Tick areas are shown on the map in figure 12.7. Haemaphysalis is found only in coastal areas of Wales. Ticks prefer coarse, uncultivated pasture, because the tufts of grass provide them with moisture and protection.

Life cycle of the tick
The life-cycle of the tick is spread over three years, as shown in figure 12.8. An egg laid in the grass in year one slowly develops over the following winter to hatch as a larva in the spring of year two. The tick larva climbs to the top of the grass or a small bush, and waits there until an animal brushes past, whereupon it attaches itself to the animal and then slowly engorges itself with blood. This takes four to six days. When full it drops onto the ground and remains there over the summer and the second winter until the spring of the third year, when it moults and emerges as a nymph. The feeding process is repeated and the nymph returns to the ground until the spring of the fourth year, when a further moult occurs, and it emerges as an adult. The adults feed, then mating takes place, either on the animal or on the ground. The males die soon afterwards, but the females live slightly longer and lay their eggs into thick matted pasture.

There are two phases of tick activity, one in the spring (May and June) and the other in the autumn (September). Ticks which hatch as larvae in the spring continue as spring-feeding nymphs and adults, whereas those hatching in the autumn continue as autumn feeders. To feed, the tick inserts its mouthparts through the animal's skin, squirts in saliva to act as an anti-coagulant and then begins to fill itself with blood. When fully engorged it drops back onto the pasture where it remains in cracks and crevices, to

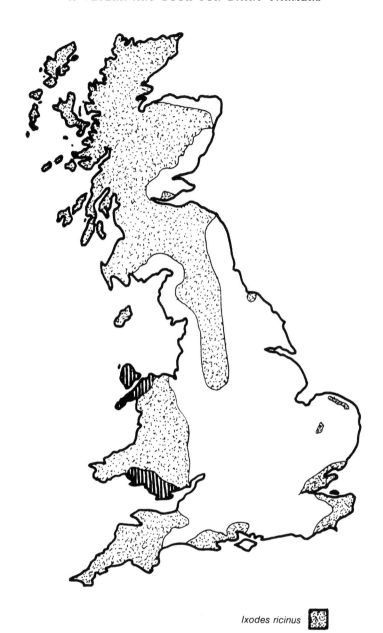

Figure 12.7   The distribution of cattle ticks in the United Kingdom.
From R. E. Purnell (1982), *Proc. Brit. Cattle Vet. Assoc.*, p. 103.

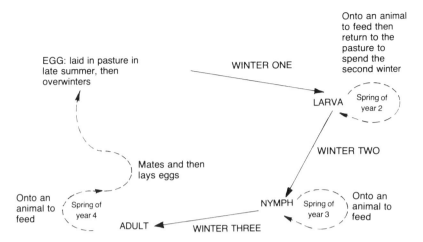

Figure 12.8   The three-year life cycle of a spring-feeding tick.

complete the moult which is the next stage of its development. It takes three years for a tick egg to become an adult, therefore, and during this time it will have only fed once each year. Most of their life is spent on the ground. Ticks can feed on most animals including sheep, cattle, deer, rabbits, dogs and even man. However, although they may transmit sheep infections to cattle and vice versa these infections never become established in the wrong species.

Disease caused by ticks is of two kinds, primary and secondary. Primary disease is related to the tick's feeding activities and consists of irritation and anaemia due to extensive blood loss. It is rare that tick burdens are ever high enough to produce significant anaemia under British conditions, however. Secondary disease is far more common and is due to the effects of the parasites carried by the ticks, the two main conditions in cattle being redwater and tick-borne fever, both of which are carried by Ixodes. Haemaphysalis carries a less important form of redwater and another blood parasite called Theileria. Ticks also carry the sheep disease louping-ill and cause tick pyaemia.

Redwater

Redwater is caused by a small single-celled protozoan parasite called *Babesia divergens*. It is related to the parasite which causes malaria in man. Babesia is carried by the tick Ixodes and it is transmitted into the cattle with the drop of saliva which is pushed down through the tick's mouthparts as an anticoagulant at the start of feeding. Once in the bloodstream Babesia starts to multiply in the red blood cells. Waves of infection occur, with the new crop of Babesia rupturing the red blood cells as they are released. Haemoglobin pigment is also liberated from the ruptured cells. It passes out in the urine and hence the name of redwater.

Clinical signs

In the early stages of the disease the animal will be standing apart from the others and running a very high temperature. This is the multiplication phase of Babesia. Within twenty-four hours and possibly sooner, the urine turns a deep port-wine red colour and froths as it lands on the floor. The animal's pulse is very fast because of the anaemia associated with the rupturing of the red cells and often you can hear the very loud heartbeat if you stand quietly beside it. In the early stages, the dung is passed under pressure due to a spasm of the anus and this produces a 'pipe stem' effect, almost as if the animal is scouring. As the effects of the anaemia develop, however, constipation sets in. If left untreated, death may occur. A proportion of animals will un- doubtedly have less serious infections and some recover without treatment, possibly without having been noticeably ill.

Treatment

There are specific drugs such as amicarbalide ('Diampron', May & Baker) which your vet can administer to affected animals to specifically kill the Babesia. If the urine is still discoloured after twenty-four hours, a repeat treatment will be needed. Iron injections and vitamins will help re-form the red cells, although if the anaemia is severe a blood transfusion may be necessary.

Immunity

Young animals have an inherent immunity (sometimes called a premunity) against redwater and the disease is unlikely to be seen in cattle less than nine months old. If they are then slowly exposed to low levels of infection they can build up their own true immunity. However, this immunity soon wanes and as only certain parts of a farm may be suitable tick habitats, and as ticks are only active during two quite short periods of the year, it is possible that even if animals stay on the same farm they may not be exposed to Babesia for two to three years or more, by which time their immunity will have waned. If the weather then becomes warm and slightly humid when the cattle are grazing rough pastures, heavy tick infestations can occur and clinical redwater may be seen. Disease can also occur when non-immune stock are introduced into a tick area. A vaccine, consisting of Babesia-infected blood which has been partly inactivated by radiation treatment, has been produced and although it is not available in Great Britain it is used in other parts of the world where ticks are a much more serious problem.

Babesia can survive inside the tick for three years as it passes from the egg through its larval, nymph and into the adult stages, despite the fact that the tick may not have fed on cattle blood over this period. It can even pass into the next generation of ticks via the ovary and tick egg. In this way pastures can remain infective for many years, even in the absence of cattle and certainly without cases of redwater being seen.

Tick-Borne Fever

This is the other important infection carried by ticks. It is caused by *Cytoecetes*. This is a rickettsial parasite, an organism with a size and characteristics part way between viruses and bacteria. Whereas Babesia attacks red blood cells, Cytoecetes destroys neutrophils. Neutrophils are one of the types of white cells in the blood. Naturally disease only occurs in tick areas and only during the periods of tick activity. Affected animals show stiffness in the joints, lethargy, a loss of appetite and they run a high temperature. Deaths would be rare, although infection can cause weight loss or a drop in milk production.

Treatment with the antibiotic oxytetracycline is usually very effective and your vet will probably use a long-acting injection to give a four-day cover. Infections are probably quite common, more so than with Babesia, but because the symptoms are mild and rather non-specific, the majority of attacks go unnoticed. With up to 50 per cent of its white blood cells destroyed, however, an animal suffering or recovering from tick fever will have lost some of its defence mechanisms and so it will be more susceptible to other diseases for the next one to two weeks.

DISEASES OF THE KIDNEYS, BLADDER AND UTERUS

Hydrops of the Uterus

The majority of the problems affecting the uterus (endometritis, metritis, torsion, prolapse, etc.) are dealt with in Chapters Five and Eight, although the condition of *hydrops* has not yet been mentioned. In the sixth to seventh month of pregnancy there is normally a marked increase in the production of allantoic fluid, but in some cows this becomes uncontrolled so that the uterus continues to accumulate fluid. Some 250–300 litres (55–66 gallons) may be present. The cow's abdomen becomes massively dilated and she loses weight rapidly. Once she becomes recumbent, slaughter is necessary, although if the condition is recognised soon enough, termination of the pregnancy, for example with prostaglandin, cortisone or a Caesarian operation may be effective. Even then the sudden loss of fluid may lead to death from shock. There was originally some confusion as to whether the fluid was accumulating in the allantoic or amniotic sacs (see page 101 for explanation of these terms), and hence the condition is sometimes referred to as 'hydrops amnion' or 'hydramnios', rather than the correct name of 'hydrops allantois' or 'hydrallantois'.

Abscesses and tumours are occasionally found in the kidneys, and sometimes the bladder may turn itself inside out and is seen as a prolapse through the vagina. This is shown diagrammatically in figure 12.9. It should not be confused with a *vaginal polyp*, which is a tumour attached to the vaginal wall by a long stalk and which may also be seen protruding through the lips of the vulva. When the cow stands up, polyps are often pulled back into the vagina.

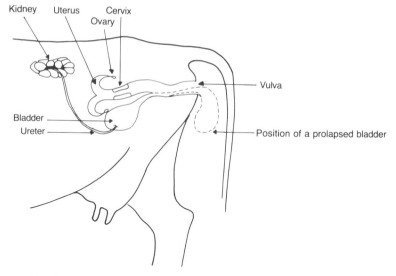

Figure 12.9   The positions of normal and prolapsed bladders.

The three most common conditions affecting the urinary system are obstruction of the penis, cystitis/pyelonephritis and leptospirosis.

Obstruction of the Penis

This can occur in any age of calf from weaning onwards and is particularly common in housed animals receiving moderate to large quantities of concentrate. Probably the first thing you will see is an animal looking rather dull and uncomfortable with a large swelling under its belly, halfway between the scrotum and the navel. The swelling will be quite hard, but it is obviously fluid because it can be pushed in with pressure from your finger. What has happened is that small mineral calculi or 'stones', have passed along from the bladder and have obstructed the penis at this point. Urine builds up under pressure, then bursts the wall of the penis and escapes under the skin.

Surgery is the only treatment. Your vet will probably amputate the penis just behind the scrotum so that urine can flow out between the hind legs. Most of these cases heal remarkably well. The calculi are thought to form initially from a combination of a highly mineralised diet and possibly an inflammation of the bladder.

Cystitis and Pyelonephritis

The word cystitis means inflammation of the bladder and pyelonephritis means inflammation and pus in the kidney. One of the common causes is infection with the organism *Corynebacterium renale*. Only cows and heifers are affected. They run a moderate temperature, will be off their food for a few days and the urine will be a red colour, due to blood leaking from the inflamed surface of the bladder. This should not be confused with the darker purple-red urine of Redwater, however. Provided that treatment is given fairly promptly, recovery rates are good. Your vet will probably use streptomycin, ampicillin, sulphonamides or some other antibacterial drug which is excreted via the urine, thus achieving a high concentration at the site of the bacterial attack. If the condition is allowed to progress, however, infection can track up the ureter towards the kidneys (see figure 12.9 and note the unusual shape and structure of kidneys in cattle). Once the kidneys become badly infected and abscesses develop, treatment is unlikely to be successful. The animal loses weight rapidly and may become toxic and die.

Leptospirosis

We have already mentioned leptospirosis in Chapter Seven as a cause of mastitis and in Chapter Eight as a cause of abortion. The strain involved in cattle is *Leptospira interrogans var. hardjo*. By measuring antibody levels in the blood it has been shown that a large proportion of cows in the British Isles have been exposed to infection, although the actual clinical disease is much less commonly diagnosed. Cows are infected by urine splashing into their eyes, mouth or cuts in their skin. The first stage of the disease is simply a raised temperature and a reduction in appetite, and this is when the leptospires are multiplying in the liver. Such mild clinical signs may not be noticed in maiden heifers and many recover in one or two days without treatment. In dairy cows however, the clinical signs can be much more pronounced and they are characterised by a sharp fall in milk production. The udder becomes quite flaccid, the milk is thick, almost like colostrum, and at first you may think that your cow has mastitis in all four quarters, but without any swelling. This is why leptospirosis is sometimes referred to as the 'milk drop' or 'flabby bag' syndrome.

The third clinical sign caused by leptospirosis is abortion. This usually occurs six to twelve weeks after the initial infection and temperature rise and is especially common if the cow is in the final third of pregnancy. It is quite possible that the earlier infection did not cause a significant milk drop and that abortion is the only clinical sign seen. Your vet could take a blood sample to check for exposure to leptospirosis. In 1983 almost forty thousand abortions were reported to the Ministry of Agriculture and in over three-quarters no cause was found. With improved diagnostic techniques, it is possible that leptospirosis will be shown to account for a significant proportion of these.

Treatment and control

If left untreated affected cows would slowly recover on their own, although they would probably never regain their full milk potential for that lactation.

The use of antibiotics, especially streptomycin, will speed recovery. Following infection, some cows rid themselves of leptospira and develop an immunity. However this lasts only one to two years, after which they are susceptible to further attacks. Other cows remain carriers with a focus of leptospira infection in their kidneys which periodically bursts out and leads to intermittent excretion in the urine. This combination of carrier cows and waning immunity leads to repeated outbreaks of disease, even in a closed herd.

There is now a good killed vaccine available for cows and heifers. Two doses are given, four weeks apart, and a booster is needed each year. This could be given in late summer just before heifers enter the herd and to give extra protection to cows during the autumn, which is the main period of risk. Unfortunately carrier animals can still occur after vaccination and so immunity has to be maintained by repeated annual boosters.

Leptospirosis in man

Although cattle are the main hosts of L. hardjo, other animals can become infected, including man. Anyone working in a milking parlour is especially at risk, because it is so easy to get splashed with urine from an infected cow. The symptoms in man include headaches, fever and aching joints, very similar to a severe attack of influenza. Occasionally cases of meningitis and even death occur.

MISCELLANEOUS CONDITIONS

Listeriosis

This is an infection caused by the bacterium *Listeria monocytogenes*. In cattle it is mainly seen as a nervous disease, although it may also cause abortion or even sudden death. In the typical case you will see one side of the animal's face droop, due to paralysis of the facial muscles and this leads to drooling. Eating is difficult, appetite is depressed and weight loss occurs. Nervous signs then start, initially with the animal walking round and round in circles. This develops into convulsions, eventually followed by coma and death. Antibiotics can be used for treatment, but many cases never recover.

Listeria is an interesting organism. It can survive for many years in dung or soil, it is a common contaminant of silage and yet disease is relatively rare. Most cases occur in silage-fed cattle in late winter and the stress of poor housing, unhygienic management and dietary changes increase the risk of disease. The organism is frequently found in man, but it rarely causes disease, although high levels of human infection in sewage sludge could be a danger to animals.

Blindness

Blindness may be present at birth, when we say that the calf has a congenital defect, or it may occur later in life, possibly as a result of an improperly treated New Forest eye. Some cows suddenly go blind however, with no other symptoms and this could be due to a localised blood clot or an abscess in the brain.

In calves the most common defect is a lens opacity or *cataract*. If you look at an eye with a cataract you see that the circle filling the centre of the pupil is blue-grey in colour and light cannot enter. This is thought to be caused by toxins or infections (e.g. BVD virus) acting on the cow in early pregnancy, at the stage when the eyes are being formed. Cataracts can be treated by making cuts on the surface of the lens with a very small 'needling' knife. The fluid of the eyeball (the aqueous humour) then dissolves away the lens. Sight is slowly restored over one to two months, but for distant vision only. Some cataracts are of genetic origin, and occasionally groups of calves are affected but no cause is found.

Blindness can also be a symptom of some other condition, for example lead poisoning, meningitis, CCN or vitamin A deficiency.

Aujeszky's Disease

This is a virus infection which occurs mainly in pigs, where it causes nervous disease, pneumonia and reproductive failure. Cases in cattle are rare, but when they do occur there is excitement, drooling and intense itching. There is no treatment. Aujeszky's disease is also called pseudorabies, because the symptoms are indistinguishable from a true rabies infection of cattle. It is a notifiable disease.

The PPH Syndrome

This is another disease of cattle which can cause intense itching. The letters PPH stand for pruritis (itching), pyrexia (raised temperature), and haemorrhage (bleeding from various sites in the body). It is a fairly rare condition, seen only in dairy cows, and often in housed animals being fed silage which has been made with a sulphuric acid/formalin additive. The early signs are intense irritation of raised patches of skin on the head, neck, tail and udder, and in mild cases this is all you will see. In more severe cases however, the cow runs a high temperature, goes off her food and may develop haemorrhagic areas inside the nose and mouth, sometimes with fresh blood being passed with the dung. These cases do not recover and the animal is best slaughtered.

The cause of PPH is not known, although recently research workers have found a fungal organism in the kidneys and it is the kidneys which show most of the damage seen at post mortem.

Electrocution and Lightning Stroke

Death from electrocution and lightning is more common in cattle than in any other species, partly because of an inherent susceptibility, partly because their four feet placed firmly on the ground makes a good earth and partly because they are often in milking parlours and other housing where free electricity can occur.

Lightning stroke

It is unlikely that you will see anything except a dead animal, or possibly a group of cattle lying together, although sometimes there are also one or two staggering around with concussion. Perhaps you will be able to see other evidence to substantiate your diagnosis, such as scorch marks on adjacent trees, broken branches, marks along the ground, or burns on the animal itself. This is not necessarily the case however. If lightning strikes damp ground, or if an overloaded power cable falls into a pool of water, there may be sufficient ground current to be fatal and there are then no marks to be seen on the carcase.

Electrocution

Waterpumps, vacuum pumps and milking machines are the most common sources of free electricity and so milking cows are commonly affected. I have seen a case where four cows dropped dead during milking and after they were released the other six were staggering around aimlessly, suffering from electrical concussion. They recovered eventually. In this instance there was a fault in the water heater, and the element had an earth which passed through the milking equipment. On another occasion the farmer thought that his cows had a low-grade grass staggers because they were unusually nervous and jumpy in the parlour. The problem was eventually traced to a fault on the lift pump which gave the cows a shock as it switched on. The farmer felt nothing himself because he was wearing rubber boots. Beef cattle can also be affected, and electrocution of animals inside a metal-framed building where the stanchions are standing in a damp area is not uncommon. I can remember seeing five from a group of ten finished beef cattle found dead from electrocution between two metal stanchions. The cause was traced to a 'short' from a 3-phase electric cable onto a metal pole some 20 metres away. The cattle had been killed by ground current: the electric cable blew against the metal pole and sent pulses of electricity along the ground to the cattle in the building.

If you wish to pursue an insurance claim, it is most important that you do not move the cattle until your vet has arrived. He will want to see them in situ, looking for scorch marks and other electrical damage. He will also want to clear them for anthrax before carrying out a post-mortem examination.

Haematomas

This is the technical name given to blood-blisters, large accumulations of free blood which develop under the skin. The most common sites are the points where a cow can bruise herself, for example, along her back (from being caught under a cubicle rail) and over her ribs (from rushing through a doorway with others). The cow in plate 12.13 is a typical example. She has a haematoma over her shoulders due to continual rubbing and bruising against a horizontal feeding barrier while stretching in for food. Outbreaks of haematomas can occur in dairy herds which have over-eaten concentrate and some of these cows present a bizarre picture. Their heads, necks or legs may be swollen to three or four times their normal size with blood.

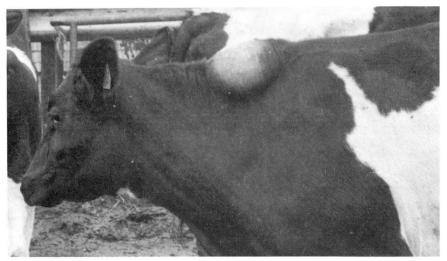

Plate 12.13   A haematoma, or blood-blister, on the neck just in front of the shoulders. This was caused by continual banging against a feeding barrier.

No treatment is necessary. If left alone the blood will slowly disperse over the course of two to three months. You ought to get your vet to check that the swelling is a haematoma and not an abscess or a rupture however, since an abscess would need lancing. Abscesses slowly increase in size and are usually hot and tense, whereas haematomas occur suddenly, do not get any larger and tend to be soft and fluctuating under the skin. Ruptures normally occur on the flank, and can be distinguished by feeling the tight edge of muscle through which a soft swelling (usually containing intestine) has passed to lie under the skin.

Chapter 13

ROUTINE TASKS AND DEALING WITH POISONS

FOR MANY years there has been a steady decline in the number of dairy units in Britain, although the total number of cows in the national herd has remained approximately constant. The effect of this is that the size of the individual dairy herd is increasing and in turn this has led to the need for a more specialised stockman. Many of the routine tasks and basic treatments which were once considered to be the province of the veterinarian are now being carried out by stockmen and I think that this trend will continue. The vet will do less routine work and instead will spend more time on preventive medicine programmes, monitoring performance and organising fertility control schemes.

Much of this book has been written with these changes in mind, that is to try to give the stockman a better understanding of the principles involved in disease control. It is more difficult to give a written description of practical techniques, however, and I would urge the reader to contact his local Agricultural Training Board officer. The ATB organises some excellent courses, where trainees are given the theory of the task as well as undertaking supervised practical training.

In the following I have tried to give guidelines on some of the more basic procedures which you may have to perform.

Giving an Injection

When giving an injection, chemicals are being administered directly into the body, and in so doing, many of the animal's normal defence mechanisms are being by-passed. If bacteria are introduced there is a risk of serious side-effects, so cleanliness and hygiene are essential. It is important that your syringes and needles are rinsed through with clean water after using them and that they are then boiled or soaked in alcohol to sterilise them. They should be stored, ready for use, in a clean, dry container with a lid. Even if a new needle and syringe are used for each course of injections it is probably very little extra expense compared to the cost of the drug or the value of the animal being treated.

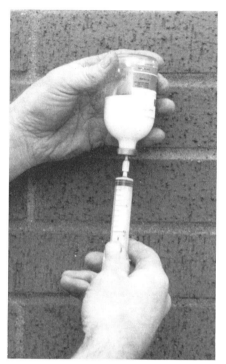

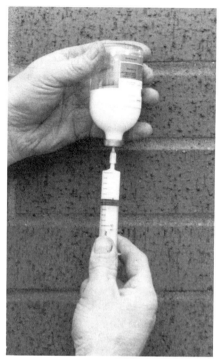

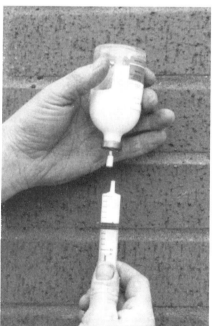

Plate 13.1 (*top left*)   Filling a syringe: invert the bottle, then insert the needle with the syringe attached.

Plate 13.2 (*top right*)   Pull the plunger back until you have the required dose.

Plate 13.3 (*left*)   If an excessive vacuum builds up, simply disconnect the needle from the syringe to allow air to enter.

To fill the syringe

First shake the bottle to make sure that the contents are thoroughly mixed. Many antibiotics are in a suspension rather than fully dissolved and if you simply inject the liquid taken from on top of the solid you will be seriously underdosing. With the syringe plunger depressed and the bottle held upside down, insert the needle through the rubber bung (plate 13.1). Then, holding the syringe at eye level, slowly pull the plunger back until you have the correct dose (plate 13.2). If this creates an excessive vacuum in the bottle, simply disconnect the syringe from the needle (plate 13.3). This allows air to enter and the filling process can then be continued. I do not like the more traditional method of first pumping in a volume of air equal to the volume of injection to be withdrawn. There is a greater risk of contaminating the drug, and it would put some bottles under so much pressure that the drug would leak out through the rubber bung.

Before giving the injection, make sure that the animal has been firmly restrained. Injections can be given in four ways, intradermal (into the skin) subcutaneous (under the skin), intramuscular (into the muscle) and intravenous (directly into the blood stream). Intradermal injections are used in the tuberculosis test (see page 284). The intravenous route gives the most prompt effect and it may have to be used for certain drugs which would cause irritation if given subcutaneously or intramuscularly. There are great dangers in giving intravenous injections too fast however, and some preparations are

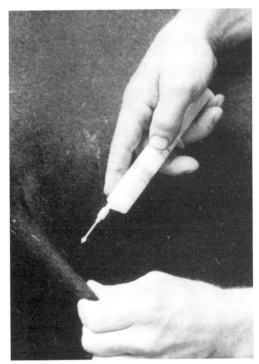

Plate 13.4 Subcutaneous injection. The best site is the loose skin just behind the shoulder.

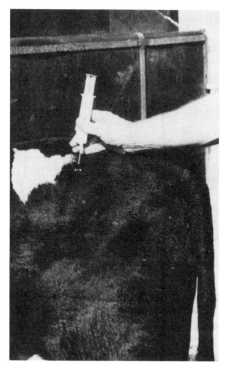

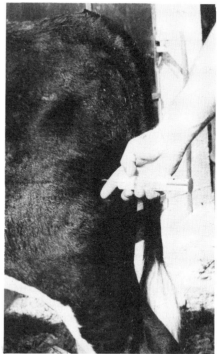

Plate 13.5 Intramuscular injection—preferred site in adult animals. The needle would be inserted first and the syringe connected afterwards.

Plate 13.6 Intramuscular injection—preferred site in younger animals.

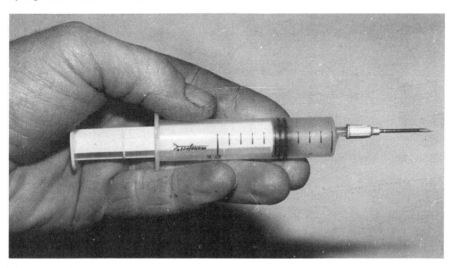

Plate 13.7 Method of holding the syringe to make a rapid injection into the hind leg.

not suitable for intravenous use. You should *always* read the instructions and consult your vet before administering any drug. Whatever the route of injection, make sure that the site chosen is clean. Ideally you should use a swab soaked in methylated spirits, but this is not usually done, and provided that the skin is not covered with mud or dung and that your needle is clean, the risk of abscess formation in cattle is very low.

Subcutaneous injections

I prefer to use the loose skin behind the shoulder. Catch hold of a fold between your finger and thumb, then push the needle forwards towards the shoulder (plate 13.4). The cow's skin is very tough (after all, it is leather!) and you will be surprised how much force is needed, even with a sharp needle. If you are dosing large numbers of animals, for example blackleg vaccination or worming, then change the needle for a clean and sharper one every ten to fifteen animals, or immediately if you think it is dirty. If you are repeatedly taking doses from the same pack *without* an automatic syringe you *must* make sure that you leave one needle in the bottle to transfer the drug into the syringe and use a second needle to carry out the injections. This avoids the risk of spreading infection by contaminating the bottle.

Intramuscular injections

In adult cattle I use the area of muscle covering the pelvis, each side of the tail (plate 13.5). Firmly grasp the needle between your forefinger and thumb, then stab it downwards with as much force as you can. Connect the syringe and inject. A one-inch needle should go in up to its butt.

In younger animals I use the fleshy part of the hind leg (plate 13.6) and hold the syringe in the palm of my hand, with the needle attached (plate 13.7). When the needle reaches its full depth in the muscle, the force from the palm of your hand propels the plunger forwards and the injection is given very quickly.

Intravenous injections

These should always be given slowly and with great care. If you are thinking of carrying out intravenous injections, discuss the technique with your vet first. The jugular vein is found in a furrow which lies between the trachea and the muscle of the neck, shown as a white chalk mark in plate 13.8. In this vein, blood is flowing from the head back to the heart, so if you obstruct the vein using finger pressure or a rope around the neck, you will see it swell up. I find it best to stab the needle into the centre of the vein first, slightly adjusting its position until blood flows. Then incline the butt of the needle towards the cow's head and push the point *down* the vein until the butt is against the skin. This is shown in plate 13.9. Once in this position the needle is far less likely to come out of the vein while the injection is being given.

Flutter valves

Many large-volume injections are now prepared in plastic packs which collapse as the liquid runs out of them (plate 13.10). These tend to be more

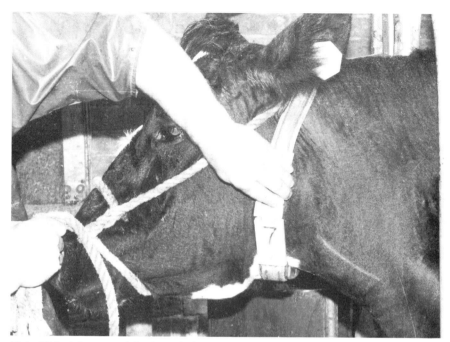

Plate 13.8   Intravenous injection—the jugular vein lies in a furrow which is indicated here as a chalk mark.

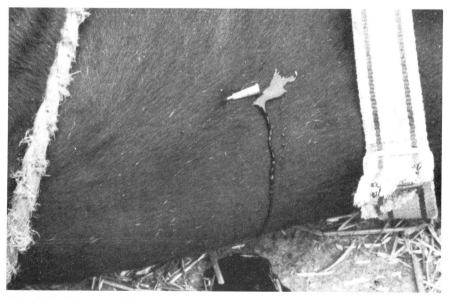

Plate 13.9   Intravenous injection—the vein has been raised using a rope and the needle has been inserted to its butt and is pointing down the vein.

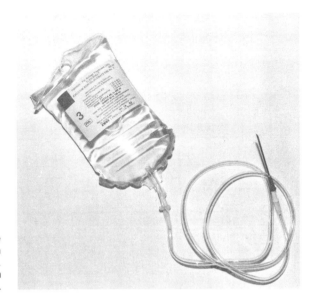

Plate 13.10   Collapsible plastic pack of calcium complete with its giving set. This is ideal for on-farm use.

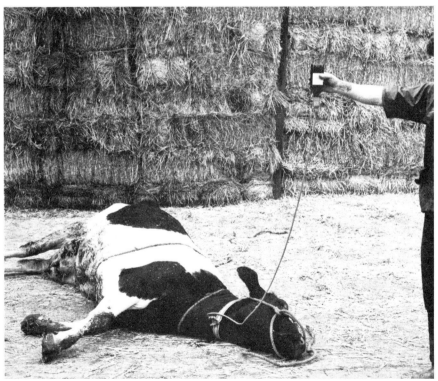

Plate 13.11   Administering calcium using the older-style rubber flutter valves.

expensive than the older-style bottles, but as there is no need to sterilise the 'giving set' each time, I think that the extra cost is well justified for on-farm use. Sometimes you have to use bottles, however, and the flutter valve is a device to allow air to enter the bottle as the injection liquid runs out. It is used as follows. First attach the head of the flutter valve to the neck of the bottle, then turn the bottle upside down and check that air is entering through the air-bleed and that liquid is flowing through the tubing. Next insert the needle into the cow; then, making sure that there is no air left in the tubing by running through a drop more fluid, connect the tubing to the needle (plate 13.11). Adjust the height of the bottle so that liquid runs in at the correct speed. You can check this by the rate at which bubbles are entering the bottle.

Giving a Drench

Drenches are best administered using a special dosing gun because the nozzle can deliver the liquid so far back over the tongue that it is virtually impossible for the animal to spit it out. Traditionally guns with short delivery tubes were used (plate 13.12) and this meant that the cow had to be restrained either by holding her nose or by wrapping your arm around her head.

Recently guns with much longer delivery pipes and a crook at one end have been introduced. Plate 13.13 shows how the device can be crooked into a cow's mouth without necessarily catching her, and animals can even be drenched in a race in this way. If a drenching bottle is to be used, choose one with a fine elongated neck which can also deliver liquid to the back of the cow's mouth. The bottle should be introduced slightly to one side of the incisor teeth and its neck then pushed back over the tongue, taking care that it stays half-way between the two rows of molar teeth. (These terms are explained on page 311.) Tilting the animal's head upwards makes it easier to pour in the drench. If it is a large volume you may need to allow them time to catch their breath half-way through. Sometimes they will not swallow: squeezing their throat over their larynx often helps them to do so.

Passing a stomach tube
See page 28.

Relieving Bloat
See pages 28 and 319.

Disbudding Calves

A cow's horn consists of two parts, the outer casing of hoof-like material and a bone in the centre. In the calf the skin around the base of the horn becomes impregnated with an extremely hard material called keratin and this grows up over the horn to form the outer casing. An extension of the skull bone then occupies the space in the centre. The object of dehorning is to destroy the area of horn-forming skin. Unless chemical cauterisation is applied during the

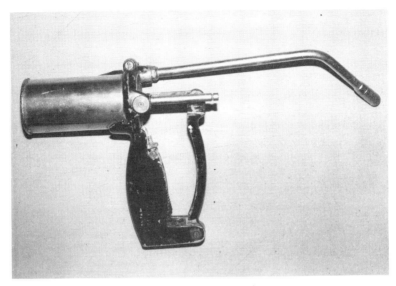

Plate 13.12   Traditional drenching gun with a short nozzle.

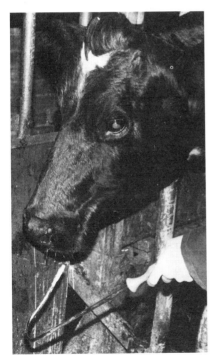

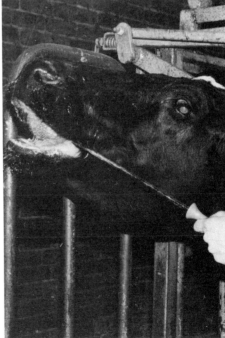

Plate 13.13   A drenching gun with a long nozzle has the advantage that the cow's head does not have to be restrained.

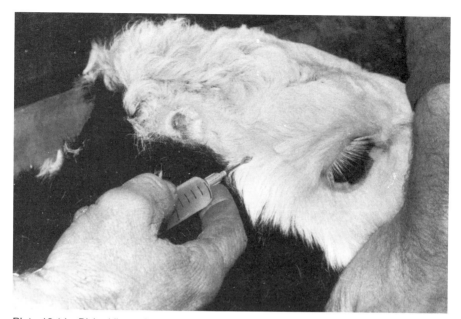

Plate 13.14   Disbudding calves: inject 2.0 ml of anaesthetic under the ridge of bone half-way between the eye and the horn.

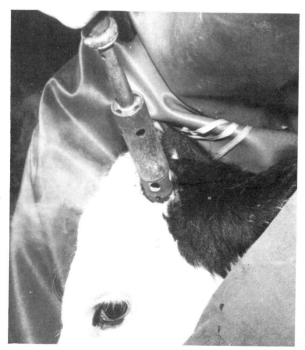

Plate 13.15   Disbudding calves: apply the hot iron firmly onto the horn bud and slowly count to ten. I prefer a gas iron to electric.

first week of life—and I would not recommend that method—the Protection of Animals Act 1911 states that calves must be given an anaesthetic before being dehorned or disbudded. The procedure is best carried out at around four to six weeks old, at an age when the horn bud can be clearly felt but before it gets so large that it cannot easily fit into the end of the disbudding iron.

The nerve to the horn runs out from behind the eye and underneath a small overhanging ledge of bone which is part of the skull. This is best seen in figure 12.1. Using a short needle (1.5 cm or less), inject 2.0 ml of anaesthetic under this ridge on each side (plate 13.14). You may find that blood flows from the injection site after you have withdrawn the needle. This is no cause for alarm. There is a vein and an artery running along beside the nerve and these can easily be punctured. It is sometimes recommended that you should slightly withdraw the plunger of the syringe before injecting the anaesthetic. If blood then appears in the syringe you know you are in a blood vessel, and the position of the needle needs altering slightly, because intravenous injection of local anaesthetic can cause collapse. This is not a procedure which I routinely follow, however.

Leave the calf for at least five to six minutes while the anaesthetic takes effect. Its action is almost immediate if you happen to have deposited anaesthetic directly onto the nerve; however if you have just missed, some time must elapse before the drug can diffuse to its target. The speed of onset of anaesthesia also varies with the anaesthetic being used. Clip the hair around the area then, with the calf's head held firmly, place the hot iron over the horn so that the bud fits into the depression at the tip of the iron (plate 13.15). Apply moderate pressure while you hold the iron in this position and count to ten, then angle the iron to scoop out the horn bud (plate 13.16). Provided that the skin around the outside of the horn has been destroyed, it is not strictly necessary to remove the bud itself. If the bud is too large to fit into the iron, first cut it off with scissors or even hoof clippers, then proceed as before. When using hoof clippers, try to remove the bud with a small ring of hair around its base. This is the horn-forming tissue and there is then no risk of regrowth. Finally apply an antibiotic/gentian violet aerosol to dry the wound and promote healing.

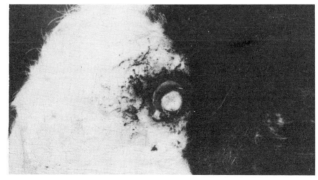

Plate 13.16 Disbudding calves—the area of skin around the horn bud has now been destroyed.

Removing Supernumerary Teats

As part of routine stockmanship you should always check for extra teats when disbudding calves which are to be retained for breeding. If left, spare teats may develop mastitis, or, even worse, when they are too close to a true teat, they interfere with milking. By law you must use an anaesthetic in calves over two months old and if the calf is over three months old the operation may only be performed by a veterinary surgeon.

In small calves it is best to hold the calf in a sitting position (the technique for turning it is shown in plate 13.17) and examine for extra teats by spreading the udder skin with your fingers. I then hold the skin beneath the teat with my finger and thumb and with one movement, amputate the teat with a pair of *sharp* scissors, which have curved blades. An alternative is to pull the teat away from the skin using a pair of forceps (as shown in plate 13.18). When you have finished, apply antibiotic or antiseptic aerosol spray.

For calves over two months old, simply inject 2 cc of local anaesthetic into the base of the teat where it joins the skin. This forms a small nodule in the skin which needs to be dispersed by rubbing between your fingers.

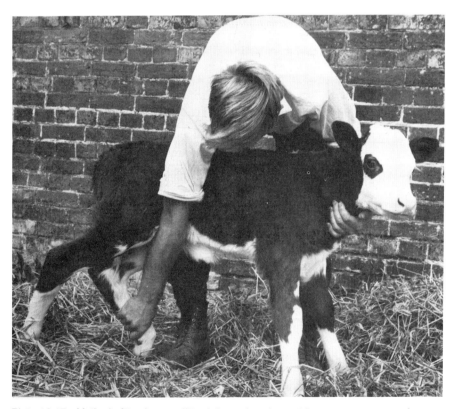

Plate 13.17   Method of turning a calf to sit it, ready to inspect for supernumerary teats.

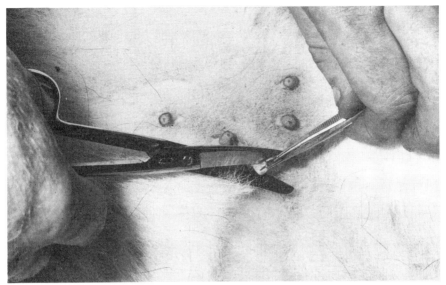

Plate 13.18   Removing supernumerary teats. If forceps are not available simply hold the skin at the base of the teat between finger and thumb before removing the teat.

Castration

There are three methods of castrating calves, namely rubber rings, the Burdizzo bloodless castrator and surgical removal of the testicles. Surgical removal is by far the most certain method, and provided that an anaesthetic is used, calves may be left entire until they are four to six months old to obtain improved growth rates and better conformation of the final carcase. From January 1983 however, it became a legal requirement that calves over two months old may only be castrated by a veterinary surgeon and I would suggest that stockmen never attempt surgical castration at any age, because at less than two months old the testicles are so small that surgical castration is quite difficult.

Use of rubber rings

These are only permitted in calves less than one week old. Hold the calf in a sitting position, make sure that both testicles are in the scrotum, then apply the ring to the base of the scrotum, as shown in plate 13.19. Remove the applicator and check for a second time that both testicles are still in the scrotum. Every year we are asked to examine groups of yearling heifers for pregnancy, because they have been running with a male which someone castrated without checking that both testicles were below the ring. If you still cannot find the second testicle, my advice would be to mark the calf and get your vet to examine it at three to four months old or more. Do not apply a ring otherwise you will overlook the possibility of a second testicle descending at a later date—possibly to the detriment of next year's heifers!

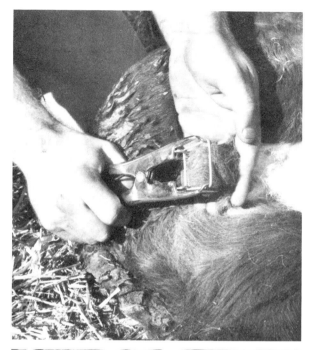

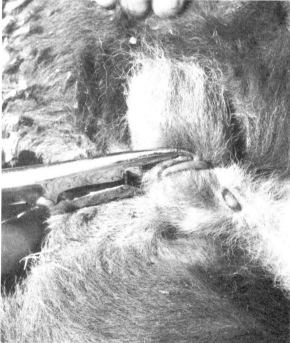

Plate 13.19 Castration using a rubber ring. After the ring has been applied it is vital to check that both testicles are still in the scrotum.

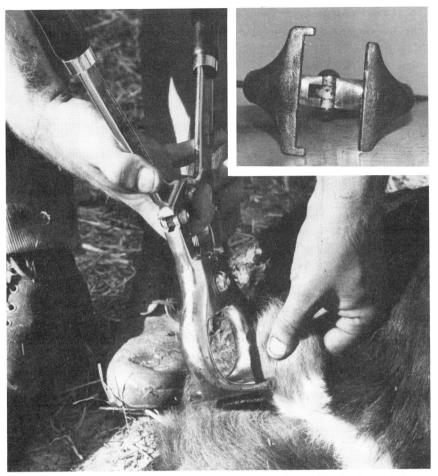

Plate 13.20 Burdizzo castration: the cord is held in place for crushing by the cord stops on the Burdizzo jaws (top right corner).

Bloodless castration

Burdizzo castration is based on the principle that crushing destroys the spermatic cord (which carries blood to the testicles) but that the skin of the scrotum remains intact. Approach the standing calf from behind and push one of the cords to the outside of the scrotum. Next apply the jaws of the Burdizzo checking that the cord is held in one place by the cord-stops (plate 13.20) and firmly close the handles. Count to five seconds. The procedure is best repeated just below the first crush (figure 13.1) and then twice on the other cord. You must make sure that the crush marks on each side to not join up to form a continuous line across the scrotum, otherwise there is a risk of the scrotum itself being destroyed. The second crush on each side should always be beneath the first, as shown in plate 13.21.

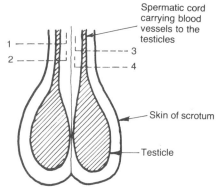

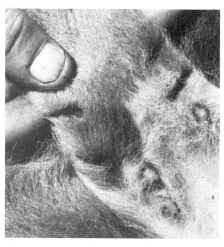

Figure 13.1   The sequence of Burdizzo castration crushing positions. Note that the first crush is always above the second, and that the crushes on each side must not be immediately opposite each other. The dotted line shows how the cord stop on the edge of one of the jaws makes sure that the cord cannot slip away.

Plate 13.21   Burdizzo castration: the crushes should be carried out toward the edge of the scrotum and should never be allowed to join up at the centre.

Taking a Temperature

A thermometer is a surprisingly difficult instrument to read and you ought to first practise holding its tip between your finger and thumb (figure 13.2) and gently rolling it until you are quite sure that you can see the thick line of mercury. Before inserting the thermometer, hold it at the end away from the mercury bulb and give it a few firm shakes. Now check that the mercury has returned towards the reservoir and that the thermometer registers 99°F or less. Apply some lubricant to the thermometer—I find saliva very effective and readily available!—hold the cow's tail up with one hand and insert the thermometer into its rectum with the other. You may find that the

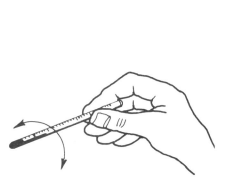

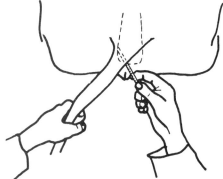

Figure 13.2   Roll the thermometer between finger and thumb until the thick line of mercury can be recognised.

Figure 13.3   Taking a temperature: deflect the thermometer to one side so that the bulb is as close to the wall of the rectum as possible.

thermometer needs to be rolled to get it to pass through the anal sphincter. At least two-thirds of its total length should be inserted and once in position, deflect the thermometer to one side (figure 13.3) so that the mercury bulb is as close to the wall of the rectum as possible. If the thermometer is left in the centre of a lump of faeces, the temperature registered may be considerably lower than the cow's actual body temperature. This is particularly important when the cow is constipated, for example with milk fever.

Withdraw the thermometer after thirty seconds, gently wipe it clean, then take the reading by again slowly rolling it between your finger and thumb until the thick line of mercury comes into view. If you are in any doubt, shake it back down and repeat the procedure.

A cow with a high temperature most probably has an infection, but this could be a viral, protozoal or bacterial infection and only the bacteria would respond to antibiotics. Temperature may also rise with excitement, for example in a cow which has been in convulsions due to hypomagnesaemia. Unfortunately the reverse is not true, that is we cannot say that a cow with an infection will always have a raised temperature, or that a cow without a temperature definitely does not have an infection. The infection may be localised, for example an abscess or a mild mastitis and although the infected area may feel hot to the touch, there is no general rise in the whole body temperature. Another possibility is that the cow may initially have had a high temperature (for example in the early stages of E. coli mastitis) but as the condition progressed, toxaemia and shock set in and body temperature fell, often to below normal. A temperature below normal (that is less than 101.5°F or 38°C) could be a bad sign—although it may simply mean that you did not have the thermometer positioned correctly in the rectum!

Dealing with Wounds

There are many different types of wounds and often they need careful treatment. If you are in any doubt you should call in your vet. He can then suture it if necessary, apply the first dressing and leave you instructions for aftercare. The following gives a broad outline on the approach to wounds in general.

Is it bleeding badly? A steady drip, drip of blood generally does no harm and usually will stop on its own. If you can see a continual pulsating squirt of blood however, this indicates that an artery has been severed and you must take action. If the legs or tail are involved it is quite easy to apply a tourniquet using a rope and stick (plate 13.22). In other areas often all you can do is to push a wad of cotton wool or a tea-towel hard against the wound until your vet arrives. Sometimes applying pressure for four to five minutes is in itself enough to stop the bleeding. A tourniquet should be applied just tight enough to arrest the bleeding and only for an hour or two. If too tight or if left on too long, it could lead to gangrene of the whole limb.

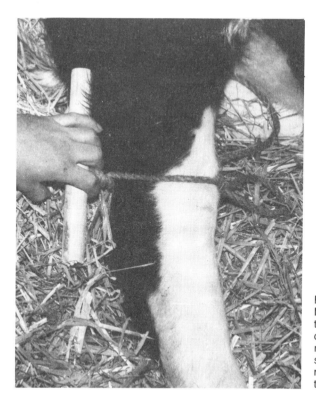

Plate 13.22   A tourniquet. Make a large loop around the leg, then use a length of wood to tighten the rope until the blood flow stops. Do not leave the rope in place for longer than necessary.

Does it need stitching? Large skin wounds and cuts on teats are best sutured, *provided* that there is sufficient loose skin available and that the wound is fairly fresh. However, suturing a cut over the knee, for example, is not worth while because any sutures are likely to pull out as soon as the animal starts walking. If the edges of the wounds are dry and healing has already started, suturing may not be successful. Also if the skin flap is very thin, feels lifeless and is 'devitalised', that is it has no feeling, suturing is probably not worth while, and on teats it is best to simply amputate the flap with scissors to prevent further skin tearing during milking (see plate 7.14).

Cleaning the wound. Infection, dirt and dead tissue seriously retard healing, so you must wash the area very carefully. If there is a skin flap, or if you are dealing with an abscess, do not be afraid to take a piece of cotton wool soaked in diluted disinfectant and wipe it deep under the skin. Repeat this with fresh swabs until they come out quite clean. Any dead tissue will have a creamy, pus-like appearance and this should also be rubbed away with your cotton wool. If the wound is an ulcer or some other lesion in the foot, then it can only be drained and cleaned by removing all the horn overlying the infected area. Abscesses may need to be lanced to allow the pus to drain, but first clean the skin, insert a needle and withdraw some of the contents of the swelling to make sure you obtain the characteristic off-white, thick, foul-smelling pus indicating that you are dealing with an abscess. If this is not found leave the swelling alone and ask your vet to look when he next comes. Abscesses should be lanced at their lowest point, as this facilitates drainage. If possible, choose a place where the skin is softening and make a bold deep cut with a scalpel blade. Squeeze out all the pus, then flush the abscess cavity with antiseptic solution as described above.

This flushing process needs repeating every two to three days. It is most important that the initial cut does not heal over for at least a week, otherwise drainage will be inhibited and the abscess may re-form. One easy but very effective way of flushing out an abscess is simply to put a cold-water hosepipe into the cavity then turn on the tap. The water pressure will help to remove all the pus and dead tissue present.

Does it need a dressing? Very large raw areas, or areas of the feet and legs which can get dirty are best covered. Apply an antiseptic ointment, then cotton wool or possibly a lint dressing and finally hold this in position with elastoplast. Abscesses are best left open for the pus to drain and should not be covered.

Ointment or spray? For many wounds, especially those on teats or other areas where the skin can crack, I prefer to use an emollient ointment, preferably one with antiseptic properties. This is especially important for severe teat chapping since teat skin lacks the sebaceous glands found on skin elsewhere in the body. Antibiotic aerosols containing gentian violet tend to dry out wounds. They are therefore very good for superficial skin cuts and following dehorning, but if applied to teat skin they may lead to excessive cracking which would retard healing.

Poulticing. Wounds caused by deep penetration, for example by a nail, cannot be washed out and cleaned with a swab. If infection develops it may be worth applying a poultice to draw pus from the deeper tissues. Hot bran or kaolin are often used. Poultices need to be changed daily and are therefore quite laborious, but they can be very effective with some of the deeper infections of the foot, especially where the tendons or navicular bone are involved.

Applying Eye Ointment

Eye infections seem to be an increasing problem, possibly because animals are being kept in larger groups and there is therefore a much greater risk of transmitting infection from one animal to another.

First hold the animal's head and tilt it to one side and then the other, to see if you can see the typical white spot of the New Forest Disease ulcer (plate 4.8). Next turn the eyelids back to make sure that no barley awns or other foreign bodies are present: only the very tip may be visible, and care is needed to make sure this is not broken off when removing it from the eye.

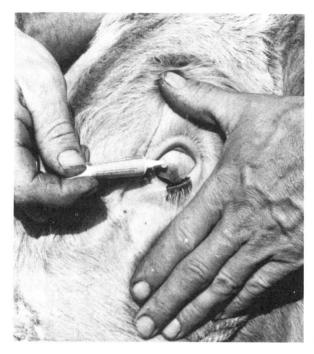

Plate 13.23   Applying eye ointment.

Finally apply a line of ointment across the front of the eyeball, holding the tube at an oblique angle to the eye as shown in plate 13.23. Some ointments provide antibiotic cover for two days. If you think an even longer period of antibiotic is needed, you could ask your vet to deposit an injection under the conjunctiva (plate 4.10). The animal needs to be held very still, because of the risk of damaging the eyeball with the needle.

Putting on a Halter

Perhaps this is hardly a veterinary task, but it surprises me how many people cannot apply a halter correctly. Lassoing a cow leads to unnecessary stress and does not restrain it particularly well because it can still move its head from side to side. The correct procedure is shown in plate 13.24. There are essentially three pieces of the halter:

- the fixed length segment which fits over the animal's nose;
- the lead rope which should come out from underneath the animal's chin;
- an adjustable loop which fits behind the animal's ears.

If possible, apply the halter in one movement, by lifting the lower loop over the animal's nose and continuing to fit the upper loop behind its ears. Finally adjust the lead rope so that it is tight under its chin and check that the side pieces are not rubbing its eyes.

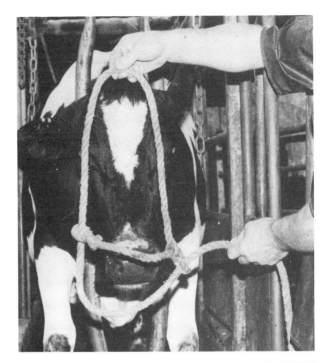

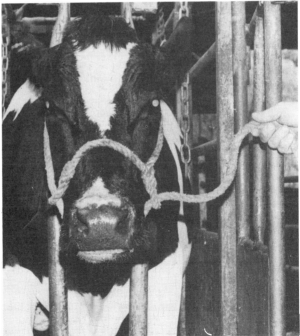

Plate 13.24 Applying a halter: the fixed-length segment runs over the cow's nose and the lead rope should come up from under its chin.

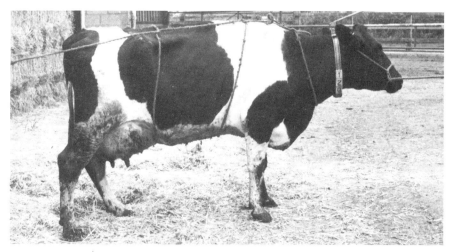

Plate 13.25 Casting a cow—Reuff's method. A long rope is looped around her neck, behind her front legs, and in front of her hind legs.

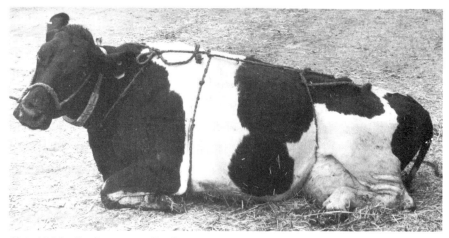

Plate 13.26 Casting a cow—Reuff's method. When the rope is tightened, the cow sinks to the ground.

Casting a Cow—Reuff's Method

Although cattle are most commonly restrained in a crush, it is sometimes useful to be able to cast them. With the help of sedation, I use the Reuff's method of casting for rolling cows to correct a displaced abomasum (see page 324) and also for casting bulls for foot trimming when they are too large to go into a crush. Steady the cow with a halter, then tie a second rope around her neck, looping it behind her fore legs then in front of her udder, hind legs and pin bones, as shown in plate 13.25. Tighten the chest loop, then pull hard on the free end to tighten the abdominal loop. Provided sufficient tension can be applied, the animal will sink to the ground (plate 13.26), and it will stay there until the rope is released. Although it will work with any cow, the procedure is much easier if the cow has been sedated first. Take care that the rear loop of rope is not catching on the udder (plate 13.25).

Ringing a Bull

For ease of handling and for safety I think it is best to ring a bull soon after six months old, so that he gets used to being led. Holding the bull's head very

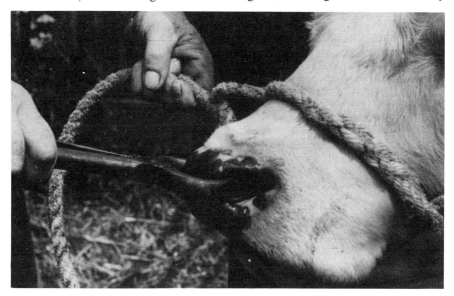

Plate 13.27 (*above*)   Ringing a bull— applying the nose-punch.

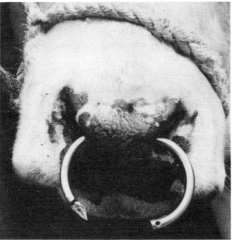

Plate 13.28 (*left*)   Ringing a bull— the ring has been inserted and now needs closing with the lock-screw.

firmly, inject a small volume (1–2 cc) of anaesthetic into the soft tissue dividing the nostrils before applying the nose punch (plate 13.27). The hole should be made as far back from the nostrils as possible for added strength, but it should not go through the harder tissue of the cartilage of the nostrils. You can easily feel this with your fingers. Having firmly closed the punch move it up and down a few times to cut the hole through completely, then insert the ring (plate 13.28). Carefully locate the locking screw into the thread, screw it up as tight as possible, then break off the protruding segment. File away any rough edges. It is best to allow two to three weeks for the hole to heal before training the bull to lead.

Hormone Implants

Recent years have seen a marked increase in the number of hormone implants used for fattening cattle and currently well over 50 per cent of all cattle slaughtered have been treated at some stage of their life. The rationale of hormone use is as follows:

- heifers and cows have ample female hormone so they are implanted with male hormones;
- steers have no hormones and are implanted with male and female products;
- bulls have ample male hormone and some female, so they are given additional female hormones.

The response to implantation is therefore greatest in steers, where a 30 per cent increase in growth rate can be anticipated, with additional improvements in carcase quality and in feed conversion efficiency. Implanted heifers and cull cows become much more muscular and some may even develop a few male characteristics. As hormone implants affect growth *rate* it is clearly most advantageous to use them when the animal's natural rate of growth is already at a high level. For example, a 30 per cent improvement in the growth rate of an animal growing at 0.3 kg per day is only 0.1 kg, whereas if the natural growth is already 1.5 kg per day, a 30 per cent improvement would give 0.5 kg per day. The relationship is by no means as simple as this, but the example serves to illustrate the point very well.

The effects in entire bulls are much less dramatic, partly because of their natural rapid growth and good carcase conformation. Implants of female hormone should still give them a 5–10 per cent increase in growth rate however, and there may be additional benefits from reduced mounting behaviour and aggressiveness.

Implants should be given under the skin of the ear, because this is the part of the carcase which is discarded and there is then no risk of large residual doses being eaten. The products used are either synthetic compounds (e.g. zeranol and trenbolone or natural hormones (e.g. oestradiol, testosterone and progesterone). It is claimed that the second group are equally as effective and have the advantage that no withdrawal period is necessary. Thus they may be more acceptable to the consumer lobby.

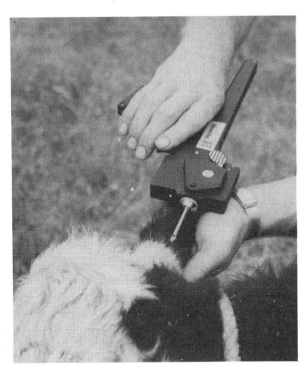

Plate 13.29 Implanting an anabolic steroid growth promoter.

There are currently five licensed products on the market, and the implanting technique for one of them, an anabolic steroid, is demonstrated in plate 13.29. It would be a good idea to get your vet to demonstrate the technique on the first few animals before doing any yourself.

Using a Mastitis or Dry-Cow Tube

Infusing intramammary antibiotic into cows for mastitis or at drying off is probably one of the most frequent veterinary tasks that the stockman has to undertake. Cleanliness is essential, otherwise infections such as E. coli or yeasts can be introduced into the udder. If dealing with a case of mastitis, thoroughly strip out the quarter, possibly leaving it for five to ten minutes then try again. Stripping is an excellent way of removing the bacteria and toxins. If they are not stripped out, the cow would have to remove them by absorbing them into her system, and this could increase the severity of the illness. If the teats are very dirty, they should be washed *and* dried. Next rub the end of the teat ten times with a piece of cotton wool soaked in meths, alcohol or antiseptic (see plate 7.6 and page 177). Only at this stage should you remove the protective cap from the nozzle of the antibiotic tube, and many herdsmen find that their teeth are the best way of achieving this!

Holding the teat in one hand, bend it slightly so that the orifice is pointing towards you. If the orifice is not clearly visible, draw a few drops of milk to act

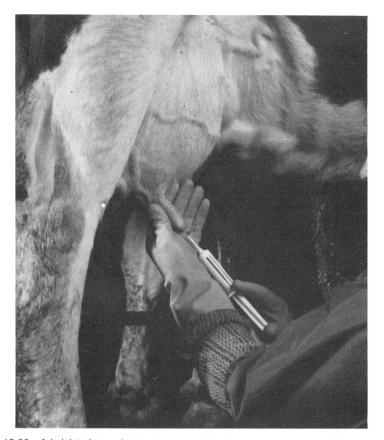

Plate 13.30   Administering an intramammary antibiotic tube (photograph: MMB).

as a marker. Holding the tube in the other hand, gently touch the nozzle against the orifice (plate 13.30) and then slowly slide it through. If the cow is nervous, use an anti-kick bar or get help from a second person rather than risk contaminating the tube and introducing infection. Withdraw the tube and, holding the tip of the teat between your thumb and forefinger, use the other hand to work the antibiotic up into the udder. Finally apply teat dip.

Taking a milk sample
This was explained in detail in Chapter Seven, on page 176.

Foot trimming
This was described in Chapter Nine under the heading of lameness prevention on page 266.

Handling a 'downer' cow
This was described in Chapter Five, page 123, including moving a cow on a gate and the use of an inflatable bag and the Bagshawe hoist as lifting aids.

Dealing with Poisons

I find dealing with poisoning a particularly frustrating subject. To start with, many poisons give the same vague symptoms of dullness, abdominal pain and possibly nervous signs, so you probably cannot diagnose on the symptoms alone. Even if you suspect a particular poison, it may be difficult to get laboratory tests to confirm that the substance is present. Then, if it is detected, it still may not be the cause of all, or of even any, of the symptoms seen. At the end of all this, being convinced that you know what is causing the illness, the treatment is often only vague and is aimed at alleviating the symptoms rather than specifically counteracting the effects of the poison!

There are a few exceptions to this of course and lead poisoning is a good example. But even with lead the symptoms can be variable, ranging from dullness and blindness, to an extreme excitement, racing around the pen and bellowing. So, often, suspicions of poisoning must rest with a history of possible access to a known toxic substance and this is why I have only listed some of the more common poisons in this chapter. I have already said that symptoms and treatment can be very variable and for this reason I have given very few details. If you suspect poisoning I would strongly recommend that you contact your vet for advice. Remember that for many poisons, small quantities are relatively harmless—they may even be beneficial. It is only when they are taken in excessive amounts—for example plants which are eaten because there is no other grazing available—that poisoning occurs.

Acorns and oak leaves
Green acorns are particularly toxic if eaten in large quantities. The poison is called tannic acid, a chemical which is used to preserve and harden hides in leather making. Initially cattle show dullness, abdominal pain and loss of appetite, but later there may be severe diarrhoea, the dung being black with blood, due to inflammation of the gut. Drenching with chlorodyne (60 g) and linseed oil or liquid paraffin (500 ml) may help, and drugs can be given by injection to alleviate the intestinal spasm and pain.

Antibiotics
Sometimes concentrates fed to cattle are contaminated with residues of antibiotics or other drugs which were perhaps being used as growth-promoters or medicants in pig or poultry rations. Although there is now a much stricter control at the feed mills when cleaning out between different mixes, mistakes can still occur. Most of the drugs involved destroy the normal bacteria in the rumen, and this makes the rumen go sour and the animal goes off its food. Quite severe reductions in milk production have been reported when contaminated feed has been given to dairy cows. The antibiotic *lincomycin* is especially dangerous because it kills ruminal protozoa as well as bacteria.

Arsenic
This was once a common constituent of sheep dips and potato sprays. It is now rarely used, but cattle may gain access to old cans and some seem to even

like its taste! Arsenic causes severe inflammation of the gut, leading to abdominal pain, colic and scouring. Badly affected animals become recumbent and die. Treatment is similar to that for acorn poisoning.

Bracken

Bracken poisoning occurs especially in late summer when grazing is sparse, although symptoms may not be seen until three weeks or more after the animals have been removed from the pasture. Although the green plant (figure 13.4) is bitter, dried bracken may be readily eaten with hay, so bracken poisoning can occur indoors in winter. There are two types of symptoms. The first is associated with gut inflammation caused by eating the fresh plant, and this leads to scouring with blood in the dung. The other syndrome is one of severe anaemia. Bracken affects the formation of certain cells, the thrombocytes (sometimes known as the blood platelets), in the bone marrow and this produces a thrombocytopenia (a deficiency of thrombocytes) which interferes with blood clotting. You may see large red haemorrhagic areas in the mouth, eyes or vulva and the urine may also turn red. There is no specific antidote, although antiscour treatments and blood stimulants will help.

Copper

This is a good example of a cumulative poison. Cattle cope with high intakes of copper by storing the excess in their liver, but eventually they reach the stage where no more can be stored and the liver literally bursts. This causes severe jaundice, abdominal pain and blood in the urine. Deaths are common. Copper poisoning usually occurs following a fairly long period of high intake, for example cattle grazing an orchard in which the trees were sprayed with copper salts, or following over-enthusiastic supplementation of rations with copper. In fact the acute toxic episode may not occur until after the cattle have been removed from the source and are then stressed in some way. Usually if one animal is affected by copper poisoning it means that the remainder of the group are at great risk of collapse and death and must be handled very carefully.

Creosote

It is surprising what cattle will drink and cases of creosote, diesel, paraffin and petrol poisoning are by no means uncommon. The early signs of poisoning are dullness, loss of appetite and abdominal pain, and these become more intense, leading to nervous signs and convulsions as the effects of severe liver damage become apparent. Often diagnosis is helped by the smell of creosote or diesel in the dung or even in the milk. At lower levels diesel may simply affect growth rate and hair formation. Plate 13.31 shows one such calf. The whole group had been affected by licking the diesel which dripped from a pipe in the enclosure. Dosing the calves with vitamin A and moving them to a new pen eventually produced a complete recovery.

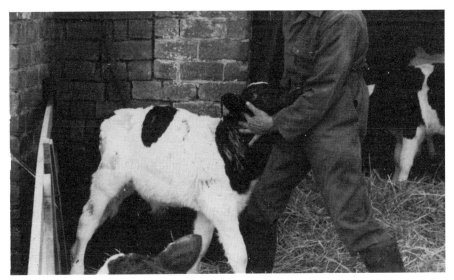

Plate 13.31 This calf had been licking diesel which was dripping from a pipe in the yard. Its growth was stunted and it was losing its coat.

Fluorine

Fluorine is emitted from a large number of industrial processes and unless precautions are taken it can contaminate the surrounding grassland. It may also be present in certain types of rock phosphate. Most of the fluorine eaten is deposited in the animal's bones and teeth, and symptoms are unlikely to be seen until there has been a continuous exposure for several months. One of its main effects is lameness, which can be due to either a fracture of the bone in the hoof (see also page 258) or to exostoses which are small sharp lumps projecting from the surface of the bone. If exostoses occur on the joints, lameness is particularly severe. Teeth abnormalities may also occur, especially in younger animals, with breaks and pitting of the enamel. Many of the symptoms of fluorosis are similar to those of rickets. Very small doses of fluorine are beneficial to the bones and teeth, as we all know from dentistry advertisements. The only treatment for poisoning is to remove the cattle from the contaminated pasture, give vitamins A and D and wait for the fluorine to be slowly excreted.

Insecticides

There are two main groups of insecticides, the organochlorines (or chlorinated hydrocarbons) and the organophosphorus compounds. Both can cause poisoning in cattle. The organochlorines include DDT, BHC (the common constituent of louse powder) and dieldrin (formerly used in sheep dips). Poisoning results from a gradual build-up of the organochlorines in the

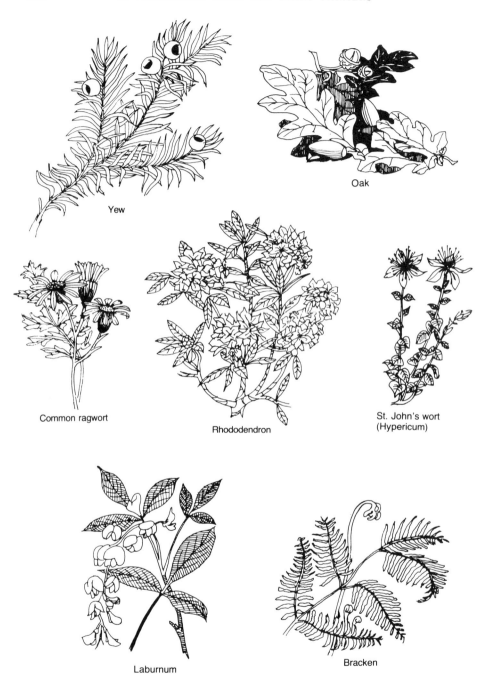

Yew

Oak

Common ragwort

Rhododendron

St. John's wort
(Hypericum)

Laburnum

Bracken

Figure 13.4   Some of the more common British poisonous plants.

animal's tissues, especially in the fat, although the onset of symptoms of excitability and muscle spasms can be quite sudden. Treatment is symptomatic only and consists of giving sedatives and muscle relaxants to control the convulsions.

Poisoning with organophosphorus compounds is far more common. This is because they are more widely used, because they can be absorbed through the skin and because they are inherently more toxic. Cattle may be exposed to sprays drifting from an adjacent field and I have seen several cases of poisoning when animals have been allowed to graze orchards immediately after spraying. Although the spray may remain on the outside of the foliage for only a few days, it can take several weeks for the organophosphorus compounds absorbed by the plants to lose their toxicity. The main symptoms of poisoning are salivation, colic, diarrhoea, difficulty in breathing and apparent blindness. Badly affected animals develop convulsions and die. Your vet will probably use atropine for treatment. This is a drug derived from Deadly Nightshade, which is in itself a poisonous plant. Atropine only counteracts some of the symptoms however and recovery will still be very slow.

Organophosphorus compounds include pour-on warble dressings, fly-repellants and some anthelmintics, as well as insecticides and sheep dips.

Kale
Overeating kale has been mentioned elsewhere in the book (page 303). There are three possible toxic syndromes. First, large intakes of kale over a short period may lead to a breakdown of the red blood cells. This is caused by a chemical in the kale called S-methyl cysteine sulphoxide (SMCO), and it is seen clinically as blood in the urine and anaemia. Frosted kale is considered to be especially dangerous. Secondly, lower intakes of kale for prolonged periods may cause problems of depressed blood formation and anaemia. Thirdly, kale interferes with thyroid function, leading to goitre. Intakes above 20 kg per day for long periods should be avoided. Cabbage, rape and other members of the brassica family can cause similar problems if fed in excess.

Laburnum
Next to yew, laburnum is the most dangerous tree grown in Britain and you would be well advised to study a plant guide to make sure that you can recognise it. All parts of the plant are poisonous, but the pods and seeds are especially toxic and produce nervous signs of excitement, incoordination, convulsions and death. There is no specific antidote, although your vet could give sedatives to help control the nervous signs until the animal overcomes and excretes the toxin itself.

Lead
This was discussed in detail in Chapter Three (page 59).

Mycotoxins
When feedingstuffs are stored under unsatisfactory conditions, especially humidity and warmth, moulds (a type of fungus) may grow. The majority of moulds are quite harmless and although they may reduce its nutritional content and palatability, the affected food can still be fed to cattle. However, some moulds produce toxic byproducts, known as *mycotoxins*, and if eaten by cattle they can produce poisoning. The symptoms seen depend on the type of mycotoxin present and this in turn depends on the species of mould which was originally growing on the food. Examples of mycotoxins include sterigmato-cystin, ochratoxin A (causes kidney damage), citrinin, trichothecene (a gut irritant) and tremorgens (pasture moulds). The most common however is called *aflatoxin*, which is a contaminant of imported groundnut and cotton-seed cakes. In 1980, over 20 per cent of the imports tested were found to contain aflatoxin, although many were below the level likely to cause symptoms. Some feedingstuff manufacturers have now stopped using ground-nut and cottonseed, and legislation exists to prohibit the incorporation of materials containing more than 50 parts per billion of aflatoxin. If fed to cattle it causes liver damage and this leads to a drop in milk yield or a reduction in growth rates in younger animals. There is also concern that a breakdown product of aflatoxin which appears in the milk may cause liver tumours in man. Such tumours are extremely rare however and aflatoxin is by no means the only cause.

Nitrates
In the rumen, nitrates are converted into nitrites. These are absorbed into the blood where they combine with haemoglobin and prevent it carrying oxygen. Symptoms of poisoning therefore include panting, gasping and trembling, followed by collapse. Death may occur in as little as half an hour from the symptoms first being seen and the blood of affected animals is very dark. In cows which recover, abortions and stillbirths may occur. It is not an easy condition to diagnose in the live animal, although the treatment, which consists of giving a 5 per cent solution of methylene blue intravenously, is quite successful.

Many plants can accumulate dangerous levels of nitrates, and grazing itself may become toxic if there have been very heavy applications of slurry and artificial fertiliser. This is especially so during periods of drought when there has been no rain to wash nitrates from the soil, or during warm, overcast weather, when nitrates accumulate in the plant but there is insufficient sunlight to complete their conversion to protein. Other sources of nitrate include effluent from silage clamps or bags of compound fertiliser which cattle sometimes tear open and eat. There is some evidence that conserved forage is more dangerous than fresh grazing and deaths have been reported within one or two hours after giving cattle a particular bale of hay. Some weed sprays lead to increased levels of plant nitrate, so always read the manufacturer's instructions before reintroducing cattle to the grazing.

Ragwort

Ragwort (figure 13.4) can cause permanent and irreversible changes in the liver and although symptoms often appear quite suddenly, it is likely that the plant has been eaten in small amounts over several months. It is particularly dangerous in hay, because then its bitter taste is not so obvious to the cattle. Symptoms include severe straining, sometimes leading to prolapse of the rectum. The abdomen becomes enlarged and swollen with excess fluid and the animal blindly wanders around appearing very dull and often bumping into things. There is no treatment and cases should be slaughtered before they lose excessive weight. Ragwort grows on marginal pastures and so cultivation and application of nitrogen are the best methods of controlling the plant. Sprays are also available.

Rhododendron

This is an interesting poison because it is one of the few occasions when you may see cattle vomiting. Other symptoms include colic, drooling, nervous signs and difficulty with breathing. Stimulants such as ephedrine are said to be useful for treatment, although the animal may still remain ill for several days during which warmth and nursing are vital.

Slug bait

I suspect that this is one of the more common poisons affecting both dogs and farm livestock, and I have had to treat several cases. The active chemical is metaldehyde and it is made attractive to slugs (and cattle!) by incorporating it into a cereal base. It is extensively used in crop husbandry. Metaldehyde causes dullness, depression, inco-ordination, staggering and colic. Eventually the animal becomes recumbent and death occurs from respiratory failure. There is also liver damage. Treatment is largely symptomatic and your vet will probably give respiratory and liver stimulants, with saline or calcium borogluconate intravenously.

St John's Wort

The toxic chemical in this plant is called hypericin. It persists even when the plant has been dried and so remains poisonous in hay. The symptoms are those of photosensitisation, and this was described on page 88.

Strychnine

Strychnine is still used on farms for the control of moles. Poisoning leads to severe muscle spasms, with the whole animal going rigid and in this respect it resembles the final stages of tetanus. Muscle relaxants are used in treatment. Fortunately cattle are relatively resistant and in fact strychnine is used in low doses, in the form of nux vomica, as an appetite stimulant.

Urea

Urea-based feedingstuffs were once very common and they are still used in fattening and rearing rations. Although cattle can tolerate quite high levels of urea, they must be slowly introduced onto a urea ration and they must continue to receive a constant intake. Even a gap of a few days could be dangerous. Ammonium sulphate fertilisers cause a similar poisoning syndrome, since most of the urea is converted into ammonia in the rumen. The symptoms are dullness and rapid breathing in early or mild cases, although nervous signs and staggering can develop and death may be accompanied by violent struggling and bellowing. Increasing the acidity of the rumen reduces the conversion of urea to free ammonia, and also decreases the rate of absorption of ammonia from the rumen so drenching a cow with 2–3 litres (half gallon) of vinegar would undoubtedly help. Your vet could also give drugs to control the nervous signs.

Warfarin

This is a dicoumarol derivative and it is a commonly used rat poison. It prevents the action of vitamin K in the animal and thus interferes with blood clotting mechanisms. This was described on page 308. Poisoning in cattle is not common, although calves sometimes gain access to large quantities of rat bait. The symptoms are colic, dullness and sometimes stiffness due to bleeding into the joints. There may be bleeding from the nose or blood in the dung. Vitamin K and iron are used for treatment.

Yew

The yew tree is the most poisonous British plant known for cattle and I suggest you carefully study a plant guide so that you can recognise it. All parts of the tree, the leaves and the berries, are toxic, the active chemical being taxine, a substance which stops the heart. It is unlikely that you will see anything except a dead animal, although there have been reports of cattle surviving for a day or so after eating the plant. The only treatment is for your vet to carry out a rumenotomy, that is to operate and empty the rumen, taking out all the yew. However, this would be an expensive procedure and not without its own risks. As it is most probable that by the time you realise that the cattle have eaten yew those which are going to be affected have already died, treatment is probably irrelevant. Some people have reported successful recovery using large quantities of black coffee, sugar and vitamin B_{12}, but this is not well documented.

APPENDICES

Appendix 1—Normal Values

Temperature   101.5°F   38.6°C
Pulse rate   45–50 per minute
Respiratory rate 15–20 per minute

The figures apply to normal healthy adult animals at rest.
Higher values will be obtained:

- from younger animals
- after exercise
- following excitement, e.g. handling or stress
- during very hot conditions
- in fevered animals, e.g. from infection and occasionally toxaemia.

Rumen contractions—twice per minute
one eructation/cud regurgitation per minute

Sleep—cattle have two types of sleep, deep sleep and drowsy sleep. The total amount of deep sleep required is very little, around thirty to sixty minutes per day and individual periods last for approximately five minutes only. Rumination ceases and brain activity is reduced, but the animal remains sitting. Drowsy sleep accounts for about one-third of the total day and can take place when the animal is standing or sitting. Rumination continues, but at a reduced rate. Younger animals need more sleep than adults.

Appendix 2—Lists of Clinical Signs

Some of the more common clinical signs of disease have been selected, together with lists of possible causes. Each cause may be referred to in more detail by consulting the index. The lists are by no means exhaustive and other diseases, apart from those mentioned, could be involved.

Abortion	brucellosis
	BVD
	fever/very high temperature
	IBR
	leptospirosis
	listeriosis
	nitrate poisoning
	salmonellosis
	summer mastitis
Anaemia	abomasal ulcer
	bracken poisoning
	coccidiosis
	copper deficiency
	EBL
	fluke
	haemorrhage—e.g. into uterus
	kale poisoning
	lice
	red water
	ticks
Blindness	cataract
	CCN
	lead poisoning
	listeriosis
	meningitis
	nervous acetonaemia
	New Forest eye
	overeating syndrome/acidosis
	spontaneous
	vitamin A deficiency
Bloat	abomasal displacement/abomasal torsion
	choke
	frothy bloat
	overeating/acidosis
	rumenal atony
	tetanus
	wire = traumatic reticulitis

Blood in Urine	bracken poisoning
	copper poisoning
	cystitis
	kale poisoning
	pyelonephritis
	red water
Coughing	calf pneumonia
	dust
	lungworm
Downer Cow	acute mastitis
	acute metritis
	debilitation and weakness
	fracture of pelvis or leg
	hypomagnesaemia
	milk fever
	obturator paralysis
	scouring
	selenium/vitamin E deficiency
	severe haemorrhage
Drooling	BVD
	choke
	diphtheria
	Foot and Mouth
	IBR
	lumpy jaw
	mucosal disease
	tooth abscess
	toxaemia
	wooden tongue
Eye Discharge	conjunctivitis
	enzootic pneumonia
	foreign body—e.g. barley awn
	fly irritation
	IBR
	MCF
	New Forest eye
	scratch on surface of eye
	tumour of third eyelid
	ultra-violet light damage
Nervous Signs	acetonaemia
	botulism

Nervous Signs   CCN
(contd)   hypomagnesaemia
                  lead poisoning
                  listeriosis
                  meningitis
                  over-eating barley or concentrates
                  poisoning—by many substances
                  tetanus
                  toxaemia
                  vitamin A deficiency

Panting   acetonaemia
                  acidosis/overeating
                  anaemia
                  calf pneumonia
                  excitement
                  fever
                  fog fever
                  haemorrhage/blood loss
                  heart defect
                  hypersensitivity reactions
                  hypomagnesaemia
                  lungworm
                  poisoning
                  scouring

Scouring   BVD
                  coccidiosis
                  cryptosporidia
                  digestive upset
                  E. coli
                  Johne's disease
                  Mucosal Disease
                  nutritional
                  Ostertagia
                  overeating
                  salmonellosis
                  toxic mastitis

Skin Conditions actinobacillosis
                   lice
                   mange
                   parakeratosis
                   photosensitisation
                   PPH
                   ringworm
                   warts

Straining (raised tail and abdominal contractions)
                  abortion
                  calving difficulty
                  coccidiosis
                  cystitis
                  intestinal obstruction
                  intussusception
                  ragwort poisoning
                  vaginal infection

Sudden Death   abomasal ulcer
                  bloat
                  heart failure
                  hypomagnesaemia
                  internal haemorrhage
                  intestinal torsion
                  mastitis
                  muscular dystrophy
                  poisoning (especially yew)

INDEX

FARMING PRESS BOOKS

Below is a sample of the wide range of agricultural and veterinary books published by Farming Press. For more information or for a free illustrated book list please contact:

Books Department, Farming Press Ltd, Wharfedale Road, Ipswich IP1 4LG, Suffolk, Great Britain.

The Principles of Dairy Farming
Kenneth Russell, revised by Ken Slater

The standard introduction to dairy farming covering the complete range of topics including buildings, farm systems, management, dairy farm crops and feed, milking techniques and milk production, breeding, calf rearing, disease control and profitability.

The New Herdsman's Book
Malcolm Stansfield

The basic manual of stockmanship for farmers and students. Covers all the essential topics to enable a herdsman to maximise his productivity and maintain the health of the herd.

TV Vet Book for Stock Farmers No. 1
Recognition and Treatment of Common Cattle Ailments
The TV Vet

Recognition and treatment of common cattle ailments completely covered in over 300 vivid action photographs with brief, to-the-point text.

TV Vet Book for Stock Farmers No. 2
Calving the Cow and Care of the Calf
The TV Vet

Calving the cow and care of the calf covered in complete details with 338 photographs. Hardback.

Cattle Footcare and Claw Trimming
E. Toussaint Raven

A detailed and highly illustrated account of the most up-to-date techniques for controlling dairy cow lameness and trimming feet. Translated from the Dutch.

Cattle Feeding
John Owen

A detailed new account of the principles and practice of cattle feeding. Includes an important section on the assessment of optimal diets and feed formulations.

Breeding Dairy Cattle
C. J. M. Hinks

A thoughtful analysis of the many factors involved in dairy cow breeding. It challenges popular assumptions and identifies the principles and rewards of an effective breeding strategy.

Grass Farming
M. McG. Cooper and D. W. Morris

The standard work on practical grassland management which unravels the complexities of pasture cultivation and cropping, and covers the features of livestock farming necessary for the successful conversion of fresh and conserved grass to meat and milk.

Forage Conservation and Feeding
W. F. Raymond, G. Shepperson and R. W. Waltham

Brings together the latest information on crop conservation, haymaking, silage making, mowing and field treatments, grass drying and forage feeding.

Dairy Farm Business Management
Ken Slater and Gordon Throup

Two leading farm business consultants take a close look at dairying. They outline the general principles of assessing profits and then describe the ways and means of improving the performance of the dairy farm.

Profitable Beef Production
M. McG. Cooper and M. B. Willis

Provides a concise account of the basic principles of reproduction, growth and development, nutrition and breeding. Emphasises production systems for dairy-bred beef.

Tackling Farm Waste
Kevin Grundey

An authoritative guide for livestock farmers to help them solve the problems of muck and slurry. Covers storing, handling, disposal and profitable utilisation of farmyard manure.

Farming Press also publish three monthly magazines: *Dairy Farmer, Pig Farming* and *Arable Farming*. For a specimen copy of any of these magazines please contact Farming Press at the address above.